Contemp and Management of

Neonatal Respiratory Diseases®

Third Edition

Thomas N. Hansen, MD

Professor and Chairman, Department of Pediatrics,
The Ohio State University,
School of Medicine and Public Health, and
Chief Executive Officer, Children's Hospital, Columbus, Ohio

Leonard E. Weisman, MD

Professor of Pediatrics, Baylor College of Medicine;
Head, Section of Neonatology, Baylor College of Medicine;
Director, Neonatal-Perinatal Medicine Fellowship Program,
Baylor College of Medicine; and Chief, Neonatology Service,
Texas Children's Hospital, Houston, Texas

Published by Handbooks in Health Care Co., Newtown, Pennsylvania, USA

International Standard Book Number: 1-931981-06-X

Library of Congress Catalog Card Number: 2002107057

Contemporary Diagnosis and Management of Neonatal Respiratory Diseases®. Copyright © 2003, 1998, 1995 by Handbooks in Health Care, a Division of AMM Co., Inc. All rights reserved. Printed in the United States of America. No part of this book may be used or reproduced in any manner whatsoever, including but not limited to electronic or mechanical means such as photocopying, recording, or using any information storage or retrieval system, without written permission, except in the case of brief quotations embodied in critical articles and reviews.
www.HHCbooks.com

Table of Contents

Contributors vii

Foreword ix

Chapter 1: Anatomy and Development of the Lung
Alveolar Development 1
Vascular Development 5

Chapter 2: Respiratory Physiology
Lung Mechanics 8
Oxygen Transport and Alveolar Ventilation 19
Ventilation-Perfusion Relationships 29
Lung and Heart Interaction 40
Surfactant 43

Chapter 3: Approach to the Patient With Respiratory Disease
History 54
Physical Examination 56
X-ray Patterns in Neonatal Lung Disease 62
Pulmonary Function Testing 68
Differentiation of Heart and Lung Disease 82

Chapter 4: Acute, Acquired Parenchymal Lung Disease
Hyaline Membrane Disease 90
Transient Tachypnea of the Newborn 108
Persistent Pulmonary Hypertension
  of the Newborn 113
Pulmonary Edema 124
Pulmonary Hemorrhage 130
Pleural Effusions 131
Meconium Aspiration Syndrome 135
Pneumonia 141

Chapter 5: Subacute and Chronic Acquired Parenchymal Lung Diseases

Air Block 152
Chronic Pulmonary Insufficiency of Prematurity . 162
Bronchopulmonary Dysplasia 163
Wilson-Mikity Syndrome 180

Chapter 6: Congenital Diseases Affecting the Lung Parenchyma

Cystic Malformations of the Lung 186
Congenital Lobar Emphysema 187
Bronchogenic Cyst 188
Neurenteric and Enteric Cyst 190
Cystic Adenomatoid Malformation 190
Other Lung Malformations 192
Pulmonary Sequestration 192
Pulmonary Arteriovenous Fistula 194
Congenital Pulmonary Lymphangiectasia 194
Pulmonary Agenesis 195
Pulmonary Hypoplasia 198

Chapter 7: Diseases Affecting the Diaphragm and Chest Wall

Diseases of the Diaphragm 203
Congenital Diaphragmatic Hernia 203
Paralysis of the Diaphragm 209
Disorders of the Chest Wall 210
Sternal Deformities 210
Thoracic Deformities 210
Muscle Weakness 211

Chapter 8: Diseases of the Upper Airway

Disorders of the Nose, Mouth, and Pharynx 214
Choanal Atresia 214
Pierre Robin Sequence 216
Macroglossia 217
Glossoptosis-Apnea Syndrome 217
Pharyngeal Incoordination 218

Disorders of the Larynx 218
  Laryngomalacia 218
  Vocal Cord Paralysis 218
  Subglottic Stenosis 219
  Laryngeal Tumors 221
  Laryngeal Webs 222
Disorders of the Trachea 222
  Esophageal Atresia
    and Tracheoesophageal Fistula 222
  Laryngotracheoesophageal Cleft 224
  Tracheal Agenesis 224
  Congenital Tracheal Stenosis 225
  Tracheobronchomalacia 225
  Vascular Rings 226

Chapter 9: Control of Breathing in Neonates

  Central Control of Respiration 230
  Airway Patency and Airway Receptors 232
  The Respiratory Pump 233
  Apnea 234

Chapter 10: Respiratory Therapy–General Considerations

  Initial Stabilization 241
  Oxygen Use and Monitoring 246
  Management of the Airway 252
  Surfactant Administration 259
Positive Pressure Ventilatory Support 263
  Continuous Positive Airway Pressure 264
  Intermittent Positive Pressure
    Ventilation 266
  Synchronized Intermittent Mandatory
    Ventilation 279
  High-Frequency Jet
    Ventilation 281
  High-Frequency Oscillatory
    Ventilation 282

Nonventilatory Management of Respiratory Failure 286

    Inhaled Nitric Oxide 286

    Extracorporeal Membrane Oxygenation 288

Chapter 11: Nutritional and Gastrointestinal Support for the Infant with Respiratory Distress

    Nutritional Support 302

    Postdischarge Nutrition 319

    Gastrointestinal Support of Feeding Problems .. 322

Chapter 12: Ethical Considerations

    Parent-Physician Communication 328

    Prenatal Counseling and Delivery Room Care .. 330

    Withholding Care 330

Chapter 13: Discharge Planning

    Discharge Criteria 333

    Special Considerations 334

    Home Apnea Monitoring 335

    Car Seats 336

    Respiratory Syncytial Virus Prophylaxis 337

    Home Nutrition 338

Index 341

Contributors

Steven A. Abrams, MD
Professor of Pediatrics, Baylor College of Medicine, Houston, Texas

James M. Adams, Jr, MD
Professor of Pediatrics, Baylor College of Medicine, Houston, Texas; Medical Director, Special Care Nurseries, Texas Children's Hospital, Houston, Texas

Diane Anderson, PhD, RD, CSP, FADA
Associate Professor of Pediatrics, Baylor College of Medicine, Houston, Texas

Carol L. Berseth, MD
Associate Professor of Pediatrics and Gastroenterology, Baylor College of Medicine, Houston, Texas

Gerardo Cabrera-Meza, MD
Associate Professor of Pediatrics, Baylor College of Medicine, Houston, Texas

Robert G. Castile, MD
Associate Professor of Pediatrics, The Ohio State University, School of Medicine and Public Health, Columbus, Ohio

Timothy R. Cooper, MD
Neonatologist, Austin, Texas

Caraciolo J. Fernandes, MD
Assistant Professor of Pediatrics, Baylor College of Medicine, Houston, Texas

Joseph A. Garcia-Prats, MD
Professor of Pediatrics and Ethics, Department of Pediatrics and Center for Medical Ethics and Health Policy, Baylor College of Medicine, Houston, Texas; Co-Director, Perinatal Outreach Program, Texas Children's Hospital, Houston, Texas

Alfred L. Gest, MD
Clinical Assistant Professor of Pediatrics, The Ohio State University, School of Medicine and Public Health, Columbus, Ohio

Michael R. Gomez, MD
Neonatologist, San Antonio, Texas

Charleta Guillory, MD
Assistant Professor of Pediatrics, Baylor College of Medicine, Houston, Texas

Thomas N. Hansen, MD
Professor and Chairman, Department of Pediatrics, The Ohio State University, School of Medicine and Public Health, Columbus, Ohio; Chief Executive Officer, Children's Hospital, Columbus, Ohio

Karen E. Johnson, MD
Assistant Professor of Pediatrics, Baylor College of Medicine, Houston, Texas

Joyce M. Koenig, MD
Assistant Professor of Pediatrics, University of Florida, Gainesville, Florida

Steven R. Leuthner, MD
Assistant Professor of Pediatrics and Bioethics, Medical College of Wisconsin, Milwaukee, Wisconsin

George T. Mandy, MD
Assistant Professor of Pediatrics, Baylor College of Medicine, Houston, Texas

Alicia A. Moïse, MD
Clinical Associate Professor of Pediatrics, The Ohio State University, School of Medicine and Public Health, Columbus, Ohio

Donough O'Donovan, MD
Assistant Professor of Pediatrics, Baylor College of Medicine, Houston, Texas

Richard J. Schanler, MD
Professor of Pediatrics and Director, Neonatal Nutrition Service, Baylor College of Medicine, Houston, Texas

Michael E. Speer, MD
Professor of Pediatrics, Baylor College of Medicine, Houston, Texas; Director of Nurseries, The Methodist Hospital, Houston, Texas; Director of Nurseries, St. Luke's Episcopal Hospital, Houston, Texas

Christina J. Valentine, MD, RD
Pediatrics Resident, Baylor College of Medicine, Houston, Texas

Mary E. Wearden, MD
Neonatologist, San Antonio, Texas

Leonard E. Weisman, MD
Professor of Pediatrics; Head, Section of Neonatology; and Director, Neonatal-Perinatal Medicine Fellowship Program, Baylor College of Medicine, Houston, Texas; Chief, Neonatology Service, Texas Children's Hospital, Houston, Texas

Stephen E. Welty, MD
Associate Professor of Pediatrics, The Ohio State University, School of Medicine and Public Health, Columbus, Ohio

Odell Wilson, MD
Assistant Professor of Pediatrics, Baylor College of Medicine, Houston, Texas

Foreword

In recent years, we have witnessed an explosion of new information about the pathophysiologic processes involved in diseases of the respiratory system of the newborn. This has led to improved treatments, such as surfactant replacement, that have markedly reduced morbidity and mortality in this vulnerable population.

In this third edition of this book, we review the epidemiology, pathophysiology, presentation, management, and outcomes of respiratory disorders affecting the newborn. In addition, we have provided updated reviews of pulmonary physiology and ventilatory and nonventilatory management of respiratory distress. Finally, we have stressed supportive care that is necessary to optimize outcome by including sections on nutritional and gastrointestinal support, communication with parents, ethical considerations, and discharge planning.

To a large extent, this book represents a compilation of lectures and handouts provided to postdoctoral fellows, pediatric residents, medical students, and nurses working in the nurseries of the Baylor College of Medicine Affiliated Hospitals, Columbus Children's Hospital, and The Ohio State University. A list of suggested readings accompanies each chapter. Although comprehensive, this book is not meant to be an exhaustive review of the literature on any topic. It simply represents a starting point, and the reader should obtain additional information where appropriate.

The authors of this text were all students of Dr. Arnold J. Rudolph, the consummate teacher of neonatology. They wish to acknowledge his immeasurable contributions to their education, lives, and careers. We would also like to acknowledge Marlane Kayfes for her technical and administrative assistance.

Thomas N. Hansen, MD
Leonard E. Weisman, MD

This book has been prepared and is presented as a service to the medical community. The information provided reflects the knowledge, experience, and personal opinions of all the contributing authors, but especially of the two co-editors, Thomas N. Hansen, MD, and Leonard E. Weisman, MD.

This book is not intended to replace or to be used as a substitute for the complete prescribing information prepared by each manufacturer for each drug. Because of possible variations in drug indications, in dosage information, in newly described toxicities, in drug/drug interactions, and in other items of importance, reference to such complete prescribing information is definitely recommended before any of the drugs discussed are used or prescribed.

Chapter 1

Anatomy and Development of the Lung

Neonatal lungs are not simply small versions of adult lungs. Respiratory disease occurs in a setting of incomplete development of the tracheobronchial system or the pulmonary vasculature, especially in the case of the preterm infant. There is a complex relationship of genetic factors, growth factors, hormones, and extracellular matrix factors that control cell proliferation and differentiation in the developing lung. Much of the respiratory physiology observed at the bedside of the sick neonate can be accounted for by underdeveloped or maldeveloped alveolar and vascular architecture.

Alveolar Development

The tracheobronchial airway system begins as an endoderm-lined, respiratory diverticulum from the foregut. This embryonic lung bud contains the pluripotent stem cells that give rise to more than 40 different cell types and more than 250 million alveoli. Appropriate development depends on mesenchymal-epithelial interactions and cell-cell communication. The lung bud continuously divides and branches, steadily penetrating the mesenchyma and progressing toward the periphery. The process is described in five phases (Figure 1).

Embryonic Phase (through week 5)
Development of proximal airways

The lung bud arises from the foregut 23 to 26 days after fertilization. Abnormal lung bud development at this early stage can result in tracheal agenesis/stenosis or in tracheo-esophageal fistula. Pulmonary sequestrations develop from

Figure 1: The five phases of the process of tracheobronchial airway development. (Adapted from Weibel ER: *Morphometry of the Human Lung.* Berlin, Springer-Verlag, 1963, p 111.)

Phase	Embryonic	Pseudoglandular	Canalicular	Terminal Sac	Alveolar
Gestation (wks)	0 → 5	6 → 16	17 → 24	25 → 37	38+
Generation (n)	0 1 2	7 8 9 20	21 → 23	24 25 26 27	
	Trachea Bronchi	Nonrespiratory bronchioles	Respiratory bronchioles	Alveolar ducts	
	Conducting Airways		**Terminal Respiratory Units**		

accessory lung buds. If an accessory lung bud develops early, the sequestration and normal lung will share a common pleura. As many as 30% of infants with congenital diaphragmatic hernia (CDH) will have pulmonary sequestrations.

Pseudoglandular Phase (weeks 6 through 16)
Development of lower conducting airways

In this phase, 20 generations of conducting airways form. The first eight generations (the bronchi) ultimately acquire cartilaginous walls. Generations 9 to 20 comprise the non-respiratory bronchioles, which do not possess cartilage. By the end of this phase, development of preacinar structures (which form the conducting airways) is largely complete. Airways are always accompanied by surrounding lymph vessels and bronchial capillaries.

The mesenchymal-epithelial interactions during the embryonic and pseudoglandular phases of branching are being worked out. The fibroblast growth factor (FGF) family is an important early mediator. Without FGF-7, there is no branching; meanwhile, excess FGF-7 leads to poor differentiation, which histologically resembles congenital cystic adenomatoid malformation (CCAM).

FGF-10 is another important factor that may affect the *Sonic hedgehog (Shh)* signaling pathway. In animal models lacking *Shh* expression, there are abnormalities in foregut development, leading to tracheal-esophageal atresia, esophageal atresia, and other tracheal and lung abnormalities.

Other important molecules expressed in the thoracic mesoderm include *Gli* genes and a group of homeobox or *Hox* genes. Mutations in *Gli3* have been observed in Pallister-Hall syndrome, causing tracheal stenosis, tracheal-esophageal fistula, or lung lobulation defects.

The origin of bronchogenic cysts detected in infancy can be traced to the formation of bronchi with dysgenic cartilage. A more common disorder, congenital lobar emphysema, may have a similar origin but is clinically characterized by partial airway closure and gas trapping in downstream alveoli.

3

Closure of the diaphragm also occurs during the pseudoglandular phase. If closure is delayed past 8 to 10 weeks' gestation, migration of bowel into the thoracic cavity is possible, resulting in CDH. The pathophysiology of CDH involves more than a space-occupying lesion with compression of the developing lung. Associated pulmonary hypoplasia is characterized by decreased numbers of tracheobronchial generations and alveoli. A decreased number of pulmonary arteries and abnormal extension of muscle into acinar arterioles account for the persistent pulmonary hypertension that often occurs with CDH. The earlier in gestation that bowel migrates into the chest, the more severe the lung hypoplasia.

Canalicular Phase (weeks 17 through 24)
Formation of gas-exchanging acini

Continued branching of the airways forms respiratory bronchioles that represent the first gas-exchanging sites (acini) within the tracheobronchial tree (generations 21 to 23). During this phase, the relative amount of connective tissue diminishes. This mesenchymal thinning involves the process of apoptosis (programmed cell death). Development of pulmonary capillaries precedes acinar development, and by the end of the canalicular phase, the capillaries have begun to appose the acini. Lung function of infants born around 24 weeks greatly depends on the degree to which acinar development and acinus-capillary coupling have occurred.

Terminal Sac Phase (weeks 25 through 37)
Development of acini

The rudimentary primary saccules divide into subsaccules and alveoli, while the interstitium continues to dissipate. Capillary invasion becomes more extensive and leads to an exponential increase in alveolar-blood barrier surface area. Positive pressure ventilation of infants born early in the terminal sac phase can result in pulmonary interstitial emphysema, a condition in which microscopic rupture of acini leads to accumulation of small bubbles of air within the relatively thick interstitium. Incomplete invasion of the acini by surrounding capillaries provides an anatomic basis for the ventilation-perfusion mismatching that contributes to hyaline membrane disease and other parenchymal diseases.

Alveolar Phase (week 38 to age 3 years)
Continued alveolar proliferation and development

This final phase begins between 30 and 37 weeks. Subsaccules become alveoli as a result of thinning of acinar walls, dissipation of interstitium, and invagination of alveoli by pulmonary capillaries. Ultimately, alveoli attain a polyhedral shape. The distal airway formation and the epithelial cell differentiation during the canalicular, terminal sac, and alveolar phases are thought to be influenced by epidermal growth factor (EGF), transforming growth factor-β (TGF-β), and platelet-derived growth factor (PDGF). Interestingly, the delayed lung maturation of males is thought to be mediated by TGF-β.

Vascular Development

The lung is supplied by the systemic bronchial circulation and the pulmonary circulation. The vasculature of the mature lung arises from the thoracic mesoderm. Systemic bronchial arteries supply the conducting airways, visceral pleura, connective tissue, pulmonary arteries, and pulmonary sequestration tissue. By contrast, the pulmonary circulation participates in gas exchange and supplies arterial blood to cystic adenomatoid malformations.

Beyond 16 weeks' gestation, preacinar pulmonary arteries increase only in length and diameter, whereas intra-acinar arteries proliferate. Muscularization of fetal pulmonary arteries is confusing but important to the understanding of persistent pulmonary hypertension, a condition caused by failure of the pulmonary vasculature to relax normally in the postdelivery period. Arteries <100 μm in diameter are nonmuscular, arteries 100 to 180 μm are transitional, and arteries >180 μm are muscular. For any given size muscular artery, wall thickness *as a fraction of total vessel diameter* is greater in the fetus than in the adult. Wall thickness as a fraction of total diameter remains constant through the second half of gestation, so as the number of vessels increases, the total amount of pulmonary vascular smooth muscle increases. This explains, in part, why persistent pulmonary hypertension is largely a phenomenon of term and near-term infants.

During the second half of gestation, the number of arteries increases 10-fold, but blood flow increases only twofold to threefold and reaches only 7% of combined ventricular output near term. The increase in smooth muscle content and hypoxic vasoconstriction together act to limit pulmonary blood flow until after delivery. At birth, oxygenation, mechanical distention of the lung, and endothelial-dependent mechanisms all contribute to a dramatic decrease in pulmonary vascular resistance and increased pulmonary blood flow.

Conclusion

The degree of vascular and alveolar development within the lung modifies the disease process in most neonatal respiratory disorders. In some circumstances, such as CDH, aberrant development is itself the primary cause of abnormal lung function.

By Steven R. Leuthner, MD

Suggested Readings

Bellusci S, Grindley J, Emoto H, et al: Fibroblast growth factor 10 (FGF10) and branching morphogenesis in the embryonic mouse lung. *Development* 1997;124:4867-4878.

Hansen TN, Corbet AJ: Lung development and function. In: Taeusch HW, Ballard RA, Avery ME, eds. *Schaffer and Avery's Diseases of the Newborn*. 6th ed. Philadelphia, WB Saunders Co, 1991.

Hislop A, Reid L: Growth and development of the respiratory system. In: Davis JA, Dopping J, eds. *Scientific Foundations of Paediatrics*. London, Heineman, 1974.

Hislop A, Reid L: Development of the acinus in the human lung. *Thorax* 1974;29:90.

Kappen C: *Hox* genes in the lung. *Am J Respir Cell Mol Biol* 1996;15:156-162.

Langston C, Kida K, Reed M, et al: Human lung growth in late gestation and in the neonate. *Am Rev Respir Dis* 1984;129:607-613.

Litingyung Y, Lei L, Westphal H, et al: *Sonic hedgehog* is essential to foregut development. *Nat Genet* 1998;20:58-61.

Motoyama J, Liu J, Mo R, et al: Essential function of *Gli2* and *Gli3* in the formation of lung, trachea, and oesophagus. *Nat Genet* 1998;20:54-57.

Murray JF: In: Murray JF, ed. *The Normal Lung*. Philadelphia, WB Saunders Co, 1986.

Nielsen HC, Martin A, Volpe MV, et al: Growth factor control of growth and epithelial differentiation in embryonic lungs. *Biochem Mol Med* 1997;60:38-48.

Chapter 2

Respiratory Physiology

Lung Mechanics

Breathing, the physical act of moving gas in and out of the lung, is affected by mechanical properties of the tissues of the lung, the chest wall, and the inspired gas (Table 1).

Elastic Forces

The lung is composed of elastic tissues that resist stretching. Consequently, the distending pressure needed to inflate the lung increases with the volume of inflation (Figure 1). The chest wall, like the lung, contains elastic tissues and also has a compliance, C_{cw}. The lung and chest wall together determine the elastic properties of the entire respiratory system (Figure 2).

The lung has no innate resting volume, and if isolated from the chest wall, it collapses completely. As distending pressure increases from zero, lung volume increases proportionally. The chest wall has a resting volume (volume at distending pressure equal to zero) that is greater than zero. This volume is determined by the fixed volume of the rib cage. Lowering the volume of the chest cage below its resting value requires a negative distending pressure to overcome this elastic recoil. Increasing the volume of the chest cage above this resting volume requires a positive distending pressure.

Together, the lung and chest wall make up the *respiratory system*. At rest, the tendency for the chest wall to expand is balanced by the tendency for the lung to collapse. The point at which these two forces are exactly equal and opposite is the resting lung volume or functional residual capacity (FRC). At this point, the distending pressure across the respiratory system is zero (Figure 3). Exhalation below FRC requires a

Table 1: Pulmonary Function in Term Newborns

Lung Volumes	Measurement
Functional residual capacity	30 mL/kg
Tidal volume	6 mL/kg
Dead space volume	2 mL/kg

Ventilatory Measurements	Measurement
Respiratory rate	35 breaths/min
Minute ventilation	210 mL/kg/min
Alveolar ventilation	140 mL/kg/min

Mechanics	Measurement
Respiratory system compliance	3 mL/cm H_2O
Lung compliance	4 mL/cm H_2O
Chest wall compliance	20 mL/cm H_2O
Total inspiratory resistance	0.069 cm H_2O/mL/s
Total expiratory resistance	0.097 cm H_2O/mL/s
Inspiratory time constant	0.2 s
Expiratory time constant	0.3 s

Figure 1: The relationship between distending pressure and volume of inflation for the lung is nearly linear over the volume range encompassed by normal breathing. At higher volumes of inflation, the curve becomes flatter as the lung reaches its elastic limit. The slope of the pressure-volume curve for the lung, $\Delta V/\Delta P$, is a measure of lung distensibility or compliance (C_L). Accordingly, the pressure (P) required to overcome lung elastic forces at any lung volume (V) is inversely related to compliance, $P = V/C_L$. A poorly compliant lung requires a large increase in pressure to produce a given change in volume.

Figure 2: The lung and chest wall are coupled at their pleural surfaces and together form the respiratory system. The pressure inside the lung is alveolar pressure (P_{alv}), while the pressure surrounding the lung is pleural pressure (P_{pl}). Therefore, the distending pressure for the lung is $P_{alv} - P_{pl}$. Similarly, the pressure 'inside' the chest wall is pleural pressure, the surrounding pressure is atmospheric pressure

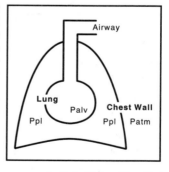

sure (P_{atm}), and the distending pressure is $P_{pl} - P_{atm}$. The distending pressure for the respiratory system is the sum of the distending pressures for the lung and chest wall or $P_{alv} - P_{atm}$.

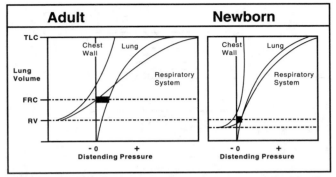

Figure 3: Idealized pressure-volume curves are plotted for the lung and chest wall separately and then for the complete respiratory system (lung + chest wall). Lung volume is normalized to total lung capacity (TLC). Other volumes shown are functional residual capacity (FRC) and residual volume (RV). The distending pressures for the lung, chest wall, and respiratory system are listed in Figure 2. (Adapted from Hansen TN, Corbet AJ: Pulmonary physiology of the newborn. In: Taeusch HW, et al, eds. *Schaffer and Avery's Diseases of the Newborn.* 6th ed. Philadelphia, WB Saunders, 1991, p 475.)

negative distending pressure (active expiration). The bony structures of the chest wall limit exhalation to a minimum volume—residual volume (RV). Inflation of the thorax above FRC initially requires that work be done only to overcome the elastic forces of the lung. However, as inflation continues beyond the resting volume for the chest wall, the distending pressure must overcome the elastic recoil of the lung and chest wall. When corrected for size of the lung, the compliance of the newborn lung is similar to that of the adult lung, but the chest wall compliance is greater. Consequently, the newborn has a lower FRC and RV.

Resistance

Resistance to breathing results from friction generated by movement of gas (airway resistance) and movement of tissues (viscous tissue resistance).

Figure 4: During laminar flow, gas molecules travel in straight lines, with the faster-moving molecules near the center of the gas stream. For laminar flow, the pressure gradient, ΔP = P_1 - P_2, is directly proportional to the rate of flow ($\dot{V}$): ΔP = $K_1 \times \dot{V}$. K_1, the resistance term, increases with length of the airway and viscosity of the gas and decreases with the fourth power of the radius of the airway. During turbulent flow, gas molecules move chaotically and the velocity of flow is the same across the stream. ΔP is proportional to the flow rate squared: $\Delta P = K_2 \times \dot{V}^2$. K_2, the resistance term, is more complicated and increases with length of the airway and density of the gas and decreases with the fifth power of the radius of the airway. (Adapted from Comroe JH, et al. *The Lung: Clinical Physiology and Pulmonary Function Tests*, 2nd ed. Chicago, Year Book Medical Publishers, 1962.)

Airway resistance

Friction develops as molecules of gas slide over one another and past airway walls. Gas flow through a tube requires a pressure gradient to overcome these friction forces. The magnitude of the pressure gradient is proportional to the rate of flow times a constant termed *resistance*. Gas flow through a tube may be *laminar* or *turbulent* (Figure 4).

Turbulent flow typically occurs at high rates of gas flow or at points where airways change size or branch. In the lung, the highest rate of gas flow is in the trachea because all of the gas entering and leaving the lung must pass through the trachea. Conversely, the lowest rates of flow will occur in small peripheral airways, because each small airway is exposed to only a fraction of the total gas flow. Therefore, flow in small airways tends to be laminar, and turbulent flow tends to occur in large central airways.

Both types of flow can occur in the lung at the same time, so the total pressure gradient required to sustain flow can be summarized by:

$$\Delta P = K_1 \times \dot{V} + K_2 \times \dot{V}^2$$

Differences between laminar and turbulent flow can be used to ascertain the site of airway obstruction. K_1 is directly related to viscosity of the gas, while K_2 is related to the density of the gas (Figure 4). Therefore, in a patient with large airway obstruction, such as croup or tracheal stenosis, decreasing the density of the inspired gas by changing from a mixture of oxygen in nitrogen to a mixture of oxygen in helium, Heli-Ox, should lower resistance to breathing and improve gas flow. Conversely, if the obstruction is in small airways, then changing gas density will not affect airway resistance and work of breathing.

Airway resistance is directly related to the length of the airway but is related to the fourth power of the airway radius. Therefore, during inspiration, as airways dilate and lengthen, the dominant effect is to lower airway resistance. Similarly, during expiration, airways are compressed and resistance increases. Consequently, expiratory airway resistance is greater than inspiratory airway resistance.

Viscous tissue resistance

Viscous tissue resistance develops because of friction between tissues in the lung and chest wall. It accounts for roughly 20% of resistive forces in the newborn.

Total resistance

The total respiratory resistance is the sum of airway resistance and tissue resistance. Approximately 80% of total resistance results from airway resistance, and in the newborn, about 50% of that is nasal resistance.

In practice, gas flow in the lung is assumed to be laminar, and tissue and airway resistances are lumped as the total resistance of the respiratory system (R). The pressure required to overcome resistive forces is expressed as the product of gas flow rate, $\dot{V}$, times resistance, R: $P = \dot{V} \times R$.

Inertance

During breathing, work must also be performed to accelerate gas and tissues. Generally, inertance losses are negligible compared with resistance losses and are ignored.

Dynamic Interaction

The *total driving pressure* required to move gas in or out of the lung is determined by the sum of the pressures needed to overcome elastic, resistive, and inertial forces of the lung and chest wall.

Spontaneous breathing

For spontaneous breathing, the driving pressure is simply alveolar pressure minus pleural pressure (the distending pressure across the lung [Figure 2]). During a spontaneous inspiration, inspiratory muscles of the chest wall and the diaphragm contract, increasing thoracic volume and decreasing intrapleural pressure. Decreased intrapleural pressure acts as a stretching force, expanding the lung and decreasing alveolar pressure. The pressure at the mouth and nares is equal to atmospheric pressure, so as alveolar pressure decreases, a pressure gradient develops and gas flows through the airways into the alveoli. As the number of gas molecules in the alveoli increases, alveolar pressure increases until it equals atmospheric pressure, at which time gas flow, hence inspiration, ceases.

During exhalation, respiratory muscles relax, thoracic volume decreases, and pleural pressure increases. The elastic recoil of the lung and chest wall compresses the lung, increasing alveolar pressure. Since alveolar pressure is greater than atmospheric pressure, gas flows out of the lung. As the number of gas molecules in the alveoli decreases, alveolar pressure decreases until it equals atmospheric pressure and gas flow, hence expiration, ceases.

Positive pressure ventilation

For positive pressure breathing, the total driving pressure is airway pressure minus atmospheric pressure (the pressure across the respiratory system [Figure 2]). During a positive pressure breath, the ventilator increases upper airway pressure above alveolar pressure, and gas flows into the alveoli. Alveolar pressure increases and provides the stretching force necessary to expand the lung and chest wall. Because the lung pushes on the chest wall, pleural pressure is positive relative to atmospheric pressure. Gas flows into the lung until alveolar pressure equals airway pressure. Exhalation is passive and similar to that for a spontaneous breath.

Equation of motion and respiratory time constant

The mechanical behavior of the respiratory system over time can be described mathematically by the *equation of motion*. This equation states that the driving pressure, P(t), required to move gas in and out of the lung at a given time (t) during the respiratory cycle is the sum of the pressures required to overcome elastic [Pel(t)], resistive [Pr(t)], and inertance forces [Pi(t)]:

$$P(t) = Pel(t) + Pr(t) + Pi(t)$$

Now, Pel(t) = V(t)/C (the volume of the respiratory system at time [t] divided by the compliance) and Pr(t) = $\dot{V}$(t) x R (the rate of gas flow at time [t] times resistance). If we ignore inertance, the equation of motion simplifies to the first order differential equation:

$$P(t) = [V(t)/C] + [\dot{V}(t) \times R]$$

Special solutions to the equation of motion

While a general solution to the equation of motion is outside the scope of this handbook, there are several special solutions that are clinically useful:

Points of no gas flow. At end expiration and end inspiration, gas flow is zero, and the equation of motion reduces to $P(t) = V(t)/C$; that is, driving pressure is affected only by elastic forces. At all other times in the respiratory cycle, driving pressure must overcome both elastic and resistive forces.

Passive exhalation. The simplified equation of motion is useful in explaining the behavior of the respiratory system during passive exhalation. During passive exhalation, airway pressure [P(t)] equals atmospheric pressure, which equals 0, and the equation of motion has the simple solution:

$$V(t) = V_o \times e^{-t/R \times C}$$

This solution allows us to calculate the volume of gas, V(t), remaining in the lung at any time (t) during a passive exhalation (Figure 5). V_o is the volume of gas in the lung at the beginning of exhalation, e is a constant roughly equal to 2.72, t is time, and R x C is the product of resistance and compliance. R x C has the units of time and is called the *respiratory time constant*.

The rate at which the lung empties during exhalation is determined by the time constant. If resistance or compliance decreases, the lung will empty more rapidly. Conversely, if resistance or compliance increases, the time constant increases and the lung empties more slowly. In particular, diseases that cause airway obstruction will increase resistance, increase the time constant, and cause the lung to empty more slowly.

During spontaneous or positive pressure ventilation, if the expiratory time is less than three time constants, the lung will not empty completely before the next inspiration. With each subsequent breath, additional gas will be trapped and the lung volume will increase. Lung overinflation secondary to this form of gas trapping often complicates the course of diseases that

Figure 5: During passive exhalation, the volume of gas in the lung at any time (t) depends on the starting lung volume (V_o) and the product of resistance and compliance, the respiratory time constant. If exhalation proceeds for a time equal to 1 time constant, $t = 1 \times R \times C$ (0.25 second in this example), this equation predicts that the volume of gas left in the lung will be roughly 0.37 x the initial volume (V_o), or that the lung will be 63% empty. After 2 time constants, the lung will be 86% empty, and after 5 time constants, it will be 99% empty. (Adapted from Hansen TN, Corbet AJ: Pulmonary physiology of the newborn. In: Taeusch HW, et al, eds. *Schaffer and Avery's Diseases of the Newborn*, 6th ed. Philadelphia, WB Saunders, 1991, p 478.)

increase airway resistance and the respiratory time constant, such as bronchopulmonary dysplasia.

Preterm infants may use this phenomenon to compensate for chest wall instability. As discussed earlier, because of a highly compliant chest wall, the preterm infant should have a decreased resting lung volume, FRC. However, when FRC is measured in spontaneously breathing preterm infants, it is of-

Figure 6: In this example, a constant airway pressure of 12 cm H$_2$O is applied to the airway. The equation predicts that at time equal to one time constant (0.25 second in this example), the lung will inflate to 63% of its maximum volume (Vmax), and if t = 5 x R x C, the lung will inflate to 99% of Vmax. (Adapted from Hansen TN, Corbet AJ: Principles of respiratory monitoring and therapy. In: Taeusch HW, et al, eds. *Schaffer and Avery's Diseases of the Newborn.* 6th ed. Philadelphia, WB Saunders, 1991, p 491.)

ten similar to that found in term infants. This discrepancy occurs because the preterm infant breathes sufficiently fast to impinge on expiration and traps enough gas to normalize FRC. Of course, during periodic breathing or apnea, this defense mechanism is lost and FRC falls.

Positive pressure inflation. Another special solution to the equation of motion occurs during inflation of the lung with a constant airway pressure; that is, the pressure in the lung over time [P(t)] equals airway pressure (Paw), which is constant. In this case, shown in Figure 6,

$$V(t) = Vmax(1 - e^{-t/R \times C})$$

Vmax is the maximum volume of lung inflation for a given airway pressure and equal to Paw x C_L. Therefore, our equation can be modified to:

$$V(t) = Paw \times C_L(1 - e^{-t/R \times C})$$

According to this relationship, the maximum volume of gas that can be instilled into the lung during an infinitely long, positive pressure breath is limited by Paw x C_L. The rate at which the lung inflates to this volume is determined by the time constant, R x C. Increases or decreases in resistance will affect the rate of inflation but will not alter the ultimate lung volume. Changes in compliance, however, will affect the ultimate lung volume and the rate of inflation to that volume. The roles of resistance and compliance in lung inflation are explained in more detail in the sections on pulmonary function tests (Chapter 3) and positive pressure ventilation (Chapter 10).

By Thomas N. Hansen, MD

Oxygen Transport and Alveolar Ventilation

Individual cells take up oxygen (O_2) continuously from their environment to support oxidative metabolism and excrete carbon dioxide (CO_2), the byproduct of this metabolism. Evolution from single-celled organisms to multicellular organisms required the development of a complex system to allow cells to exchange gas with the environment (Figure 7).

Lungs: Alveolar Ventilation

The lung consists of a *preacinar* compartment, containing the conducting airways to the level of the terminal bronchiole, and an *acinar* compartment, containing respiratory bronchioles, alveolar ducts, and alveoli. The total volume of gas moving in and out of the lung with each breath is the *tidal volume*. The product of tidal volume and respiratory rate is the *minute ventilation*. The conducting airways do not exchange gas with blood and represent the *dead space volume* (Figure 8). The acinar compartment does exchange gas with the blood and rep-

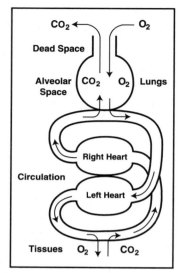

Figure 7: Oxygen uptake and delivery can be broken down into three components: (1) an intake and exhaust component—the lungs; (2) a delivery system—the circulation; and (3) an O_2 reservoir—the blood. Oxygen is extracted from the atmosphere by the lungs and delivered by the circulation to the tissues to support oxidative metabolism. Carbon dioxide generated by the tissues is transported back to the lung for excretion into the atmosphere. (Adapted from Hansen TN, Corbet AJ: Pulmonary physiology of the newborn. In: Taeusch HW, et al, eds. *Schaffer and Avery's Diseases of the Newborn*, 6th ed. Philadelphia, WB Saunders, 1991, p 479.)

resents the *alveolar volume* (Figure 8). Alveolar volume equals the tidal volume minus the dead space volume. Effective ventilation or *alveolar ventilation* is the product of the alveolar volume and the respiratory rate (Table 1).

Alveolar ventilation is intermittent, while tissue O_2 consumption and CO_2 production are continuous. Removal of O_2 from alveoli by the blood during expiration and addition of CO_2 decreases alveolar O_2 tension and increases alveolar CO_2 tension. Arterial blood O_2 and CO_2 tensions are in equilibrium with those of alveolar gas and change similarly. Fortunately, the lung is provided with a buffer—the functional residual capacity—that is large (30 mL/kg body weight) compared with the tidal volume (5 to 7 mL/kg body weight). During expiration, this large buffer continues to provide O_2 to capillary blood and acts as a sump for CO_2 so that alveolar, hence arterial, gas tensions remain relatively constant over the respiratory cycle.

Figure 8: Alveolar and dead space ventilation are depicted as delivery of packets of atmospheric gas (white) to the lung. During inspiration, the packet of gas residing in the dead space (shaded) moves into the alveolar volume. This packet has gas tensions similar to alveolar gas and no net gas exchange occurs. As inspiration continues, packets of fresh gas move into the lung. These packets deliver O_2 to the alveolus and remove CO_2. Of the three packets of gas entering the lung from the atmosphere (the tidal volume), only two participate in gas exchange. The last packet of fresh gas occupies the dead space. At end inspiration, dead space gas tensions are identical to those of atmospheric gas. With expiration, the first packet of gas to leave the lung exits from the dead space and has gas tensions identical to atmospheric gas. As expiration continues, packets with gas tensions similar to those of alveolar gas exit the lung and the CO_2 tension of expired gas increases while its O_2 tension decreases. The last packet of expired gas fills the dead space so that at end exhalation the dead space gas tension is identical to that of alveolar gas. Measurement of end expired CO_2 and O_2 tensions provides a reasonable approximation of alveolar gas tensions.

Alveolar ventilation is coupled to tissue O_2 consumption and CO_2 production. If alveolar ventilation increases so that O_2 uptake and CO_2 elimination by the lungs are greater than O_2 consumption and CO_2 production, the stores of O_2 in the lung and blood will increase and those of CO_2 will decrease. This is called *hyperventilation*. It will be reflected as an increased alveolar O_2 tension and decreased alveolar CO_2 tension. Conversely, a decrease in alveolar ventilation relative to O_2 con-

Table 2: Calculations of Alveolar Oxygen Tension, P_{AO_2}

Ventilation	$Paco_2$	R	Fio_2	BMP	P_{AO_2}
Hyperventilation	20	0.8	0.21	760	125
Normal	40	0.8	0.21	760	100
Hypoventilation	80	0.8	0.21	760	50
Hypoventilation	80	0.8	0.40	760	185
Normal	40	0.8	0.21	630	72

Using arterial CO_2 tension ($Paco_2$) as an index of alveolar ventilation, alveolar O_2 tension (P_{AO_2}) can be calculated using a simplified alveolar-air equation:

$$P_{AO_2} = Fio_2 (BMP - P_{H_2O}) - Paco_2/R.$$

Fio_2 is the fraction of inspired O_2, BMP is the barometric pressure (760 torr at sea level), P_{H_2O} is the partial pressure of water in alveolar gas (47 torr at 37°C), and R is the respiratory exchange ratio, usually 0.8 to 1.0, depending on the relative amount of fat versus carbohydrate being used as fuel. Since arterial O_2 tension is never greater than alveolar O_2 tension, this equation predicts the maximum arterial O_2 tension obtainable for any given Fio_2 and level of ventilation. Hyperventilation increases alveolar O_2 tension at any given Fio_2. Hypoventilation decreases alveolar O_2 tension, hence arterial O_2 tension, and causes hypoxia when Fio_2 is 0.21 (room air). Supplemental O_2 (eg, Fio_2 = 0.40) relieves hypoxia secondary to hypoventilation. Ascending to an altitude of 5,000 ft (eg, Denver, CO) lowers the barometric pressure to 630 torr and decreases the alveolar oxygen tension and the arterial O_2 tension.

sumption and CO_2 production is called *hypoventilation* and is reflected as a decreased alveolar O_2 tension and increased alveolar CO_2 tension. Generally, changes in arterial O_2 and CO_2 tensions are proportional to changes in alveolar O_2 and CO_2. Therefore, measurements of arterial CO_2 tension can be used to estimate changes in alveolar ventilation (Table 2).

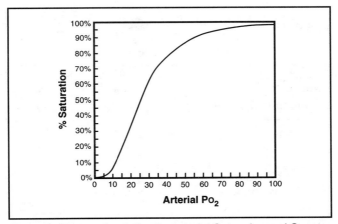

Figure 9: The graph relating the arterial O_2 tension and O_2 saturation is called the oxyhemoglobin dissociation curve. The flat upper portion of the curve ensures that blood passing through the lungs will be near fully saturated with O_2 over a wide range of alveolar O_2 tensions, while the steep middle portion of the curve allows a large volume of O_2 to be unloaded to the tissues while still maintaining mixed venous O_2 tension above the critical level for O_2 tension.

The Circulation

Blood in the alveolar capillary bed equilibrates with alveolar gas, then returns to the heart via the pulmonary veins and left atrium, and is finally pumped to the tissues of the body by the left ventricle through the systemic arterial circulation (Figure 7). In the systemic capillary bed, O_2 is removed by the tissues to support oxidative metabolism. In the tissues, O_2 diffuses out of the capillaries, into the cells, and finally into the mitochondria along a gradient of partial pressures. The minimal O_2 tension necessary to maintain this diffusion gradient is the *critical O_2 tension*. End capillary Po_2 or mixed venous Po_2 helps maintain the driving pressure for tissue oxygenation, so mixed venous Po_2 must be maintained

Table 3: Factors Affecting the Position of the Oxyhemoglobin Dissociation Curve

Shift Curve to the Left and $\Downarrow P_{50}$ (Impair Oxygen Delivery)	Shift Curve to the Right and $\Uparrow P_{50}$ (Improve Oxygen Delivery)
• Alkalosis	• Acidosis
• $\Downarrow$ Temperature	• $\Uparrow$ Temperature
• $\Downarrow$ 2,3-DPG concentrations	• $\Uparrow$ 2,3-DPG concentrations
• $\Uparrow$ Fetal hemoglobin	• $\Uparrow$ Adult hemoglobin

above the critical O_2 tension to ensure delivery of O_2 into the cells and mitochondria. Blood is then returned to the heart via the systemic venous circulation and right atrium and is pumped to the lungs by the right ventricle through the pulmonary arteries. In the lungs, CO_2 is excreted and additional O_2 is taken up by the blood.

The Blood-Oxygen Reservoir
Oxygen content

Oxygen is transported in the blood bound to hemoglobin. One gram of hemoglobin can carry roughly 1.34 mL O_2. The binding of O_2 to hemoglobin is usually expressed as a percentage saturation, Sao_2, the ratio of oxygenated hemoglobin to total hemoglobin. The percentage saturation is a non-linear function of the Pao_2 (Figure 9).

The position of the oxyhemoglobin dissociation curve is affected by changes in type of hemoglobin, pH, temperature, and concentrations of 2,3-diphosphoglycerate (2,3-DPG). Fetal hemoglobin binds O_2 more avidly than does adult hemoglobin and tends to shift the curve to the

Figure 10: The total O_2 content of blood is the sum of the O_2 bound to hemoglobin (1.34 mL O_2/g Hb x [Hb] x Sao_2) plus the dissolved O_2 (0.003 mL O_2/torr x Pao_2), where [Hb] is the hemoglobin concentration of blood in g/dL. The relationship between Po_2 and O_2 content is curvilinear because of the shape of the oxyhemoglobin dissociation curve. A change in Po_2 in the steep part of the curve from 40 to 80 torr results in a large change in content, while a large change in Pao_2 on the flat part of the curve from 80 to 400 torr has much less effect. Note the profound effect of changes in [Hb] and the small effect of changes in dissolved O_2 on O_2 content.

left. As a result, the Pao_2 at which hemoglobin is 50% saturated (P_{50}) is decreased. This shift benefits the fetus since it favors O_2 uptake at the low O_2 tensions in the placenta. However, in the newborn, this left shift may impair O_2 delivery to the tissues because mixed venous O_2 tension will decrease, decreasing tissue Po_2 and the gradient favoring diffusion of O_2 into cells (Table 3). During the first months after birth, the oxyhemoglobin dissociation curve begins to shift to the right, and between 4 and 6 months of age it is similar to that of the adult.

A small amount of O_2 is also carried dissolved in plasma (0.003 mL for each torr of PaO_2). The volume of dissolved O_2 is linearly related to the PaO_2 (Figure 10).

Oxygen delivery

Oxygen delivery to the tissues is the product of arterial oxygen content and cardiac output, and it is directly affected by changes in PaO_2, hemoglobin concentration (Hb), and cardiac output. A decrease in any one of these components can be offset to some extent by increases in the others (Figure 11).

Oxygen consumption is equal to the cardiac output times the difference between arterial O_2 content and venous O_2 content. Oxygen consumption can be affected by O_2 delivery and by the ability of the tissues to extract O_2 from blood. The difference between arterial O_2 content and venous O_2 content is a measure of effectiveness of O_2 delivery to tissues. An increase in the gradient between arterial and venous O_2 contents infers that delivery is inadequate and that the tissues are increasing extraction to maintain O_2 consumption. The ability to lower the mixed venous O_2 tension and increase extraction is limited, because a minimum gradient of oxygen tension must be maintained to facilitate diffusion of oxygen into cells and mitochondria. If mixed venous O_2 tension falls too low, O_2 delivery to mitochondria will be compromised and O_2 consumption will decrease as the cell switches from aerobic to anaerobic metabolism. Anaerobic metabolism is much less efficient, generating only 2 mol of adenosine triphosphate (ATP)/mol glucose compared with 38 mol of ATP/mol glucose for aerobic metabolism. This inefficiency results in ATP depletion and ultimate cell death. In addition, anaerobic metabolism generates two molecules of lactic acid for every molecule of glucose metabolized, resulting in tissue lactic acidosis. Therefore, the appearance of significant amounts of lactic acid in blood (>3 mmol/L) is indicative of inadequate O_2 delivery to the cellular mitochondria.

Figure 11: At top left is a plot of O_2 delivery as a function of O_2 tension for a fixed cardiac output of 200 mL/kg/min, a hemoglobin concentration of 15 g/dL, and an O_2 consumption of 10 mL/kg/min. At the arterial point A, an arterial O_2 tension of 60 torr results in an O_2 delivery to the tissues of nearly 35 mL/kg/min. If 10 mL/kg/min of O_2 is removed by the tissues, then the delivery of O_2 back to the heart from the tissues is roughly 25 mL/kg/min. This removal of O_2 decreases the O_2 tension at the venous point (V) to roughly 30 torr. In the top right figure, O_2 delivery is plotted as a function of O_2 tension for a constant cardiac output (200 mL/kg/min) and varying hemoglobin (g/dL) concentrations. On the bottom figure, O_2 delivery is plotted at a constant hemoglobin concentration and varying cardiac outputs (mL/kg/min). At arterial O_2 tensions over 50 torr, hemoglobin concentration and cardiac output have the most profound effects on O_2 delivery. Also note that at a constant arterial O_2 tension (A), as O_2 delivery decreases, the O_2 tension of venous blood (V) decreases.

Figure 12: The relationship between Pco_2 and CO_2 content of blood is nearly linear. Mixed venous Pco_2 is about 6 torr higher than arterial Pco_2. The CO_2 content of reduced blood is greater than that of oxygenated blood.

Carbon Dioxide Transport

Oxygen transport evolved to optimize oxygen-carrying capacity in room air. Carbon dioxide transport, however, evolved so that large amounts could be excreted continuously from high body concentrations to low atmospheric concentrations. Carbon dioxide can be carried by the body in several forms: dissolved in plasma, carried as bicarbonate in equilibrium with dissolved CO_2, or carried by amino acid groups in hemoglobin. The largest fraction of CO_2 is in the form of plasma or red cell bicarbonate. Carbon dioxide is 20 times more soluble in blood than oxygen, and its dissociation curve is nearly linear over physiologic ranges. As a result, large amounts of CO_2 can be carried in blood and removed from the body with relatively small changes in blood CO_2 tension (Figure 12).

Carbon dioxide and oxygen interact in the blood to enhance each other's loading and unloading capabilities where concentration extremes exist. The binding of CO_2 to hemo-

Table 4: Causes of Hypoxemia

Cause of Hypoxemia	Pa_{CO_2}	Hypoxemia Relieved by ⇑ F_{IO_2}
Hypoventilation	⇑	Yes
Diffusion block	⇒	Yes
Ventilation-perfusion mismatch	⇒ ⇓	Yes
Right-to-left shunt	⇒ ⇓	No

globin in the tissues augments unloading of oxygen from capillary blood—the *Bohr effect*. On the other hand, the binding of O_2 to hemoglobin in the alveolar capillary bed augments CO_2 unloading from capillary blood into the alveolar space—the *Haldane effect*.

By Thomas N. Hansen, MD

Ventilation-Perfusion Relationships

The four causes of arterial hypoxemia in infants are hypoventilation, diffusion block, ventilation-perfusion mismatch, and right-to-left shunt (Table 4). Hypoxemia secondary to hypoventilation is discussed in the previous section. Hypoxemia secondary to diffusion block is virtually nonexistent in the newborn and will not be addressed further. Therefore, the rest of this chapter will focus on hypoxemia secondary to ventilation-perfusion ($\dot{V}_A/\dot{Q}$) mismatch (Figure 13) and right-to-left shunt.

Ventilation-Perfusion Mismatch
Distribution of ventilation and alveolar gas tensions

In the simplest form of $\dot{V}_A/\dot{Q}$ mismatch, the lung is divided into two ventilatory compartments. One is normal or *well ventilated*, while the other is abnormal secondary to parenchymal lung disease and is *poorly ventilated*. The well-ventilated compartment receives a disproportionate share of each tidal vol-

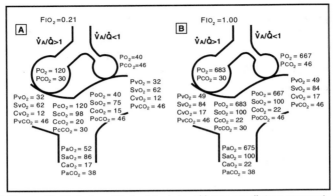

Figure 13: Both A and B depict a lung with two ventilatory compartments—one normal ($\dot{V}_A/\dot{Q}$ >1) and the other severely underventilated ($\dot{V}_A/\dot{Q}$ <1). In Figure A, the F_{IO_2} is room air, and in B, it is 100% O_2. Barometric pressure is 760 mm Hg, respiratory exchange ratio is 1.0, cardiac output is 200 mL/kg/min, hemoglobin concentration is 15 g/dL, and O_2 consumption is 10 mL/kg/min. In each figure, 50% of the total blood flow goes past each compartment. The abbreviations are defined below. See text for discussion.

Measurement	Units	Compartment Mixed Venous	Ideal Capillary	Poorly Ventilated	Mixed Arterial
O_2 Tension	mm Hg	PvO_2	PcO_2	PoO_2	PaO_2
O_2 Saturation	%	SvO_2	ScO_2	SoO_2	SaO_2
O_2 Content	mL O_2/100 mL blood	CvO_2	CcO_2	CoO_2	CaO_2
CO_2 Tension	mm Hg	$PvCO_2$	$PcCO_2$	$PoCO_2$	$PaCO_2$

ume, and the minute ventilation exchanges gas predominantly with this compartment. If blood flow to each compartment is equal, the well-ventilated compartment is ventilated out of proportion to its level of perfusion. It has a high ventilation-to-perfusion ratio ($\dot{V}_A/\dot{Q}$ >1) and is analogous to a single hyperventilated lung unit. It has a low alveolar CO_2 tension

(P_{CO_2}) and a high alveolar O_2 tension (P_{O_2}) (see *Oxygen Transport and Alveolar Ventilation* section, this chapter). The poorly ventilated compartment is perfused out of proportion to its level of ventilation and has a low ventilation-to-perfusion ratio $(\dot{V}_A/\dot{Q} <1)$. It is hypoventilated relative to its level of perfusion and has a high alveolar CO_2 tension and low alveolar O_2 tension.

Effects of $\dot{V}_A/\dot{Q}$ Mismatch on Blood Gas Tensions

Well-ventilated compartment

In the capillary bed of the well-ventilated compartment, mixed venous blood equilibrates with alveolar gas, and its O_2 tension increases and CO_2 tension decreases. The increased O_2 tension increases O_2 saturation and content. Blood flowing through this compartment is termed *idealized capillary blood*.

Poorly ventilated compartment

In the capillary bed of the poorly ventilated compartment, mixed venous blood also equilibrates with alveolar gas. However, alveolar gas tensions are similar to those of mixed venous blood, so O_2 tension increases only slightly, while CO_2 tension remains virtually unchanged. In fact, mixed venous gas tensions form the limits for alveolar gas tensions in this compartment. Alveolar O_2 tension cannot be lower than the O_2 tension of mixed venous blood, nor can alveolar CO_2 tension be higher than the CO_2 tension of mixed venous blood, no matter how severely ventilation is impaired.

Mixed arterial O_2 tension

Blood from the well-ventilated and poorly ventilated compartments combines to form *mixed arterial blood*. The O_2 content of mixed arterial blood is determined by the O_2 content and the relative blood flow through each compartment. Because the oxyhemoglobin dissociation curve is nonlinear, the O_2 content of mixed arterial blood must be calculated before calculating mixed arterial O_2 tension. Mixed arterial O_2 content is equal to the fraction of blood flowing past normal alveoli times its O_2 content plus the fraction of blood flowing past poorly ventilated alveoli times its O_2 content. Mixed arterial P_{O_2} is determined from plots of arterial O_2 tension vs content and O_2 saturation from the oxyhemoglobin dissociation curve (see *Oxygen Transport and Alveolar Ventilation* section, this chapter).

Mixed arterial CO_2 tension

Since the plot of blood CO_2 tension vs CO_2 content is roughly linear, mixed arterial CO_2 tension can be calculated from the capillary CO_2 tensions and relative blood flows of each compartment.

Mixed venous O_2 tension

Since $\dot{V}A/\dot{Q}$ mismatch decreases arterial O_2 content, it must also decrease mixed venous O_2 content, if O_2 consumption and cardiac output remain constant (see *Oxygen Transport and Alveolar Ventilation* section, this chapter). In Figure 13, mixed venous oxygen content can be calculated from O_2 consumption and calculated O_2 delivery.

Venous admixture

In infants with $\dot{V}A/\dot{Q}$ mismatch, the severity of hypoxemia is determined by the relative proportion of blood flow through the open, poorly ventilated lung compartment. The contribution of $\dot{V}A/\dot{Q}$ mismatch to arterial hypoxemia can be calculated as the venous admixture. The venous admixture is that fraction of mixed venous return that is not oxygenated above mixed venous levels on passing through the lung. It is calculated using the values for ideal pulmonary capillary O_2 content (CcO_2), mixed arterial O_2 content (CaO_2), and mixed venous O_2 content (CvO_2):

$$\text{Venous admixture} = [(CcO_2 - CaO_2)/(CcO_2 - CvO_2)] \times 100\%.$$

In the example in Figure 13A, the venous admixture is 38%.

Effect of Increased F_{IO_2} on Venous Admixture

Because the poorly ventilated alveoli are open to the airway, increasing the inspired O_2 tension should increase their alveolar P_{O_2} (Figure 14). In Figure 13B, increasing F_{IO_2} to 1.00 dramatically increases the P_{O_2} in the open but poorly ventilated lung units.

Figure 14: Alveolar P_{O_2} is plotted as a function of F_{IO_2} for normal alveoli $\dot{V}_A/\dot{Q} = 1$ and for alveoli that are progressively underventilated with respect to their perfusion, $\dot{V}_A/\dot{Q} < 1$. As ventilation decreases relative to perfusion, more O_2 is removed from the alveolus by the blood than can be replaced by alveolar ventilation, and the alveolar P_{O_2} decreases. For severely underventilated units, $\dot{V}_A/\dot{Q} < 1$, alveolar P_{O_2} increases only when F_{IO_2} approaches 1.00. The dramatic increase in alveolar P_{O_2} occurs because of nitrogen washout (Table 5). (Adapted from Hansen TN, Corbet AJ: Disorders of the transition. In: Taeusch HW, et al, eds. *Schaffer and Avery's Diseases of the Newborn.* 6th ed. Philadelphia, WB Saunders, 1991, p 500.)

The O_2 content of the blood perfusing these units increases 30%, while the O_2 content of the blood perfusing the well-ventilated units increases only 10%. As a result, the O_2 content of mixed arterial blood increases. The calculated venous admixture is now near zero. Note that most of the increase in mixed arterial O_2 content was the result of increased O_2 content in the open but poorly ventilated alveoli. This example demonstrates an important concept. The cause of hypoxemia in infants with $\dot{V}_A/\dot{Q}$ mismatch is perfusion of poorly ventilated but open alveoli. The only way to increase the arterial P_{O_2} in these infants is to increase the P_{O_2} in these poorly ventilated alveoli (Table 5).

Table 5: Distribution of Gas Pressures*

	$F_{IO_2} = 0.21$	$F_{IO_2} = 1.00$
P_{O_2} (mm Hg)	40	667
P_{CO_2} (mm Hg)	46	46
P_{N_2} (mm Hg)	627	0
P_{H_2O} (mm Hg)	47	47
Total (mm Hg)	760	760

*The sum of the partial pressures of all gases in an alveolus that is communicating with the airway must equal atmospheric pressure (760 mm Hg). In a poorly ventilated lung unit exposed to an $F_{IO_2} = 0.21$, alveolar N_2 tension accounts for most of this partial pressure. If the lung unit is ventilated with pure O_2 for several hours, all of the gaseous N_2 is washed out and the alveolar $P_{N_2} = 0$. Since the P_{CO_2} is fixed by the mixed venous P_{CO_2}, and P_{H_2O} is determined by body temperature, the alveolar P_{O_2} must increase to make up the difference or the alveolus will collapse.

Right-to-Left Shunt

Blood that flows from the venous circulation (the right side of the circulation) to the arterial circulation (the left side of the circulation) without flowing past an open lung unit results in a *right-to-left shunt*. There are three pathways through which right-to-left shunt may occur:

- through the lung, past areas of atelectasis or through vessels that develop before alveoli form;
- through persistent fetal circulatory pathways such as the foramen ovale or ductus arteriosus;
- through abnormal structures resulting from congenital abnormalities of the heart and great vessels.

Right-to-left shunt represents a special case of $\dot{V}_A/\dot{Q}$ mismatch where ventilation equals zero, hence $\dot{V}_A/\dot{Q} = 0$ (Figure 15).

Figure 15: A and B each depict a lung with a well-ventilated compartment and right-to-left shunt. In A, the $FIO_2 = 0.21$, and in B, the $FIO_2 = 1.00$. The modifier 's' refers to blood flowing through the shunt. In both figures, half of the mixed venous return flows through the shunt and half past normal lung units. The other abbreviations and assumptions are the same as for Figure 13.

Effects of Shunt on
Mixed Arterial Blood Gas Tensions
Mixed arterial O_2 tension

In infants with right-to-left shunt (Figure 15), mixed venous blood returns to the lung poorly oxygenated. A portion of this blood flows past normal alveoli where it equilibrates with alveolar gas and becomes well oxygenated *(ideal capillary blood)*. The remainder, the true right-to-left shunt, flows from the mixed venous to the arterial circulation without passing an open lung unit and remains poorly oxygenated *(shunt blood)*.

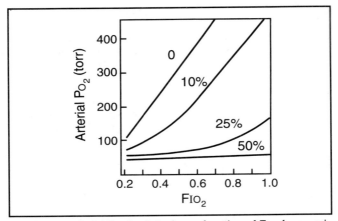

Figure 16: Arterial P_{O_2} is plotted as a function of F_{IO_2} for a variety of right-to-left shunts. When the total right-to-left shunt exceeds 50%, there is little effect of increasing F_{IO_2} on arterial P_{O_2}. (Adapted from Benatar SR, et al: The use of iso-shunt lines for control of oxygen therapy. *Br J Anaesth* 1973;45:722.)

These two streams of blood mix before returning to the heart. The O_2 content of this mixed arterial blood is determined by the O_2 content and relative blood flows through each compartment. The effects of right-to-left shunt on mixed arterial O_2 content, O_2 saturation, and O_2 tension can be calculated as described in the section on $\dot{V}_A/\dot{Q}$ mismatch. Since shunt decreases arterial O_2 content, it also decreases mixed venous O_2 content if O_2 consumption and cardiac output remain constant.

Mixed arterial CO_2 tension

Mixed arterial CO_2 tension is calculated as described for $\dot{V}_A/\dot{Q}$ mismatch. The normal lung compartment is relatively hyperventilated, while the ventilation in the shunt compartment equals zero.

Shunt equation

Using the values for ideal pulmonary capillary O_2 content (C_cO_2), mixed arterial O_2 content (C_aO_2), and mixed venous

O_2 content (CvO_2), we can calculate the percentage for the shunt: $[(CcO_2 - CaO_2)/(CcO_2 - CvO_2)] \times 100\%$. In the example in Figure 15, the shunt is 50%.

Effect of Increased FIo₂ on Right-to-Left Shunt

Arterial hypoxemia secondary to right-to-left shunt cannot be completely relieved by administration of supplemental O_2 (Figure 15B). Increasing FIO_2 increases the O_2 content of blood flowing through the normally ventilated compartment but does not affect the O_2 content of the blood flowing through the shunt. While mixed arterial O_2 tension will increase slightly because of the small increase in O_2 content of blood flowing past normal alveoli, this increase is relatively small compared to that found with $\dot{V}A/\dot{Q}$ mismatch (Figure 13B). More importantly, the calculated shunt remains 50%. The effects of right-to-left shunt on arterial O_2 tension are shown graphically in Figure 16.

Combination V̇A/Q̇ Mismatch and Right-to-Left Shunt Disorders

In most clinical conditions, hypoxemia is a result of a combination of $\dot{V}A/\dot{Q}$ mismatch and right-to-left shunt (Figure 17). Well-oxygenated blood flowing past well-ventilated alveoli mixes with poorly oxygenated blood flowing past open poorly ventilated alveoli and blood flowing through the right-to-left shunt. The mixed arterial O_2 content depends on the O_2 content and the relative amounts of blood flowing through each of these three compartments. The *venous admixture* is that fraction of blood returning to the left side of the heart that is not oxygenated above mixed venous O_2 content. For values of FIO_2 <1.00, blood flowing past poorly ventilated alveoli and blood flowing through the right-to-left shunt contribute to the venous admixture. When FIO_2 equals 1.00, any contribution to the venous admixture from open, poorly ventilated alveoli disappears (Figure 13B). Therefore, when $FIO_2 = 1.00$, the size of the venous admixture is determined only by the size of the right-to-left shunt; that is, percent venous admixture = percent shunt. This phenomenon is the basis for the hyperoxia test. If an infant breathes 100% O_2, any contribution from the perfusion

Figure 17: In this example of a combination disorder, hypoxemia is the result of perfusion of poorly ventilated alveoli and right-to-left shunt. See text for discussion.

of poorly ventilated alveoli to arterial hypoxemia is abolished, and any remaining hypoxemia must be the result of right-to-left shunt. Failure to increase arterial O_2 content, saturation, or tension while breathing 100% O_2 is strongly suggestive of anatomic right-to-left shunt and congenital heart disease.

Arterial-Alveolar Gas Tension Gradients

In the simple one-compartment model of the lung used to describe alveolar ventilation, it was assumed that capillary blood equilibrated completely with alveolar gas so that arterial blood gas tensions were identical to alveolar gas tensions. This is also true for the multicompartment lung, provided that all compartments are equally well ventilated and well perfused; that is, all have $\dot{V}_A/\dot{Q} = 1$. In the face of $\dot{V}_A/\dot{Q}$ mismatch, however, alveolar gas tensions are not equal to arterial gas tensions (Figure 17).

Table 6: Calculation of Alveolar and Mixed Arterial Gradients from the Example in Figure 17

	Alveolar (mm Hg)	Mixed Arterial (mm Hg)	Gradient (mm Hg)
O_2	120	40	$A\text{-}aDo_2 = 80$
CO_2	30	41	$a\text{-}ADco_2 = 11$
N_2	563	595	$a\text{-}ADN_2 = 32$

A-a: Alveolar to arterial; a-A: Arterial to alveolar

In lungs with unequal ventilation, most of each tidal volume enters and leaves the well-ventilated compartment ($\dot{V}A/\dot{Q} > 1$). Therefore, the composition of end tidal expired gas is determined predominantly by the alveolar gas composition in the well-ventilated compartment (Table 6 and Figure 17). The three commonly used alveolar-arterial gas gradients, $A\text{-}aDo_2$, $a\text{-}ADco_2$, and $a\text{-}ADN_2$, are calculated in Table 6.

$A\text{-}aDo_2$

The alveolar to arterial gradient for O_2 is used to estimate the severity of arterial hypoxemia. It is increased by increased perfusion of poorly ventilated alveoli and by increased blood flow through the right-to-left shunt. In patients breathing pure O_2, the $A\text{-}aDo_2$ is determined solely by the size of the right-to-left shunt. In patients with a right-to-left shunt, the $A\text{-}aDo_2$ increases with increasing Fio_2 and as such is a poor estimate of lung disease severity (Figure 16).

$a\text{-}ADco_2$

The arterial to alveolar gradient for CO_2 arises because some alveoli are ventilated out of proportion to their perfusion. These hyperventilated alveoli with low alveolar CO_2 tensions determine the CO_2 tensions of end tidal gas. The CO_2 tension of mixed arterial blood is determined by the CO_2 tensions in all lung compartments. An increased a-$ADCO_2$ implies that some alveoli are ventilated out of proportion to their perfusion *(physiologic dead space)* and as such is an estimate of wasted ventilation.

a-ADN_2

The arterial to alveolar gradient for N_2 is the result of perfusion of open but poorly ventilated alveoli. Alveolar or end-tidal N_2 tension is determined by the N_2 tension in well-ventilated lung units. Mixed arterial N_2 tension is determined by the N_2 tension in blood from all lung compartments. In severely underventilated alveoli, the alveolar O_2 tension is reduced because O_2 extraction by blood exceeds its replacement by alveolar ventilation. Alveolar PCO_2 is fixed by mixed venous PCO_2, and PH_2O is determined by body temperature. If the alveolus is open to the airway, the sum of partial pressures must equal 760 mm Hg. As a result, alveolar N_2 tension increases. The N_2 tension of blood perfusing these alveoli also increases; and, when this blood mixes with blood from both the well-ventilated compartment and from the right-to-left shunt, mixed arterial N_2 tension increases. N_2 is neither produced nor consumed in the tissues, so mixed arterial N_2 tension is equal to mixed venous N_2 tension. Therefore, the N_2 tension of blood from the right-to-left shunt is equal to that of mixed venous blood (mixed arterial N_2 tension), and the a-ADN_2 is not affected by the size of the right-to-left shunt. The a-ADN_2 only increases if the volume of blood flow past open but poorly ventilated alveoli increases. As a result, the a-ADN_2 is a measure of the contribution of the open but poorly ventilated alveoli to the venous admixture.

By Thomas N. Hansen, MD, and James M. Adams, MD

Lung and Heart Interaction

Pleural Pressure

The lungs, heart, and great vessels all share the thoracic cavity. As a result, changes in pleural pressure (Ppl) directly affect the heart and great vessels as well as the lungs (Figure 18).

Figure 18: Effects of pleural pressure on blood return to the right atrium (RA) via the superior vena cava (SVC) and inferior vena cava (IVC) and ejection of blood from the left ventricle (LV) into the aorta.

Table 7: Conditions Causing Sustained Increases in Pleural Pressure	
Lung Overinflation	**Distention of the Pleural Space**
Overzealous mechanical ventilation	Pneumothorax
Pulmonary interstitial emphysema	Chylothorax
Cystic lung diseases	Pleural effusion

Decreased Ppl reduces the pressure surrounding the heart and literally sucks blood from systemic veins into the right atrium, increasing venous return and right ventricular output. However, the same decrease in Ppl impedes left ventricular contraction and impairs left ventricular output. In infants with hyaline membrane disease, Ppl decreases markedly with inspiration. Consequently, left ventricular stroke volume and systolic blood pressure decrease with inspiration. If blood pressure is continuously monitored via an in-

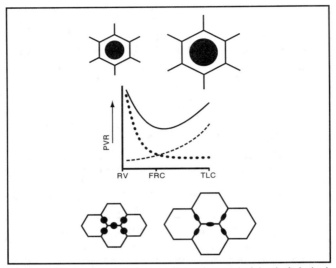

Figure 19: There are two types of blood vessels (shaded circles) in the lung: (1) Extra-alveolar vessels (top) that course in the extra-alveolar interstitium with airways and lymphatics; and (2) intra-alveolar vessels (bottom) that course through the intra-alveolar septa. During lung inflation, mechanical forces dilate extra-alveolar vessels, while the intra-alveolar vessels are compressed within the alveolar walls. Therefore, vascular resistance (PVR) of extra-alveolar vessels decreases with lung inflation (dotted line), while that of intra-alveolar vessels increases (dashed line). The net result is that total pulmonary vascular resistance (solid line) is lowest at resting lung volume, FRC, and increases at lung volumes above or below FRC (graph in middle). (Adapted from Hansen TN, Corbet AJ: Pulmonary physiology of the newborn. In: Taeusch HW, et al, eds. *Schaffer and Avery's Diseases of the Newborn*. 6th ed. Philadelphia, WB Saunders, 1991, p 483.)

dwelling arterial catheter, this 'fluctuating blood pressure' is apparent. The magnitude of the decrease in systolic blood pressure with inspiration is proportional to the decrease in Ppl, hence, it is a marker of the severity of the lung disease.

Increased Ppl compresses the heart, impairs venous return, and decreases right ventricular output. Sustained increases in Ppl may occur secondarily to lung overinflation or space-occupying lesions of the pleura (Table 7).

Conversely, cyclical increases in Ppl also compress the left ventricle, transiently augmenting ventricular systole and increasing left ventricular output. This phenomenon explains the maintenance of the circulation during external cardiac massage.

Alveolar Volume

Lung inflation directly affects the resistance to blood flow across the lung (Figure 19). Alveolar overdistention secondary to gas trapping or overzealous mechanical ventilation compresses intra-alveolar vessels and markedly increases pulmonary vascular resistance. If Ppl becomes positive, a decrease in systemic venous return occurs, and the increase in resistance results in severe hypotension. In addition, the compression of vessels in alveolar walls will increase pulmonary vascular resistance and shunt blood away from the lung through fetal pathways (see *Persistent Pulmonary Hypertension of the Newborn*, Chapter 4, and $\dot{V}_A/\dot{Q}$ *Mismatch*, this chapter), resulting in hypoxia refractory to increases in F_{IO_2}. *By Thomas N. Hansen, MD*

Surfactant

Surface Tension

The internal surface area of the human lung occupies approximately 1 m^2/kg body weight. This surface is lined by a layer of fluid that creates an air-liquid interface. At this interface, water molecules are attracted to other water molecules in the liquid phase. This attraction minimizes the surface area exposed to the air phase. These same forces cause water to form beads on a glass surface. In the lung, the net result is a tendency of alveoli to collapse according to the Pierre Simon de Laplace equation: $P = 2 \times T/R$, where P is the pressure needed to resist collapse, T is the surface tension, and R is the radius of the alveolus. According to this equation, as sur-

Figure 20: Two bubbles of unequal size are connected by a tube. When the tube is closed (top), there is no gas flow. When the tube is open (bottom), according to the Laplace equation, the pressure will be greater in the smaller bubble (radius r_s) than in the large bubble (radius r_b). As a result, gas will flow from the small bubble into the large bubble.

face tension increases, the amount of pressure needed to overcome surface tension forces also increases. Calculations suggest that if the alveoli were lined only by water, it would take pressures exceeding 55 cm H_2O to inflate the lungs. Furthermore, since the pressure needed to resist collapse is inversely proportional to the radius, the Laplace equation predicts that small alveoli would tend to empty into large alveoli and that the lung would proceed to complete collapse at end exhalation (Figure 20). Of course, individuals breathe using far less inflation pressure because of the presence in the alveolar lining liquid of *surfactant*, which lowers surface tension forces. This substance is pulmonary surfactant.

Surfactant Function

Surfactant is produced in type II alveolar epithelial cells. It is composed of phospholipid with small amounts of neutral fat, cholesterol, and protein (Figure 21). The primary active molecule is saturated dipalmitoyl phosphatidylcholine (DPPC) (Figure 22). Other components of surfactant, including unsaturated phosphatidylcholine and phosphatidylglycerol, are important in making surfactant more fluid and fa-

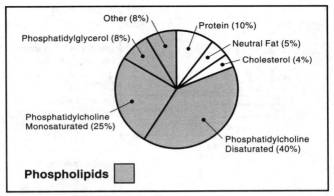

Figure 21: The composition of surfactant.

cilitating respreading. Surfactant lowers surface tension by adsorbing to the surface and displacing water molecules (Figure 23).

Surfactant Proteins

Four different proteins are associated with the pulmonary surfactant: SP-A, SP-B, SP-C, and SP-D.

SP-A

SP-A is the most abundant of the surfactant proteins, constituting nearly 5% by weight of the surfactant. It is a water-soluble protein composed of 228 amino acids in its monomeric state. The active protein consists of 18 monomeric units. SP-A reacts with SP-B, calcium, and surfactant to form *tubular myelin*, a latticelike network of lipoprotein that is highly surface active and increases adsorption of the surfactant lipids to the air-liquid interface. SP-A plays a role in surfactant recycling by enhancing the phospholipid uptake by alveolar type II cells and inhibiting phospholipid secretion. Some evidence suggests that SP-A may take part in protecting the lung from oxidative stresses. Finally, SP-A plays a role in host defense in the lung. SP-A is not present in any of the surfactants now available for clinical use.

Figure 22: DPPC consists of two molecules of palmitic acid and one molecule of phosphocholine attached to a glycerol backbone. DPPC has a hydrophobic end (fatty acids) and hydrophilic end (nitrogenous base) and aligns itself in the air-liquid interface with the hydrophobic end in the gas phase and the hydrophilic end in the water phase.

SP-B

SP-B is a hydrophobic protein whose 381 amino acid precursor protein is proteolytically processed in the cell to a 79 amino acid active protein. It is important in the formation of tubular myelin, and relatively small amounts (<1% by weight) dramatically alter spreading and adsorption of the surfactant. SP-B also enhances uptake of surfactant by alveolar type II cells and may play a role in recycling of surfactant. The importance of SP-B in the lung has recently been underscored from the case reports of several term infants with congenital SP-B deficiency. These infants presented with severe respiratory distress progressing to respiratory failure. Treatment consisted of prolonged extracorporeal membrane oxygenation (ECMO) support followed by lung transplantation. SP-B is found in all currently available natural surfactants.

SP-C

SP-C is a hydrophobic protein that constitutes roughly 0.4% of the surfactant by weight. Its 197 amino acid precursor protein is processed in the cell to a 35-36 amino acid active protein. It enhances the rate of adsorption and spreading of the surfactant. In addition, it enhances uptake of phospho-

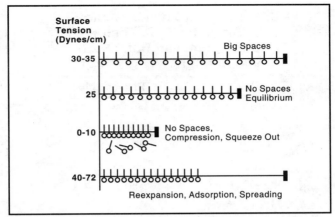

Figure 23: At equilibrium, surfactant displaces water molecules from the surface and lowers the surface tension from 72 dynes/cm to roughly 25 dynes/cm. At low lung volumes, DPPC resists compression and lowers surface tension to near zero, further ensuring alveolar stability. During compression of the surface, some surfactant molecules are squeezed out into the bulk phase. With reexpansion of the lung, any lag in returning these molecules to the surface will result in increased surface tension.

lipid vesicles by type II cells and may also play a role in surfactant recycling. SP-C is found in all currently available natural surfactants.

SP-D

SP-D is the most recent of the surfactant proteins to be described. It constitutes only 0.2% by weight of the surfactant and is similar to SP-A in structure. Its functions are most likely related to host defense mechanisms in the lung. Like SP-A, SP-D may protect surfactant phospholipids and macrophages from oxidative damage.

Surfactant Synthesis

DPPC and other lipids are synthesized in the smooth endoplasmic reticulum of the type II alveolar epithelial cell. The

Table 8: Risk of HMD as a Function of Amniotic Fluid Lecithin/ Sphingomyelin Ratio (L/S) and Phosphatidylglycerol (PG)

Amniotic Fluid	Risk of HMD
L/S >2.0 *	<0.5%
L/S <1.0	100%
L/S 1.0 to 2.0	⇓ as L/S ⇑
PG present	<0.5%
L/S <2.0; PG absent	>80%
L/S >2.0; PG present	0

* In pregnancies complicated by diabetes or Rh isoimmunization, the risk of hyaline membrane disease with an L/S between 2 and 3 is roughly 13%.

lipids are transported in vesicles along microtubules and are stored in the lamellar bodies. The surfactant proteins are synthesized outside the rough endoplasmic reticulum, glycosylated in the Golgi apparatus, and then incorporated into the lamellar bodies. Lung inflation activates β receptors in the type II cells to mobilize intracellular calcium, and the contents of the lamellar bodies are excreted into the air space. The secreted lipoprotein is converted into tubular myelin, a specialized form of surfactant, which rapidly moves to the surface of the air-liquid interface. After secretion, surfactant phospholipids can be taken back up into the type II cells by endocytosis and rapidly converted back into lamellar bodies for resecretion. The turnover time for surfactant is roughly 10 hours.

Type II alveolar epithelial cells begin to appear in the lung between 20 and 24 weeks' gestation. DPPC can be measured in whole lung extracts about this time and increases after 24 weeks. The presence of surfactant in the alveolar fluid lags considerably behind its appearance in lung tissue. Corticosteroids and thyroid hormone increase the rate of synthesis by increasing the rate of transcription and the synthesis of important rate-limiting enzymes.

The lung of the fetus is not collapsed but is filled with a fluid that is secreted by cells of the alveolar/airway epithelium. Throughout the latter part of gestation, this fluid wells up through the trachea and is either swallowed or excreted into the amniotic cavity. As a result, the fetal lung fluid contributes to the overall amniotic fluid volume and composition. Any substances, such as surfactant, secreted into the fetal alveolar space will eventually wind up in the amniotic fluid. It is possible to estimate fetal lung maturity by measuring the concentration of components of the pulmonary surfactant in the amniotic fluid. Usually, this is done by measuring the concentration of phosphatidylcholine or lecithin on samples of amniotic fluid obtained at amniocentesis. Because changes in amniotic fluid volume can change the lecithin concentration, these measurements are compared to the concentration of sphingomyelin, which remains relatively constant during gestation. The L/S ratio increases slowly between 24 and 32 weeks' gestation to about 1 and then surges at 34 to 35 weeks' gestation to greater than 2. Phosphatidylglycerol secretion into the lung, hence into amniotic fluid, also increases dramatically after 35 weeks' gestation. Its presence or absence also reflects lung maturity.

The risk of hyaline membrane disease can be predicted from individual studies or combinations of studies as depicted in Table 8.

An adequate amount of surfactant in the air-liquid interface is crucial to alveolar stability. Surfactant deficiency results from an imbalance between the production and utilization of surfactant. Since surfactant production and secretion are developmentally regulated processes, the most common cause of deficiency is early or preterm delivery (see *Hyaline Membrane Disease*, Chapter 4).

Indications

The most frequent and well-studied indication for surfactant therapy is respiratory distress syndrome secondary to surfactant deficiency or hyaline membrane disease (see *Hyaline Membrane Disease* section, Chapter 4, for treatment strategies and administration).

Several pulmonary disorders in the newborn have surfactant dysfunction or inactivation as a component of the disorder. There is some evidence that surfactant administration improves oxygenation and reduces the need for subsequent interventions. Several studies have shown that infants with meconium aspiration syndrome treated with natural surfactants have improved oxygenation, less need for assisted ventilation, or shorter hospitalizations.

There are a few reports in small numbers of patients that the lung dysfunction associated with pneumonia may be improved by exogenous surfactant administration.

The benefits of surfactant in treating patients with congenital diaphragmatic hernia are not clear. However, several small reports suggest benefit, and several report improved survival when surfactant replacement is included in a protocol for the management of infants with congenital diaphragmatic hernia.

Surfactant Preparations and Administration

See *Hyaline Membrane Disease* section, Chapter 4.

By Alicia A. Moïse, MD, and Thomas N. Hansen, MD

Suggested Readings

Lung Mechanics

Bhutani VK, Sivieri EM, Abbasi S, et al: Evaluation of neonatal pulmonary mechanics and energetics: a two factor least mean square analysis. *Pediatr Pulmonol* 1988;4:150-158.

Bryan AC, England SJ: Maintenance of an elevated FRC in the newborn: paradox of REM sleep. *Am Rev Respir Dis* 1984;129:209.

Cook CD, Sutherland JM, Segal S, et al: Studies of respiratory physiology in the newborn infant. III. Measurements of mechanics of respiration. *J Clin Invest* 1957;36:440.

Gerhardt T, Bancalari E: Chestwall compliance in full-term and premature infants. *Acta Paediatr Scand* 1980;69:359.

Lesouef PN, England SJ, Bryan AC: Passive respiratory mechanics in newborns and children. *Am Rev Respir Dis* 1984;129:552.

McCann EM, Goldman SL, Brady JP: Pulmonary function in the sick newborn infant. *Pediatr Res* 1987;21:313.

McIlroy MB, Tierney DF, Nadel JA: A new method for measurement of compliance and resistance of lungs and thorax. *J Appl Physiol* 1963;18:424.

Nelson NM: Neonatal pulmonary function. *Pediatr Clin North Am* 1966;13:769.

Nunn JF: *Nunn's Applied Respiratory Physiology*, 4th ed. Oxford, Butterworth Heinemann, 1993.

Perez-Fontan JJ, Heldt GP, Gregory GA: Resistance and inertia of endotracheal tubes used in infants during periodic flow. *Crit Care Med* 1985;13:1052-1055.

Polgar G, Promadhat V: *Pulmonary Function Testing in Children: Techniques and Standards.* Philadelphia, WB Saunders Co, 1971.

Richardson P, Pace WR, Valdes E, et al: Time dependence of lung mechanics in preterm lambs. *Pediatr Res* 1992;31:276-279.

Oxygen Transport and Alveolar Ventilation

Comroe JH, Forster RE II, Dubois AB, et al: *The Lung: Clinical Physiology and Pulmonary Function Tests.* 2nd ed. Chicago, Year Book Medical Publishers Inc, 1962, p 27.

Cook CD, Cherry RB, O'Brien D, et al: Studies of respiratory physiology in the newborn infant. I. Observations on normal premature and full-term infants. *J Clin Invest* 1955;34:975.

Nelson NM: Respiration and circulation after birth. In: Smith CA, Nelson NM, eds. *The Physiology of the Newborn Infant.* Springfield, Charles C Thomas, 1976.

Slonim NB, Hamilton LH: *Respiratory Physiology.* 5th ed. St Louis, CV Mosby, 1987, p 52.

Ventilation-Perfusion Relationships

Corbet AJ, Ross JA, Beaudry PH, et al: Effect of positive-pressure breathing on $aADn_2$ in hyaline membrane disease. *J Appl Physiol* 1975;38:33-38.

Corbet AJ, Ross JA, Beaudry PH, et al: Ventilation-perfusion relationships as assessed by $aADn_2$ in hyaline membrane disease. *J Appl Physiol* 1974;36:74-81.

Farhi LE: Ventilation-perfusion relationship and its role in alveolar gas exchange. In: Caro CG, ed. *Advances in Respiratory Physiology.* Baltimore, Williams and Wilkins, 1966.

Hansen TN, Corbet AJ, Kenny JD, et al: Effects of oxygen and constant positive pressure breathing on arterial alveolar difference for CO_2 in hyaline membrane disease. *Pediatr Res* 1979;13:1167-1171.

Landers S, Hansen TN, Corbet AJ, et al: Optimal constant positive airway pressure assessed by arterial alveolar difference for CO_2 in hyaline membrane disease. *Pediatr Res* 1986;20:884-889.

Markello R, Winter P, Olszowka A: Assessment of ventilation-perfusion inequalities by arterial-alveolar nitrogen differences in intensive-care patients. *Anesthesiology* 1972;37:4.

Nelson NM: Respiration and circulation after birth. In: Smith CA, Nelson NM, eds. The *Physiology of the Newborn Infant*. Springfield, Charles C Thomas, 1976.

Nunn JF: *Nunn's Applied Respiratory Physiology*, 4th ed. Oxford, Butterworth Heinemann, 1993.

Thibeault DW, Poblete E, Auld PA: Alveolar-arterial oxygen difference in premature infants breathing 100 per cent oxygen. *J Pediatr* 1967;71:814-824.

West JB: *Ventilation Blood Flow and Gas Exchange*. London, Blackwell Scientific, 1970.

Lung and Heart Interaction

Fishman AP: Pulmonary circulation. In: Fishman AP, Fisher AB, Geiger SR, eds. *Handbook of Physiology*. I. Bethesda, American Physiological Society, 1986, p 93.

McGregor M: Current concepts: pulsus paradoxus. *N Engl J Med* 1979;301:480.

Niemann JT, Rosborough J, Hausknect M, et al: Cough-CPR: documentation of systemic perfusion in man and in an experimental model: a "window" to the mechanism of blood flow in external CPR. *Crit Care Med* 1980;8:141.

Perlman J, Thach B: Respiratory origin of fluctuations in arterial blood pressure in premature infants with respiratory distress syndrome. *Pediatrics* 1988;81:399.

Surfactant

Auten RL, Notter RH, Kendig JW, et al: Surfactant treatment of full-term newborns with respiratory failure. *Pediatrics* 1991;87:101.

Avery ME, Mead J: Surface properties in relation to atelectasis and hyaline membrane disease. *Am J Dis Child* 1959;97:517.

Bangham AD, Morley CJ, Phillips MC: The physical properties of an effective lung surfactant. *Biochim Biophys Acta* 1979;573:552.

Bos AP, Tibboel D, Hazebroek FW, et al: Surfactant replacement in high-risk congenital diaphragmatic hernia. *Lancet* 1991;338:1279.

Bridges JP, Davis HW, Damodarasamy M, et al: Pulmonary surfactant proteins A and D are potent endogenous inhibitors of lipid peroxidation and oxidative cellular injury. *J Biol Chem* 2000;275:38848-38855.

Clements JA, Tooley WH: Kinetics of surface active material in the fetal lung. In: Hodson WA, ed. *Development of the Lung*. New York, Marcel Dekker Inc, 1977.

Clements JA: Surface phenomena in relation to pulmonary function (Sixth Bowditch Lecture). *Physiologist* 1962;5:11.

Fetter WP, Baerts W, Bos AP, et al: Surfactant replacement therapy in neonates with respiratory failure due to bacterial sepsis. *Acta Paediatr* 1995;84:14.

Findlay RD, Taeusch HW, Walther FJ: Surfactant replacement therapy for meconium aspiration syndrome. *Pediatrics* 1996;97:48-52.

Finer NN, Tierney A, Etches PC, et al: Congenital diaphragmatic hernia: developing a protocolized approach. *J Pediatr Surg* 1998;33:1331.

Glick PL, Leach CL, Besner GE, et al: Pathophysiology of congenital diaphragmatic hernia. III: exogenous surfactant therapy for the high-risk neonate with CDH. *J Pediatr* Surg 1992;27:866.

Gluck L, Kulovich MV, Borer RC, et al: Diagnosis of the respiratory distress syndrome by amniocentesis. *Am J Obstet Gynecol* 1971;109:440.

Goerke J: Lung surfactant. *Biochim Biophys Acta* 1974;344:241.

Hallman M, Gluck L: Development of the fetal lung. *J Perinat Med* 1977;5:3.

Hawgood S: Surfactant: composition, structure, and metabolism. In: Crystal RG, West JB, Barnes PJ, eds. *The Lung*. New York, Raven Press Ltd, 1991, p 247.

King RJ: Pulmonary surface active material: basic concepts. In: Bloom RS, Sinclair JC, Warshaw JB, eds. *The Surfactant and the Neonatal Lung*. Evansville, Mead Johnson and Co, 1979.

Smith BT: Pulmonary surfactant during fetal development and neonatal adaption: hormonal control. In: Robertson B, VanGolde LMG, Batenburg JJ, eds. *Pulmonary Surfactant*. Amsterdam, Elsevier Press, 1984.

Somaschini M, Locatelli G, Salvoni L, et al: Impact of new treatments for respiratory failure on outcome of infants with congenital diaphragmatic hernia. *Eur J Pediatr* 1999;158:780.

Van Golde LM, Batenburg JJ, Robertson B: The pulmonary surfactant system: biochemical aspects and functional significance. *Physiol Rev* 1988;68:374-455.

Whitsett JA: Pulmonary surfactant and respiratory distress syndrome in the premature infant. In: Crystal RG, West JB, Barnes PJ, eds. *The Lung*. New York, Raven Press Ltd, 1991, p 1723.

Chapter 3

Approach to the Patient With Respiratory Disease

As in other areas of medicine, a good history and a thorough physical examination are essential to making an accurate diagnosis and rendering the most appropriate management in newborns with respiratory disease. A systematic and complete maternal history is essential to anticipate problems and optimize care to high-risk newborns. In particular, antenatal and perinatal conditions may affect the risk and severity of respiratory distress (Tables 1 and 2).

History

The following is a suggested list of items to include in a complete history.

Maternal History

- Health before this pregnancy (including during previous pregnancies)
- Prenatal care (including date of first visit, number of visits, weight gain, and laboratory and ultrasound studies)
- Family illnesses, including father's family
- Pregnancy-related illnesses (eg, diabetes, pregnancy-induced hypertension, sexually transmitted diseases, or infections)
- Maternal medications (including vitamins and iron) and substance abuse (eg, cigarettes, alcohol, street drugs)
- Time and reason for maternal admission to the hospital
- Time of labor onset
- Maternal evaluation and treatment since admission (eg, antibiotics, corticosteroids, tocolytics, narcotics)

Table 1: Risk Factors Associated With Hyaline Membrane Disease

Increased risk	Decreased risk
Male sex	Female sex
White race	Black race
L/S ratio <2.0 in prematures	L/S ratio >2.0
Previously affected sibling	Maternal toxemia
Maternal diabetes (class A, B, or C)	Maternal diabetes (class D, F, or R)
Maternal hypotension	Maternal drug abuse
C-section without labor	Maternal antenatal corticosteroids
Third-trimester hemorrhage	Chronic abruption
Second twin	Prolonged rupture of membranes
Hydrops fetalis	Intrauterine growth retardation
Fetal depression	

- Fetal status, including time of rupture of membranes, description of amniotic fluid (clear, foul smelling, or meconium stained), maternal bleeding (timing and amount), and evidence of fetal distress
- Method of delivery (cesarean [C-section] or vaginal)
- Gestational age at delivery and the method of determination

Infant History
- Condition at delivery (resuscitation, Apgar score, and Silverman score)
- Admission vital signs
- Observations, evaluations, and treatment during the period of neonatal transition and before consultation

By Charleta Guillory, MD, and Gerardo Cabrera-Meza, MD

Table 2: Risk Factors Associated With Other Diseases

Associated With Other Lung Diseases

Congenital pneumonia	Male sex Maternal fever Chorioamnionitis Preterm labor Prolonged labor Maternal colonization with group B streptococci Tracheoesophageal fistula
Meconium aspiration syndrome	Meconium-stained amniotic fluid Fetal depression Postmaturity
Transient tachypnea of the newborn	Term infants Delivery by C-section Rapid labor Perinatal depression

Physical Examination

Examination of the respiratory system of the newborn includes inspection, palpation, and auscultation.

Inspection
Nutrition

A wasted appearance suggests placental insufficiency and an infant at risk for persistent pulmonary hypertension, while a large-for-gestational-age infant may be an infant of a diabetic mother and be at risk for hyaline membrane disease (HMD).

Associated With Other Lung Diseases

Persistent pulmonary hypertension of the newborn	Meconium aspiration syndrome
	Perinatal depression
	Pneumonia
	Polycythemia
	Congenital diaphragmatic hernia
	Maternal aspirin therapy
	Hyaline membrane disease
	Cold stress

Associated With Congenital Anomalies

Polyhydramnios	Diaphragmatic hernia
	Tracheoesophageal fistula
Oligohydramnios	Pulmonary hypoplasia
	Prolonged rupture of membranes
	Renal agenesis

Skin

The presence and distribution of cyanosis should be determined by examination while the infant is quiet and in a well-lighted area. Cyanosis of only the hands and feet (acrocyanosis) is a normal finding during the first days after birth. Central cyanosis (cyanosis of the tongue, mucous membranes, and skin) is abnormal in the noncrying infant after the first few minutes of age; it occurs when the concentration of deoxygenated hemoglobin exceeds 3 g/dL and strongly suggests hypoxemia. The presence of pallor suggests shock, cu-

Table 3: Causes of Changes in Chest Volume

Bilateral change in chest volume

Increased chest volume	*Decreased chest volume*
Transient tachypnea	Hyaline membrane disease
Meconium aspiration pneumonia	Pulmonary hypoplasia
Persistent pulmonary hypertension of the newborn	Chest wall restriction
Cystic lung diseases	

taneous vasoconstriction, obstruction of cardiac output (eg, aortic stenosis), or anemia. Plethora, meconium staining, or exanthems suggest polycythemia, meconium aspiration syndrome, or pneumonia, respectively, as the etiology of respiratory distress.

Nose

The alae nasae is the first muscle activated during inspiration. Nasal flaring represents an attempt to decrease airway resistance and is a sign of air hunger.

Chest: Size, shape, and symmetry

A barrel-shaped chest suggests increased lung volume, while a bell-shaped chest may be seen with reduced lung volume. Chest wall asymmetry results from volume differences between the two sides of the thoracic cavity. While the side that appears to bulge may be either normal or abnormal (Table 3), the normal side of the chest will usually rise and fall the most with spontaneous respirations.

Retractions

The chest wall of the infant, especially the extremely low-birth-weight infant (≤1,000 g), is extremely compliant. With spontaneous breathing, the pleural pressure (Ppl) decreases

Unilateral increase in chest volume	
Pathology on the low-volume side	*Pathology on the high-volume side*
Atelectasis	Pneumothorax
Unilateral pulmonary hypoplasia	Unilateral interstitial emphysema
	Cystic lung disease
	Diaphragmatic hernia
	Chylothorax

during inspiration. Infants with parenchymal disease, such as HMD or transient tachypnea of the newborn (TTN), must produce a more negative Ppl than normal. The highly compliant chest wall may cave inward as a result of these more negative pressures. Moderate decreases in Ppl result in intercostal and xiphoid retractions, while marked decreases result in collapse of the entire upper chest. This collapse, coupled with the outward displacement of the abdominal contents by the descending diaphragm, results in the characteristic see-saw breathing pattern of severe respiratory distress. Retractions are an external estimate of Ppl and are predictive of the severity of respiratory distress. While airway obstruction can cause retractions, the most common cause is reduced lung compliance, usually from HMD.

Respiratory rate

The respiratory rate should be counted for 1 full minute. Tachypnea, a resting rate >60 breaths/min, is the most sensitive single sign of respiratory distress.

Respiratory pattern

Many normal premature (and some term) infants exhibit periodic breathing, which consists of bursts of respirations followed by cessation of respiratory efforts (apnea) lasting 5 to 10 seconds (see *Apnea* section, Chapter 9).

Heart

The point of maximum impact (PMI) of the heart is often visible. The PMI will shift away from a space-occupying lesion or toward an area of volume loss.

Abdomen

A scaphoid, empty abdomen is a classic presentation for the infant with congenital diaphragmatic hernia or for the asphyxiated infant who has passed meconium in utero. A distended abdomen may signal a tracheoesophageal fistula, particularly in infants receiving positive pressure ventilation.

A shift of the umbilicus toward one side during inspiration, the 'belly dancer's sign,' suggests a paralyzed diaphragm on the side of the shift. As the functioning diaphragmatic leaf descends, the other leaf is pulled up by the falling Ppl into the chest, pulling the abdominal contents and umbilicus with it.

Palpation

Overinflated lungs can displace the liver and spleen from beneath the rib margins and make them more easily detectable by abdominal palpation. An enlarged, tense abdomen or a large abdominal mass can compromise the diaphragm's descent.

In newborns, capillary refilling time (CRT), the speed at which the cutaneous microcirculation resumes after a blanching pressure is applied, represents a clinical test evaluating the hemodynamic status or quality of the cutaneous vascularization. CRT is a noninvasive, easy-to-perform test that does not require extensive clinical experience. Echocardiographic evaluations used to support the validity of the CRT test in newborns revealed that the CRT was significantly linked to the cardiac index but that it remained dependent on modifications in hemodynamic status of the patent ductus arteriosus. Therefore, CRT measured at the subductal sites must be taken into consideration for proper analysis of systemic output.

It has been recommended, for reliable results, that the CRT be measured on the midpoint of the forehead and sternum and that pressure time vary from 3 to 7 seconds. Normal CRT in newborns has been reported to be <2 to <3 seconds.

Auscultation

Grunting

Infants with respiratory distress often grunt by opposing their vocal cords at the end of expiration. The grunt produces a positive end-expiratory pressure that splints small airways open and improves the distribution of ventilation. The louder the grunt, the more severe the respiratory distress.

Stridor

Stridor suggests large airway obstruction. With intrathoracic airway obstruction, expiration tends to narrow the airway, making the expiratory component of stridor worse. Conversely, with extrathoracic airway obstruction, *inspiratory* stridor is usually worse.

Breath sounds

Breath sounds can be evaluated for strength, duration, and symmetry as well as for rales, rhonchi, or wheezes. Breath sounds may be symmetrically decreased in diseases with poor air entry, such as HMD or pulmonary hypoplasia. The duration of audible, expiratory breath sounds provides information about the expiratory time constant and expiratory airway resistance. If expiration visibly ceases after one to two time constants, the observed expiratory time may be used to estimate the time constant for expiration and expiratory resistance (see *Lung Mechanics* section, Chapter 2). In asymmetric lung diseases, breath sounds are usually loudest over the normal side of the chest (Table 3).

While rales and rhonchi are nonspecific in the infant with respiratory distress, wheezing, which is more common in older infants with bronchopulmonary dysplasia or pneumonia, usually indicates significant airway obstruction.

Silverman Score

This scoring system (Table 4) may be used to quantitate the severity of respiratory distress. An infant with mild res-

Table 4: The Silverman Score			
Sign	**0**	**1**	**2**
Upper chest	Synchronized with lower chest	Lag on inspiration	See-saw
Lower chest retractions	None	Just visible	Marked
Xiphoid retraction	None	Just visible	Marked
Nasal flaring	None	Minimal	Marked
Expiratory grunt	None	Heard only with stethoscope	Audible with naked ear

piratory distress scores 2 to 4, while one with severe distress scores 8 to 10.

Transillumination

Transillumination can be valuable for detecting asymmetries of the chest. An increase in transillumination on one side suggests a pneumothorax in an acutely deteriorating infant (see *Air Block* section, Chapter 5).

By Charleta Guillory, MD, and Gerardo Cabrera-Meza, MD

X-ray Patterns in Neonatal Lung Disease: Phases of Chest X-ray

The clinical presentation of many respiratory and nonrespiratory diseases may appear similar; accurately diagnosing the etiology is difficult without chest radiographs. Careful, methodic evaluation of the radiograph is essential. Important clues or unsuspected complications can be overlooked if the clinician focuses on only a portion of the chest radiograph.

The single best view to obtain is the anteroposterior view. A cross-table lateral or lateral decubitus view can be helpful to diagnose a pneumothorax or to confirm chest tube position.

Evaluation

Proper technique and positioning

Check for proper penetration and symmetry and for proper positioning of the x-ray tube over the infant. Penetration may be evaluated by comparing the densities of the vertebral bodies and the interspace between them. Rotation of the infant may be manifested by asymmetric clavicles or spine and the anterior projection of the ribs. Improper angling of the x-ray tube nonperpendicular to the plane of the infant can produce bizarre rib patterns: with lordotic positioning, the x-ray tube is aimed toward the head, and the subsequent radiograph will display horizontal ribs and a tetralogy-like cardiac silhouette. If the tube is aimed toward the feet, the ribs can take on a bizarre, fanlike appearance.

Noncardiopulmonary features

Common normal findings and variations should be noted (Table 5).

Systematically evaluate the bones, soft tissues, and visible portions of the abdomen before concentrating on the heart and lungs. With each radiograph, check for catheter and tube position because these may not remain constant during the neonatal intensive care unit course. Skin folds, the most common artifact, result from the folding of redundant skin. They may be mistaken for pneumothoraces, especially if they lie parallel to the chest wall and do not cross outside the thorax. This may be differentiated from a pneumothorax by the presence of vascular markings and the absence of the hyperlucent field lateral to the edge of the collapsed lung seen in a pneumothorax. Radiographs taken through the walls of an incubator may show the hole in the incubator as a pseudocyst. Of course, this marking will be entirely symmetric and smooth-edged and will not be found in previous or subsequent radiographs. In infants with respiratory distress and suprasternal

Table 5: Common Chest Radiograph Findings and Variations

Normal findings	Normal variations
Uniform lung fields	Pleural fissures
Hilar markings less prominent than in child	Tracheal buckling and indentations
Eighth-ninth rib expansion	Mediastinal lines
Right-sided deviation of trachea	Pseudohyperlucent lung
Air bronchograms	Intercostal or apical herniation
Cardiac silhouette <60% of chest	Suprasternal fossa

retractions, the suprasternal fossa can appear as a radiolucency, which may be difficult to distinguish from the proximal esophageal pouch of an infant with esophageal atresia.

Airway features

The trachea and major bronchi are well distended with deep inspiration or positive pressure ventilation. Because of the increased flexibility of the neonate's trachea, compared with that of the older child, normal variations in the trachea are common and include narrowing of the trachea (which may appear striking) or anterior buckling of the airway (which may mimic the presence of a retropharyngeal mass). The trachea will usually deviate toward the right. Air bronchograms may be present, especially behind the cardiac silhouette. While airway abnormalities may be visible on plain radiographs, definitive radiographic diagnosis usually requires magnetic resonance imaging, computed tomography, or bronchography.

Gastrointestinal features

Air is commonly seen within the esophagus; however, persistent or prominent esophageal air collections may be seen with an H-type tracheoesophageal fistula or esophageal reflux. In infants with esophageal atresia, an enlarged, air-filled proximal pouch is usually found.

Cardiopulmonary features

The clinician should evaluate the heart and lungs for overall lung expansion and symmetry, for degree of pulmonary vascularity, for general parenchymal pattern (eg, clear, hazy, streaky, nodular, cystic), and for the presence of abnormal masses or extraparenchymal collections of air. Normal pulmonary parenchyma has symmetric, uniform, radiolucent-appearing fields with perihilar markings increasingly present over the medial portion of the lung field. Over the lateral lung fields, pulmonary vasculature usually is barely noticeable. Evaluating for overall lung expansion is difficult. With a good inspiration, the normal lung expands to the level of the posterior aspect of the eighth to ninth ribs. The posterior aspect of the ribs projects downward.

Normal variations of the lungs are commonly found. Visualization of the interlobar fissures, especially the right minor fissure, is reported in as many as 70% of cases. The right, posterior reflection of the pleura is sometimes visualized as a mediastinal line. This is best seen on overpenetrated radiographs. Rotation of the chest may result in a pseudohyperlucent hemithorax.

Abnormalities in expansion and parenchymal patterns are helpful in limiting the differential diagnosis under consideration (Table 6). In particular, it is helpful to evaluate the lungs for general radiodensity (dark or hazy), for variations in density (diffuse patchy infiltrates, increased density appearing to be composed of grainlike particles, or bubbly areas of hyperlucency), and for distribution of abnormalities (perihilar, peripheral, or lobar).

When evaluating streaky lungs with radiating, linear densities, differentiate air bronchograms (dark lines projected on

Table 6: Differential Diagnoses of Abnormal Radiograph Patterns

Clear or dark lungs with respiratory distress	Metabolic causes Central nervous system injury Cardiac disease Persistent pulmonary hypertension Hypoplastic lungs
Grainy lungs	Hyaline membrane disease (HMD) Poorly ventilated lungs Transient tachypnea of the newborn Pneumonia Partial anomalous pulmonary venous return with obstruction
Hazy or patchy lungs	Pulmonary hemorrhagic edema Pneumonia (usually viral) Chronic pulmonary insufficiency of the premature Early bronchopulmonary dysplasia, Northway stage II
Increased vascular markings	Transient tachypnea of the newborn Meconium aspiration Congenital heart disease with congestive heart failure Pulmonary edema Pulmonary lymphangiectasia Viral pneumonitis

a gray background, especially common over the cardiac silhouette, and generally seen only in the perihilar area) from exaggerated vasculature (light lines on a gray background, often with a lacy distribution, and extending farther to the periphery). Air bronchograms, normal if involving only the tra-

Reticulonodular lungs	Pneumonia
	Meconium aspiration
	Wilson-Mikity syndrome
	Early bronchopulmonary dysplasia
Bubbly lungs	
Small bubbles	HMD
	Pulmonary interstitial emphysema
	Bronchopulmonary dysplasia, early
Large bubbles	Bronchopulmonary dysplasia, late
	Pneumatoceles with pneumonia
	Cystic adenomatoid malformation
	Congenital lobar emphysema
	Bronchogenic cysts
	Congenital diaphragmatic hernia
Opaque lungs	Expiratory phase of HMD
	Primary atelectasis
	Pulmonary agenesis
	Massive pulmonary hemorrhagic edema—rare
	Bilateral chylothorax or hydrothorax—rare
	Weak, depressed infant with poor respiratory effort

chea and major bronchi, are common with primary parenchymal disease. Exaggerated vasculature is often seen secondary to engorged lymphatic vessels from transient tachypnea of the newborn (TTN) or pulmonary edema.

By Timothy R. Cooper, MD

Pulmonary Function Testing

Measurements of respiratory mechanics, including resistance, compliance, lung volumes, and forced expiratory flows, have been used primarily for research. However, pulmonary function tests can be clinically useful, both during and after an infant's stay in the neonatal nursery. During an infant's stay, measurements of the mechanical determinants of tidal ventilation (pressure, volume, and flow and calculations of resistance and compliance) are useful for assessing respiratory pump function and for guiding changes in mechanical ventilation. After discharge from the intensive care unit, measurements of forced expiratory flows and fractional lung volumes can be useful for assessing progress in infants with residual chronic lung disease. Clinical interpretation of these tests requires an understanding of their physiologic basis.

Measurements of Compliance and Resistance
Static compliance

In infants, *static compliance* is measured by instilling a known volume of gas into the lung through a face mask or endotracheal tube (ETT) and measuring the change in distending pressure (Table 7):

$$\text{Compliance} = \Delta \text{ volume}/\Delta \text{ pressure}$$

Alveolar pressure cannot be measured directly but is equal to airway pressure when there is no gas flow in or out of the lung (see *Lung Mechanics* section, Chapter 2). For measurements of *static lung compliance*, alveolar pressure is measured by occluding the airway until gas flow ceases and then measuring airway pressure with a pressure transducer connected to the upper airway via a face mask or ETT. This occlusion may last several seconds. Ppl is estimated using a pressure transducer connected to a balloon-tipped catheter placed in the distal esophagus. Measurements of distending pressure are repeated at multiple inflation volumes, and pressure-volume curves are constructed (Chapter 2, Figures 1 and 3). Compli-

Table 7: Distending Pressures for Measurements of Compliance

Compliance	Distending Pressure	Simplified Distending Pressure *
Lung	Alveolar - Pleural pressure	Airway - Pleural pressure
Chest wall	Pleural - Atmospheric pressure	Pleural pressure
Respiratory system	Alveolar - Atmospheric pressure	Airway pressure*

* The distending pressures can be simplified using the following assumptions:
  Airway pressure equals alveolar pressure when there is no gas flow in or out of the lung.
  Atmospheric pressure, the reference pressure, equals zero.

ance is calculated from the slope of the curve over the linear tidal breathing range. This technique can be used in intubated, paralyzed infants but is difficult to perform in spontaneously breathing infants. A method for measuring full pressure-volume curves in spontaneously breathing, sedated infants has recently been reported.

Weighted spirometer technique

The weighted spirometer technique can also be used to measure compliance in spontaneously breathing infants. The infant is connected to a spirometer, and several weights of increasing magnitude are placed on top of the spirometer bell. The increasing weights apply increasing pressures to the respiratory system, and the infant responds with increases in end-expiratory breathing level above baseline. The slope of these increases in end-expiratory volume plotted vs the corresponding step increases in spirometer pressure provide an estimate of respiratory system compliance. Other clinically useful methods for estimating compliance in the tidal breathing range have been developed.

Passive single-breath compliance and resistance

The single-breath or passive exhalation technique (Figure 1) measures compliance and resistance of the *respiratory system.* For this measurement, the infant's airway is occluded at the end of either a spontaneous or positive pressure breath. Sudden occlusion of the airway evokes the Hering-Breuer reflex and produces a brief period of apnea. The passive distending pressure of the respiratory system is measured using a pressure transducer connected to the upper airway via a face mask or ETT. The airway is then opened and the lungs are allowed to passively deflate, while exhaled gas flow rate is measured using a pneumotachometer in line with the face mask or endotracheal tube. The pneumotachometer has a fixed internal resistance; as gas flows out of the infant's lung across this resistance, a pressure differential is created. The magnitude of this pressure differential is directly proportional to the rate of flow. These *measurements of flow* can be electronically integrated to give *measurements of volume* of gas entering and leaving the lungs.

In intubated, paralyzed infants, lung volume declines after release of the occlusion until flow equals zero and ΔV equals the actual volume exhaled. Spontaneously breathing infants interrupt expiration and inspire before exhaled flow reaches zero. Therefore, ΔV is measured by extrapolating the slope of the flow-volume curve downward through zero flow on the volume axis. *Compliance* of the respiratory system is calculated by dividing the exhaled volume (or extrapolated exhaled volume) by the airway pressure measured at the end of the airway occlusion. Since the length of the airway occlusion during this maneuver may not be long enough to ensure cessation of gas flow and a true measurement of alveolar pressure, this is a measurement of *quasistatic lung compliance.* The res-

Figure 1: In the passive single-breath technique, the airway is occluded at end inspiration, and airway pressure rises to a plateau (in this example, 5 cm of H_2O [not shown]). After release of the occlusion, expiratory flow ($\dot{V}$) is plotted as a function of lung volume (V) above functional residual capacity. During expiration, lung volume decreases. Gas flow out of the lung is negative by convention. The slope of the flow-volume curve is the negative reciprocal of the time constant ($\Delta\dot{V}/\Delta V = -[R \times C]^{-1}$). Compliance ($\Delta V/\Delta P$) can be calculated from measurements of exhaled volume (ΔV) extrapolated downward through zero flow, based on the slope of the flow-volume curve and the airway pressure measured immediately before the exhalation (ΔP). $\Delta\dot{V}$ can be measured by extrapolating the slope of the flow-volume curve upward through the $\dot{V}$ axis at the end-inspiratory occlusion volume. Resistance equals $\Delta P/\Delta\dot{V}$ or can be calculated as the inverse product of the compliance and the slope of the flow-volume curve ($R = [C \times Slope]^{-1}$). In this example, respiratory system compliance = 5 mL/cm H_2O and resistance = 0.05 cm H_2O/mL/s. (Adapted from Hansen TN, Corbet AJ: Pulmonary physiology of the newborn. In: Taeusch HW, Ballard RA, eds. *Avery's Diseases of the Newborn*, 7th ed. Philadelphia, WB Saunders, 1998, p 565.)

piratory time constant is calculated from the slope of the line (-1/R x C). *Respiratory system resistance* can be measured directly (Figure 1) or calculated by dividing the time constant by the compliance.

Respiratory system compliance in the tidal range can also be measured by performing occlusions at different lung volumes during multiple exhaled breaths and plotting the pressures measured vs the occlusion volumes relative to end-expiratory volume. This is referred to as the *multiple occlusion technique*.

Dynamic compliance and resistance

Compliance and resistance can be calculated from measurements of pressure, flow, and volume (Figure 2). Since measurements are made while the infant is breathing or being mechanically ventilated, these tests are referred to as *dynamic compliance and resistance. Transpulmonary pressure (Ptp)* is the difference between Ppl estimated using a balloon-tipped esophageal catheter and pressure measured at the airway opening. During tidal ventilation, transpulmonary pressure has an elastic component (Pel) and a resistive component (Pres). At end inspiration and end expiration, both gas flow and the resistive component equal zero. Thus, the difference in Ptp between end inspiration and end expiration measures only the change in the elastic distending pressure of the lung (ΔPel).

In spontaneously breathing and mechanically ventilated infants (Figure 2), *lung compliance* can be calculated by dividing the volume of gas entering the lungs during a tidal breath (ΔV) by the change in distending pressure (ΔPel).

Resistance is calculated by picking points of equal inspiratory and expiratory mid-volume on a tracing similar to Figure 2 and measuring gas flow and transpulmonary pressure at these points. Since the elastic components of driving pressure at points of equal inspiratory and expiratory lung volume are equal and opposite, they cancel out and leave only the resistive components of the pressure differences (ΔPres). *Dynamic lung resistance* is equal to the driving pressure at the inspiratory point minus the driving pressure at the expiratory point divided by the sum of the inspiratory and expiratory flow rates (ΔV) at these points.

Dynamic lung compliance and resistance can also be calculated by continuously measuring transpulmonary pres-

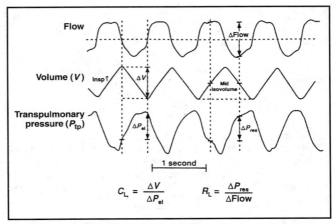

Figure 2: Measurement of dynamic compliance and resistance. Flow and volume are measured with a pneumotachometer. Transpulmonary pressure (Ptp), the difference between pleural pressure (Ppl) and pressure at the airway opening, is measured using a balloon-tipped catheter placed in the esophagus. Compliance is measured between points at which flow equals zero (ie, at end inspiration and end expiration). Between points at which flow equals zero, pressure differences represent only the elastic component of the change in transpulmonary pressure (ΔPel). *Dynamic compliance of the lung* (CL) = ΔV/ΔPel. Resistance is measured between mid-tidal points of isovolume. At these points, the elastic components of transpulmonary pressure are equal and opposite and thus cancel. The differences in transpulmonary pressure between successive isovolume points thereby represent only the resistive components of change in transpulmonary pressure (ΔPres). *Dynamic resistance of the lung* (R_L)= ΔPres/ΔFlow. (Adapted from Davis GM, Stocks J, et al: Measurement of dynamic lunge mechanics in infants. In: Stocks J, et al. eds. *Infant Respiratory Function Testing*. John Wiley and Sons, 1996, p 270.)

sure, gas flow, and volume, and then fitting these values to the equation of motion [P(t) = V(t)/C + $\dot{V}$(t) x R] using multiple linear regression techniques to derive the constants 1/C and R.

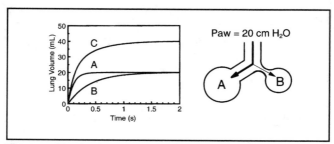

Figure 3: The figure on the right depicts a two-compartment lung (see table). The lung is being ventilated with a peak airway pressure of 20 cm H_2O. The table describes the functional characteristics of each lung compartment. The figure graphically represents the volume-time relationships of these compartments.

The two lung compartments have equal lung compliances. Compartment B has a much higher airway resistance than compartment A, and the time constant for compartment B is four times that of compartment A. Consequently, the rate of gas flow into compartment B is much less than for compartment A. Since lung compliance and airway pressure are the same for both compartments, both will eventually inflate to the same maximum lung volume (Vmax); Vmax = compliance x peak airway pressure. However, it will take four times as long for compartment B to reach Vmax as it does for compartment A. The total amount of gas in the lung at any time is equal to the sum of the volumes of gas in each compartment. Volume in C = Volume in A + Volume in B.

Compartment	Compliance (mL/cm H_2O)	Resistance (cm H_2O/mL/s)	Time Constant (s)	Vmax (mL)
A	1.0	0.10	0.10	20
B	1.0	0.40	0.40	20

Specific lung compliance

Measured compliance is markedly affected by lung size. For example, a 2.5-kg infant with a lung compliance of 2 mL/cm

H_2O requires a 10 cm H_2O distending pressure to deliver a tidal volume of 20 mL. In an adult, the same 10 cm H_2O distending pressure delivers a tidal volume of 500 mL and results in a lung compliance of 50 mL/cm H_2O. In fact, the elastic properties of the adult and newborn lung are almost equal, but the adult lung is much larger. To correct for lung size, the *specific compliance* is calculated by dividing measured compliance by the functional residual capacity (FRC; 80 mL for a 2.5-kg infant and 2,000 mL for an adult). With this correction, the infant and adult both have compliances of about 25 mL/cm H_2O/L lung volume.

Frequency dependence of lung compliance

Measurements of dynamic lung compliance rely on the assumption that at end inspiration and expiration, gas flow in the lung ceases and alveolar pressure equals airway pressure. In the presence of ventilation inhomogeneities, this assumption is not true (Figure 3). In Figure 3, the lung is composed of two ventilatory compartments—one well ventilated (A) and the other poorly ventilated (B).

This lung is ventilated with an airway pressure of 20 cm H_2O, a fixed inspiratory to expiratory time ratio of 1:1, and progressively greater respiratory rates (RR). As RR increases, inspiratory time (IT) decreases (Table 8). The volume of gas entering the well-ventilated lung compartment (A) is not affected by decreasing IT. However, as IT decreases, the volume of gas entering the poorly ventilated compartment (B) decreases, decreasing the total volume of gas entering the lung. In this example, dynamic compliance is calculated by dividing the total volume of gas in the lung at end inspiration by the peak airway pressure of 20 cm H_2O. Dynamic compliance decreases with increasing RR (decreasing IT). The decrease in dynamic compliance measured with increasing respiratory rates is termed *frequency dependence of lung compliance*.

Alveolar pressure can be calculated for each compartment by dividing the volume of gas in the compartment by its compliance. In the well-ventilated compartment (A), alveolar pressure is equal to airway pressure, but in the poorly ventilated

Table 8: Distribution of Alveolar Volumes and Pressures With Increasing Respiratory Rate

RR/ min	IT (sec)	Volume A (mL)	Alveolar Pressure A (cm H_2O)
20	1.5	20	20
30	1.0	20	20
60	0.5	20	20
75	0.4	20	20

Volumes are determined from graphs in Figure 3.

compartment (B), alveolar pressure equals airway pressure only at the slowest RR chosen.

Static compliance could have been measured at an RR of 60 breaths/min by occluding the airway at end inspiration for 2 to 3 seconds. During this occlusion, gas would actually flow from the well-ventilated compartment (A) along the alveolar pressure gradient into compartment (B) until the volumes in each compartment were equal at 17 mL. This redistribution of gas within the lung is called *pendelluft*. After this redistribution, the alveolar pressures in A and B would be equal, and the measured airway pressure would be 17 cm H_2O. Static lung compliance would then be calculated by dividing total lung volume (C) by the airway pressure (34 mL/17 cm H_2O = 2 mL/cm H_2O). This static lung compliance differs from the dynamic lung compliance because of pendelluft.

The phenomenon of frequency dependence of compliance often results in measurements of dynamic lung compliance that are less than measurements of static lung compliance. In fact, measurements of dynamic lung compliance are often

Volume B (mL)	Alveolar Pressure B (cm H_2O)	Total Volume (mL)	Total Compliance (mL/cm H_2O)
20	20	40	2.0
18	18	38	1.9
14	14	34	1.7
12	12	32	1.6

more affected by airway dysfunction than they are by changes in lung elasticity.

Measurements of Functional Residual Capacity

FRC can be determined by helium dilution, nitrogen washout, or whole body plethysmography. The helium dilution and nitrogen washout methods measure the communicating gas volume of the thorax. The plethysmographic method measures all gas contained in the chest, even the noncommunicating gas trapped behind closed airways. The helium dilution and nitrogen washout methods are easiest to accomplish in the neonatal nursery.

The helium dilution method is shown in Figure 4A. In this method, the infant is connected to a spirometer of known volume (V) containing air and a known initial concentration of the inert gas helium ($He_{initial}$). When the child is turned in to the spirometer, the concentration of helium in the system falls until the helium is equally distributed between the spirometer system and the infant's lungs. At equilibration, the final helium concentration (He_{final}) has been diluted in

Figure 4: A. Measurement of functional residual capacity (FRC) by helium dilution. At end exhalation, the infant breathes from a spirometer system of known volume (V) and helium concentration ($He_{initial}$) in air. The gas in the infant's lung dilutes the helium-air mixture to a lower concentration (He_{final}). FRC = V x ($He_{initial}$ - He_{final})/He_{final}. **B.** Measurement of FRC by plethysmography. The infant breathes spontaneously in a sealed body plethysmograph. At end exhalation, a shutter is closed, causing airway obstruction. As the infant attempts to inspire against the shutter, the volume of the thorax increases and airway pressure decreases. The increase in volume of the thorax can be measured from the change in pressure inside of the plethysmograph (Pbox). By Boyle's Law: P x FRC = (P - ΔP) x (FRC + ΔV), where P is atmospheric pressure, (P - ΔP) is airway pressure during the occlusion, and (FRC + ΔV) is the volume in the thorax during the occlusion. Therefore, FRC = (P - ΔP) x $\Delta V/\Delta P$. Because ΔP is very small compared to P, the equation can be simplified to FRC = P x $\Delta V/\Delta P$. (Adapted from Hansen TN, Corbet AJ: Pulmonary physiology of the newborn. In: Taeusch HW, Ballard RA, eds. *Avery's Diseases of the Newborn*, 7th ed. Philadelphia, WB Saunders, 1998, p 566.)

direct proportion to the volume of air added to the system by the infant's lungs. $FRC = V \times (He_{initial} \times He_{final})/He_{final}$.

In the nitrogen washout method, a one-way bias flow of 100% oxygen is used to wash out all of the nitrogen from the infant's lungs. Nitrogen is present in the lung in a concentration that is known (approximately 80%). Thus, the total volume of nitrogen washed from the lungs provides a measure of the infant's FRC. Classically, the infant is switched to breathing 100% oxygen, and the volume of expired gas (Vexp) required to wash out all of the nitrogen from the lungs is measured. This volume multiplied by the concentration of nitrogen in this expired volume (N_2 exp) equals the infant's FRC multiplied by the known starting concentration of nitrogen in the lungs. Thus, $FRC = (Vexp \times N_2 exp)/(\sim 80\%)$. This method has been simplified for use in the neonatal nursery. If the bias flow rate of oxygen is constant, the nitrogen concentration signal can be continuously integrated to obtain an index of the total volume of air expired. The system is calibrated by injecting a known amount of air approximating the infant's FRC through the bias flow system and obtaining an integrated nitrogen value. The infant is then washed out and the FRC obtained by dividing the infant's integrated nitrogen value by the calibration value.

The plethysmographic method (Figure 4B) requires placement of the infant in a closed box and is practical only for spontaneously breathing infants. Airway resistance can be measured plethysmographically, but the method is complicated, and the results provide information similar to that obtained from the methods previously described in this section.
By Robert G. Castile, MD, and Thomas N. Hansen, MD

Measurements of Forced Expiratory Flows

A method for producing partial expiratory flow-volume (PEFV) curves in infants has been available for some time. Recently, methods have been developed to obtain full adult-type maximal expiratory flow-volume (MEFV) curves in sedated infants. These methods are most useful for evaluating the effects of therapeutic interventions and following the courses of infants with chronic lung problems after discharge from the neonatal nursery. A diagram of the equipment needed to obtain measures of forced flow-volume curves in infants is shown in Figure 5. Flow is measured with a pneumotachometer attached to a face mask and volume obtained as an integral of the flow. An inflatable vest attached to a positive pressure reservoir is used to rapidly compress the chest and abdomen to produce forced flow. PEFV maneuvers are produced by inflating the vest at end inspiration. Forced flow is routinely measured at FRC ($\dot{V}$maxFRC). To produce full MEFV curves, it is first necessary to control the infant's breathing and induce a brief apneic pause. This is done by applying positive pressure (30 cm H_2O) via the face mask synchronously during several spontaneous inspiratory breaths. This is accomplished by occluding the downstream end of the bias flow system (Figure 5) with the pop-off valve set at 30 cm H_2O. The combined effects of overventilation and the Hering-Breuer reflex produce a pause in ventilation. The infant is then reinflated to 30 cm H_2O, and an MEFV curve is produced by rapid compression of the chest and abdomen using the inflatable vest. Standard spirometric measurements similar to those used in adults and older children can be obtained. Combining a measurement of FRC with measurements of vital capacity and expiratory reserve volume obtained by this technique permits the calculation of fractional lung volumes. Normal values for measurements made from PEFV and MEFV curves are available for infants.

Forced expiratory flow can also be measured in intubated, paralyzed infants using the forced deflation method. In this method, the infant's lungs are inflated to 30 to 40 cm H_2O and then rapidly deflated by the application of negative pressure at the end of the ETT. This method has been used primarily for research.

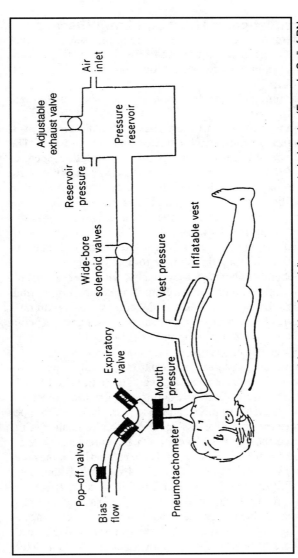

Figure 5: Diagram of equipment used for making forced flow measurements in infants. (From LeSoëuf PN, Castile RG, et al: Forced expiratory maneuvers. In: Stocks J, et al, eds. *Infant Respiratory Function Testing.* John Wiley and Sons, 1996, p 398.)

Differentiation of Heart and Lung Disease

Differentiating between heart and lung disease in a cyanotic newborn is a frequent and sometimes difficult problem that requires systematic evaluation.

Cyanosis

The clinician must determine if cyanosis is pathologic or physiologic.

Central cyanosis will present as a blue discoloration of the tongue, mucous membranes, extremities, and skin. The appearance of cyanosis depends on the absolute concentration of reduced hemoglobin in the blood, not the ratio of reduced to oxygenated hemoglobin. Three grams or more of reduced hemoglobin are required to produce visible cyanosis. Central cyanosis is abnormal in the quiet newborn after 20 minutes of age. However, it may be seen in normal infants with crying for several days after birth secondary to right-to-left shunting through the foramen ovale.

Peripheral cyanosis (acrocyanosis), which is blue discoloration of the skin of the extremities, is common in normal newborns for days to weeks. Peripheral cyanosis with cold extremities in a warm environment could suggest vasoconstriction in a septic infant or an infant in heart failure.

Causes of Hypoxemia

When central cyanosis is present on physical examination, pulse oximetry is the quickest and least invasive method of confirmation and quantification. For this reason, pulse oximetry is useful in the delivery room and in the immediate newborn period. Other methods of assessing an infant's oxygenation status are transcutaneous oxygen monitoring, measurement of arterial oxygen tension, and co-oximetry. These methods are more time-consuming or require an arterial blood sample, making them less useful as initial tests. Determination of arterial oxygen tension is not useful because the stressful process of obtaining an arterial sample by peripheral puncture may increase the degree of right-to-left shunting through the foramen ovale, leading to more cyanosis in the newborn infant. Intermittent deter-

Table 9: Causes of Hypoxemia

Cause of Hypoxemia	Associated Disorders
Hypoventilation	Loss of respiratory drive Mechanical interference with lung inflation

Ventilation/perfusion
  mismatch
	Parenchymal lung
	  disease

Right-to-left shunt	Congenital heart disease Persistent pulmonary hypertension
Methemoglobinemia	Abnormal hemoglobin Nitrate toxicity

mination of arterial oxygen tension is also of limited use because it provides information about the oxygenation status of the infant only for that moment in time; continuous measurement methods that show trends are much more useful.

Central cyanosis will be accompanied by arterial hypoxemia except when there is abnormal transport of oxygen by hemoglobin, as in methemoglobinemia and sulfhemoglobinemia. Potential causes of hypoxemia/cyanosis are listed in Table 9. Diffusion impairment is a cause of cyanosis in older children and adults but has not been described in neonates.

Diagnostic Approach
History

Infants with hypoxemia secondary to hypoventilation usually are premature or are depressed at birth secondary to maternal medications, such as narcotics or magnesium, or difficult delivery. Infants with parenchymal lung disease have a history compatible with the underlying disorder (eg, prematurity, meconium staining). Infants with persistent pulmonary hypertension of the newborn (PPHN) often have a history of meconium staining, perinatal asphyxia, or risk factors for sepsis/pneumonia. Interestingly, infants with cyanotic congenital heart disease often present in the newborn nursery after an uncomplicated labor and delivery. Finally, infants with methemoglobinemia may have a history of exposure to nitrates.

Physical Examination
Respiratory pattern

Infants with central hypoventilation will have shallow respirations and may have periodic breathing with apneic pauses. Chest wall abnormalities that interfere with lung expansion should be obvious. Infants with parenchymal lung disease will have tachypnea, grunting, and signs of altered lung compliance such as chest wall retractions and see-saw respirations. The presence of rapid breathing and cyanosis without any other evidence of respiratory distress, such as use of accessory respiratory muscles or nasal flaring ('happy tachypnea'), should always raise the suspicion of cyanotic congenital heart disease. However, infants with PPHN and little parenchymal lung involvement may have a similar presentation. Infants with cyanotic congenital heart disease will usually present without tachypnea or the appearance of respiratory distress. Infants with PPHN and little parenchymal lung involvement may have a similar presentation.

Auscultation

Breath sounds are often decreased in infants with hypoventilation or parenchymal lung disease. Infants in the latter category may also have rales. The value of asymmetric breath sounds is covered in detail in the section on physical examination at the beginning of this chapter. The presence or absence of a murmur may help alert the physician to the possibility of congenital heart disease.

Laboratory
General

A hematocrit should be obtained to rule out polycythemia. A serum glucose level should be obtained to determine the presence of hypoglycemia, which may be primary but more

Table 10: Arterial Blood Gas Tensions in Infants with Hypoxemia

Cause of Hypoxemia	Typical Arterial Blood Gas Findings
Hypoventilation	Increased Pa_{CO_2}
	Supplemental O_2 increases Pa_{O_2}
Ventilation/perfusion mismatch	Pa_{CO_2} normal to decreased
	Breathing 100% O_2 increases Pa_{O_2}
	Increased MAP increases Pa_{O_2}
Right-to-left shunt	Pa_{CO_2} normal to decreased
	Breathing 100% O_2 does not increase Pa_{O_2}
	Increased MAP does not increase Pa_{O_2}
	For infants with PPHN, hyperventilation and increased arterial pH may increase Pa_{O_2}
Methemoglobinemia/ sulfhemoglobinemia	Pa_{O_2} normal
	O_2 saturation decreased
	Arterial blood remains brown upon direct exposure to O_2*

* A spot of blood placed on a piece of paper that remains chocolate brown should raise suspicions of methemoglobinemia.

often accompanies either cyanotic congenital heart disease or parenchymal lung disease.

Arterial blood gases

Measurements of arterial blood gas tensions are often helpful in discerning the cause of hypoxemia (Table 10). The measurements may be obtained using one of the noninvasive methods examined in Chapter 10 or by obtaining samples of arterial blood. Co-oximetry and measurement of methemoglobin and sulfhemoglobin concentrations are needed in cyanotic infants with normal arterial oxygen tension but decreased hemoglobin saturation.

Chest radiograph

The chest radiograph is sometimes useful in distinguishing congenital heart disease from primary parenchymal lung disease. A large heart with clear lung fields suggests congenital heart disease but could also accompany PPHN. On the other hand, while primary lung disease will usually have a normal-size heart and abnormal lung fields, certain types of congenital heart disease, notably transposition of the great vessels and anomalous pulmonary venous return, may present with pulmonary edema.

Other tests

If congenital heart disease cannot be definitely ruled out using the tests outlined above, an electrocardiogram, echocardiogram, and cardiology consultation should be obtained. If there is still not a definitive diagnosis, then cardiac catheterization should be performed.

By Alicia A. Moïse, MD, and Alfred L. Gest, MD

Suggested Readings

History and Physical Examination

Ballard JL, et al: A simplified assessment of gestational age. *Pediatr Res* 1977;11:374.

Bates B: *A Guide to Physical Diagnosis and History Taking*. 4th ed. Philadelphia, JB Lippincott, 1987.

Jones KL: *Smith's Recognizable Patterns of Human Deformation*. 5th ed. Philadelphia, WB Saunders Co, 1997.

Oski F, DeAngelis C, Feigin R, et al: *Principles and Practice of Pediatrics*. Philadelphia, JB Lippincott, 1990.

Scanlon J: *A System of Newborn Physical Exam*. Baltimore, University Park Press, 1979.

Strozik KS, Pieper CH, Cools F: Capillary refilling time in newborns-optimal pressing time, sites of testing and normal values. *Acta Paediatr* 1998;87:310-312.

Wodey E, Pladys P, Betremieux P, et al: Capillary refilling time and hemodynamics in neonates: a Doppler echocardiographic evaluation. *Crit Care Med* 1998;26:1437-1440.

Heart and Lung Interaction

Adams JM: Neonatology. In: Garson A, Bricker JT, McNamara DG, eds. *The Science and Practice of Pediatric Cardiology*. Philadelphia, Lea & Febiger, pp 2477-2490, 1990.

Bancalari E, Jesse MJ, Gelband H, et al: Lung mechanics in congenital heart disease with increased and decreased pulmonary blood flow. *J Pediatr* 1977;90:192.

Dudell GG, Gersony WM: Patent ductus arteriosus in neonates with severe respiratory distress. *J Pediatr* 1984;104:915.

Fisher DJ: Oxygenation and metabolism in the developing heart. *Semin Perinatol* 1984;8:217.

Goldman HI, Maralit A, Sun S, et al: Neonatal cyanosis and arterial oxygen saturations. *J Pediatr* 1973;82:319-324.

Johnson GL: Clinical examination. In: Long WA, ed. *Fetal & Neonatal Cardiology*. Philadelphia, WB Saunders Co, pp 223-235, 1990.

Chest Radiographs

Avery ME, Gatewood OB, Brumley G: Transient tachypnea of the newborn. Possible delayed resorption of fluid at birth. *Am J Dis Child* 1966;111:380.

Ellis K, Nadelhaft J: Roentgenographic findings in hyaline membrane disease in infants weighing 2,000 grams and over. *Am J Roentgenol Radium Ther Nucl Med* 1957;78:444.

Emery JL: Interstitial emphysema, pneumothorax, and "air-block" in the newborn. *Lancet* 1956;1:405.

Loher E, Giedion A: Radiological aspects of massive pulmonary hemorrhage in the newborn (report of three surviving cases). *Ann Radiol* 1971;14:147.

Mikity VG, Hodgman JE, Tatter D: The radiologic findings in delayed pulmonary maturation in premature infants. In: Kaufman HJ, ed. *Pediatric Radiology*. Chicago, Year Book, p 149, 1967.

Northway WH Jr, Rosan RC: The radiographic features of pulmonary oxygen toxicity in the newborn: bronchopulmonary dysplasia. *Radiology* 1968;91:49.

Swischuk LE: Bubbles in hyaline membrane disease. Differentiation of three types. *Radiology* 1977;122:417.

Swischuck LE: Radiology of pulmonary insufficiency. In: Thibeault DW, Gregory GA, eds. *Neonatal Pulmonary Care*. 2nd ed. Appleton-Century-Crofts, 1986, pp 235-280.

Thibeault DW, Grossman H, Hagstrom JWC, et al: Radiologic findings in the lungs of premature infants. *J Pediatr* 1969;74:1.

Vollman JH, Smith WL, Ballard ET, et al: Early onset group B streptococcal disease: clinical, roentgenographic and pathologic features. *J Pediatr* 1976;89:199.

Wesenberg RL, Graven SN, McCabe EB: Radiological findings in wet-lung disease. *Radiology* 1971;98:69.

Wesenberg RL, Wax RE, Zachman RD: Varying roentgenographic patterns of patent ductus arteriosus in the newborn. *Am J Roentgenol Radium Ther Nucl Med* 1973;114:340.

Wolfson SL, Frech R, Hewitt C, et al: Radiographic diagnosis of hyaline membrane disease. *Radiology* 1969;93:339.

Pulmonary Function Testing

Castile R, Filbrun D, Flucke R, et al: Adult-type pulmonary function tests in infants without respiratory disease. *Pediatr Pulmonol* 2000;30:215-227.

Cook CD, Sutherland JM, Segal S, et al: Studies of respiratory physiology in the newborn infant. III. Measurements of mechanics of respiration. *J Clin Invest* 1957;36:440.

England SJ: Current techniques for assessing pulmonary function in the newborn infant advantages and limitations. *Pediatr Pulmonol* 1988;4:48-53.

Gerhardt T, Hehre D, Bancalari E, et al: A simple method for measuring functional residual capacity by N_2 washout in small animals and newborn infants. *Pediatr Res* 1985;19:1165-1169.

Gerhardt T, Bancalari E: Chestwall compliance in full-term and premature infants. *Acta Paediatr Scand* 1980;69:359.

Jones M, Castile R, Davis S, et al: Forced expiratory flows and volumes in infants. Normative data and lung growth. *Am J Respir Crit Care Med* 2000;161:353-359.

Krieger I: Studies on mechanics of respiration in infancy. *Am J Dis Child* 1963;105:439.

Lesouef PN, England SJ, Bryan AC: Passive respiratory mechanics in newborns and children. *Am Rev Respir Dis* 1984;129:552.

McCann EM, Goldman SL, Brady JP: Pulmonary function in the sick newborn infant. *Pediatr Res* 1987;21:313.

McIlroy MB, Tierney DF, Nadel JA: A new method for measurement of compliance and resistance of lungs and thorax. *J Appl Physiol* 1963;18:424.

Nelson NM, Prod'hom LS, Cherry RB, et al: Pulmonary function in the newborn infant. V. Trapped gas in the normal infant's lung. *J Clin Invest* 1963;42:1850.

Nelson NM: Neonatal pulmonary function. *Pediatr Clin North Am* 1966; 13:769.

NHLBI Workshop Summary: Assessment of lung function and dysfunction in studies of infants and children. *Am Rev Respir Dis* 1993;148:1105-1108.

Orlinsky A, Bryan AC, Bryan MH: A simple method of measuring total respiratory system compliance in newborn infants. *S Afr Med J* 1976;50: 128-130.

Polgar G, Promadhat V: *Pulmonary Function Testing in Children: Techniques and Standards.* Philadelphia, WB Saunders Co, 1971, pp 1-273.

Respiratory mechanics in infants: physiologic evaluation in health and disease. American Thoracic Society/European Respiratory Society. *Am Rev Respir Dis* 1993;147:474-496.

Tepper RS, Pagtakhan RD, Taussig LM: Noninvasive determination of total respiratory system compliance in infants by the weighted-spirometer method. *Am Rev Respir Dis* 1984;130:461-466.

Tepper RS, Reister T: Forced expiratory flows and lung volumes in normal infants. *Pediatr Pulmonol* 1993;15:357-361.

Tepper R, Williams T, Kisling J, et al: Static compliance of the respiratory system in healthy infants. *Am J Respir Crit Care Med* 2001;163:91-94.

Differentiation of Heart and Lung Disease

Park CM, Nagel RL: Sulfhemoglobinemia. Clinical and molecular aspects. *N Engl J Med* 1984;310:1579-1584.

Chapter 4

Acute, Acquired Parenchymal Lung Disease

Hyaline Membrane Disease

Hyaline membrane disease (HMD), also called respiratory distress syndrome (RDS), causes severe progressive respiratory distress in preterm infants.

Epidemiology

HMD occurs in approximately 40,000 infants each year and in about 14% of low-birth-weight infants in the United States. The incidence increases with decreasing gestational age and reaches 60% to 80% in infants born at <28 weeks' gestation. Numerous factors have been identified as either increasing or decreasing the risks of HMD (Tables 1 and 2).

Pathophysiology

The primary cause of HMD is surfactant deficiency, which results when the rate of use of surfactant exceeds the rate of production. Surfactant production and secretion are developmentally regulated, so the most common cause of deficiency is delivery before term (see *Surfactant* section, Chapter 2).

Lung Function
Mechanics

Insufficient surfactant at the alveolar air-liquid interface increases surface tension and decreases lung compliance. As a result, the pressure required to inflate the lung is increased (Figure 1). This means that during a spontaneous inspiration, the infant must generate a large, negative intrapleural pressure to inflate its lungs. This large, negative

Table 1: Factors Increasing Risk of HMD

- Prematurity
- Male sex
- White race
- Cesarean section delivery
- Gestational diabetes
- Second-born twin
- Family history of HMD

Table 2: Factors Decreasing Risk of HMD

- Pregnancy-induced hypertension
- Chronic maternal hypertension
- Subacute placental abruption
- Maternal narcotic addiction
- Premature rupture of membranes
- Prenatal corticosteroids

pressure results in marked chest wall retractions and paradoxical or see-saw respirations. Overall, the work of breathing is increased.

Laplace's law states that the pressure (P) required to maintain an airspace at a given radius of curvature (r) is equal to twice the surface tension (T) divided by the radius ($P = 2 \times T/r$) (see *Surfactant* section, Chapter 2). At the end of exhalation, as the radius of curvature of the infant's airspaces decreases, the pressure required to keep them expanded increases, and the tendency is toward collapse. The

Figure 1: Lungs obtained at postmortem from an infant with HMD (lower curve) require far more pressure to achieve a given volume of inflation than do those obtained from an infant dying of a nonrespiratory cause. The arrows depict the inspiratory and expiratory limbs of the pressure volume curves. (Gribetz I: *J Clin Invest* 1959;38:2168.)

highly compliant chest wall of the premature infant is unable to resist this tendency to collapse. Therefore, the infant develops progressive atelectasis, and resting lung volume or functional residual capacity decreases. The expiratory grunt and tachypnea characteristic of the infant with HMD represent attempts to prevent lung collapse. The expiratory grunt increases end-expiratory lung volume by applying end-expiratory pressure to the lungs, while tachypnea shortens expiratory time and prevents complete emptying of the lungs during exhalation.

While total airway resistance increases only slightly in infants with HMD, regional increases in resistance may be large.

Figure 2: In infants with HMD, the lung can be divided into three ventilatory compartments: (1) A well-ventilated compartment that has normal compliance and airway resistance, hence a normal to high alveolar P_{O_2}. The bulk of the gas flow in and out of the lung occurs through this compartment. (2) An open, yet poorly ventilated compartment with decreased lung compliance and increased airway resistance. Because this compartment is severely underventilated, O_2 delivery to alveoli from the atmosphere is much less than the rate of O_2 removal by the blood, so alveolar P_{O_2} is markedly decreased. (3) Atelectatic lung units that are not ventilated (not shown in this figure).

Infants with HMD have increases in airway resistance because small airways

- are also affected by surface tension, and their radius decreases in the face of surfactant deficiency;
- are compressed by interstitial edema (see *Pulmonary Edema* section, this chapter); and
- are damaged by the large shear forces generated by attempts to expand the poorly compliant air sacs.

Figure 3: A shows the two ventilatory compartments of the lungs with HMD described in Figure 2: well-ventilated lung units in which the alveolar P_{O_2} is normal or increased, and open, severely underventilated lung units in which the alveolar P_{O_2} is markedly reduced. Blood flowing through each of these two compartments is shown by the arrows, as is blood flowing through the right-to-left shunt. **B** shows the effect of increasing the inspired oxygen tension on the lung of the infant with HMD.

Despite the small increase in total airway resistance, the decrease in total lung compliance dominates measurements of pulmonary function, and the time constant for the whole lung remains very short, on the order of 0.1 second.

Distribution of ventilation

HMD is a heterogeneous disorder, with some airspaces more affected than others. This results in three distinct populations of airspaces (Figure 2).

Hypoxemia

In infants with HMD, hypoxemia is the result of right-to-left shunting of blood through shunt vessels in the lung, past atelectatic airspaces, and through the ductus arteriosus and foramen ovale.

In infants with HMD, most of the right-to-left shunt occurs in the lung through vessels that have formed before formation of alveoli. Right-to-left shunting of blood past atelectatic alveoli is limited by hypoxic vasoconstriction in these lung units. Right-to-left shunt across the foramen ovale and ductus arteriosus is unusual after the first 24 hours. In fact, left-to-right shunts across the ductus arteriosus often complicate the later course of HMD.

Right-to-left shunting occurs because blood vessels perfusing open but poorly ventilated lung units constrict in response to the marked reduction in alveolar Po_2 (Figure 3). Poorly oxygenated blood flowing through the right-to-left shunt and past underventilated lung units mixes with well-oxygenated blood flowing through the well-ventilated portion of the lung. The Po_2 of this mixture, and hence the ultimate arterial Po_2, is determined by the relative volume of blood flowing past each compartment. Since little blood flows past the open, severely underventilated lung units, the chief contributor to arterial hypoxemia is the right-to-left shunt. However, the magnitude of blood flow through the shunt is determined by the extent of hypoxic vasoconstriction in the underventilated lung and by the size of the underventilated compartment relative to the rest of the lung. With increases in Fio_2, alveolar oxygen tensions increase in both ventilated lung compartments. Blood flowing past well-ventilated lung units is nearly saturated, regardless of the Fio_2, so that increases in the alveolar Po_2 of these units result in little change in O_2 content (see $\dot{V}a/\dot{Q}$ section, Chapter 2). Increasing Fio_2 will have little effect on alveolar Po_2 in severely underventilated lung units until the Fio_2 becomes quite high, approaching 1.00. At this point, a nitrogen washout occurs and alveolar Po_2 increases dramatically, leading to relief of hypoxic vasoconstriction in the poorly ventilated part of the lung, increased blood flow past these now well-oxygenated lung units, decreased right-to-left shunt, and relief of arterial hypoxemia. Increasing airway pressure by administration of continuous positive air pressure (CPAP) or by intermittent mandatory ventilation (IMV) increases oxygenation in infants with HMD by improving ventilation to poorly ventilated lung units, increasing alveolar P_{O_2} at each F_{IO_2} (see *Positive Pressure Ventilatory Support* section, Chapter 10).

Dead space

In infants with HMD, most of the gas flow in and out of the lung occurs in well-ventilated lung units. However, a substantial amount of the blood flows through the right-to-left shunt or past severely underventilated lung units. Therefore, the well-ventilated units are ventilated out of proportion to their perfusion and, as such, they effectively increase the total physiologic dead space in the lung. Because dead space is increased, these infants often have an increased minute ventilation with normal or only slightly reduced arterial P_{CO_2}.

Pulmonary edema invariably complicates the course of HMD. Diversion of blood away from poorly ventilated lung units results in increased blood flow to normal lung units. This will result in higher vascular pressures and a higher filtration pressure (see *Pulmonary Edema* section, this chapter). In addition, overdistention of more normal lung units can injure the capillary endothelium and increase permeability to fluid and protein. The transport of interstitial fluid into airspaces (alveolar flooding) is potentiated by injury to terminal lung units from the distending pressures generated to inflate the lung. With alveolar flooding, plasma proteins enter the airspaces, further inactivating surfactant and also forming the hyaline membranes characteristic of this disorder.

Infants with HMD also develop marked peripheral edema that increases over the first 48 to 72 hours after birth and then resolves with a brisk diuresis as pulmonary function begins to improve. With surfactant replacement therapy, lung function often improves before the diuresis occurs, suggesting that the two are not functionally related. The etiology of this edema is not clear.

Pathology

Grossly, the lungs are poorly aerated and congested. Microscopic examination reveals diffuse atelectasis of distal airspaces and distal airways that are overdistended. The airspaces are lined with necrotic epithelium and plasma proteins. The protein lining the airspaces appears pink on microscopic sections stained with hematoxylin and eosin. HMD gets its name from this hyalinelike appearance. Injury to the airway epithelium is a universal accompaniment to HMD. Presumably, overdistention of airways proximal to areas of collapse results in damage to airway epithelium, with sloughing and exudation of plasma into the airways and airspaces.

Presentation

History

The typical history is that of a premature infant with symptoms of respiratory distress at birth. Respiratory distress increases in severity over 24 to 72 hours, then begins to resolve spontaneously. Improvement is heralded by a diuresis.

Physical examination

Infants are tachypneic, with retractions and expiratory grunting. Breath sounds are decreased bilaterally. The infants have cyanosis in room air, peripheral pallor, and edema.

Chest radiograph

The chest radiograph reveals a low volume lung (Figure 4). The lung parenchyma has a diffuse, reticular, granular, *ground-glass* appearance with air bronchograms. Occasionally, the disease process may appear worse in one lung than in the other. If the infant has already received positive pressure, the chest x-ray may appear better expanded and less granular.

Laboratory

Arterial blood gases demonstrate hypoxemia in room air that is relieved by breathing oxygen. The arterial P_{CO_2} may be normal or decreased initially but increases as the disease progresses. If the baby has retained significant fetal lung fluid in addition to having a surfactant deficiency, the P_{CO_2} may be elevated at birth.

Because infants with HMD are oliguric early in their course, serum Na^+ will decrease if fluid is not restricted until the diuresis occurs. Serum glucose should be monitored because these stressed premature infants are at risk for hypoglycemia.

Figure 4: Chest radiograph of an infant with HMD. Lung volumes are low despite application of positive pressure through the endotracheal tube. The lungs have a homogeneous, reticular, granular appearance.

Differential Diagnosis
Bacterial pneumonia

Bacterial pneumonia, especially secondary to infection with group B streptococci, is difficult to distinguish from HMD. The clinical presentation and chest radiograph findings can be identical. Sometimes, the lungs of babies with pneumonia may initially be more compliant than those with HMD. Treatment with antibiotics of infants with abnormal radiographs and persistent or worsening oxygen requirements may be warranted until cultures are negative.

Transient tachypnea of the newborn

Transient tachypnea of the newborn (TTN) may present with a similar clinical picture of tachypnea, oxygen requirement, and increased work of breathing. Classically, infants with TTN will be sickest shortly after birth, with gradual improvement over hours to days. Infants with TTN will have a lower O_2 requirement (usually less than 50%) and a higher $Paco_2$. The chest x-ray is helpful in differentiating TTN from HMD. Infants with TTN have a relatively high volume lung with lacelike densities emanating from the hilum, while infants with HMD have very low volume lungs with a more homogeneous appearance.

Pulmonary edema

Pulmonary edema from primary cardiovascular anomalies, especially patent ductus arteriosus (PDA), may mimic HMD or complicate the course of established HMD. These infants may not have obvious symptoms of a PDA, and the diagnosis may only be made by echocardiogram. Infants with obstructed anomalous pulmonary venous return may have an initial clinical course similar to HMD but fail to improve over time and usually have a fixed right-to-left shunt. They do not improve even transiently with oxygen. Finally, congenital abnormalities of the lymphatic system, pulmonary lymphangiectasia, can mimic HMD initially and can also be distinguished by the infant's failure to improve over time.

Aspiration pneumonia

Aspiration pneumonia, from either meconium or amniotic fluid, may present like HMD but is unusual in premature infants and demonstrates a different radiographic appearance.

Prevention

Because HMD is a disease of premature infants, prevention of preterm delivery will prevent HMD. However, for those infants who are destined to deliver prematurely, multiple controlled trials have shown that the risk of HMD can be reduced substantially by administering corticosteroids to their mothers before delivery (Table 3). Despite these trials, before 1994 only 15% of eligible mothers in the United States received antenatal glucocorticoids. In the spring of 1994, the

Table 3: Effects of Antenatal Corticosteroids and Prophylactic Surfactant on the Outcome of Premature Infants

	Corticosteroids		No Corticosteroids	
	Surfactant (n = 58)	No surfactant (n = 46)	Surfactant (n = 557)	No surfactant (n = 567)
Birth weight	992 ± 200	1013 ± 226	1012 ± 284	1021 ± 281
Gest age	27.4 ± 1.8	27.5 ± 1.8	27.2 ± 2.6	27.1 ± 2.6
% males	62%	63%	57%	53%
RDS deaths	0	6.5%	7.2%	19.6%
All deaths	0	15.2%	17.7%	24.9%
Air leaks	1.7%	13%	11%	23%
BPD	48%	55%	61%	62%
PDA	27%	22%	47%	44%
IVH	8%	9%	22%	21%

Summary data from combined prophylaxis (infants 23 to 29 weeks' gestation) and rescue (infants between 600 and 1,750 g) trials of Survanta. Jobe et al: *Am J Obstet Gynecol* 1983;168:508.

National Institutes of Health convened a Consensus Conference to evaluate the role of antenatal corticosteroids in prevention of HMD. This panel recommended that:

- The benefits of antenatal administration of corticosteroids to women at risk of preterm delivery vastly outweigh the potential risks. These benefits include not only a reduction in the risk of HMD, but also a substantial reduction in mortality and intraventricular hemorrhage (IVH).

- All mothers with fetuses between 24 and 34 weeks' gestation at risk of preterm delivery should be considered candidates for antenatal treatment with corticosteroids.
- The decision to use antenatal corticosteroids should not be altered by fetal race or gender or by the availability of surfactant replacement therapy.
- Patients eligible for therapy with tocolytics should also be eligible for treatment with antenatal corticosteroids.
- Treatment consists of two doses of 12 mg of betamethasone given intramuscularly 24 hours apart, or four doses of 6 mg of dexamethasone given intramuscularly 12 hours apart. Optimal benefit begins 24 hours after initiation of therapy and lasts 7 days.
- Because treatment with corticosteroids for less than 24 hours is still associated with significant reductions in neonatal mortality, in RDS, and in IVH, antenatal corticosteroids should be given unless immediate delivery is anticipated.
- In preterm premature rupture of membranes at less than 30 to 32 weeks' gestation in the absence of clinical chorioamnionitis, antenatal corticosteroid use is recommended because of the high risk of IVH at these early gestational ages.
- In complicated pregnancies where delivery before 34 weeks' gestation is likely, antenatal corticosteroid use is recommended unless there is evidence that corticosteroids will have an adverse effect on the mother or unless delivery is imminent.

Since the Consensus Conference, the administration of antenatal corticosteroids to eligible women has increased to almost 60% in most centers, and many centers report even greater compliance. The safety and efficacy of repeated courses of antenatal steroids after the initial course have not been established. Because of concerns about the effects of repeated courses on fetal growth and development, a recent National Institutes of Health Consensus Conference has recommended that rescue therapy or repeated doses of antenatal steroids be reserved for patients enrolled in clinical trials.

Recent double-blind, placebo-controlled studies have not identified any additional benefit of antenatal thyroid-releasing hormone to antenatal corticosteroids used to mature the neonate's lung.

Management

HMD is a transient, self-limited disease. The stress of preterm birth rapidly matures the surfactant system so that the lung can produce adequate surfactant within 48 to 72 hours of birth. Therefore, the goal of management is to support the infant without inducing further lung injury until the disease resolves.

Surfactant

Surfactant replacement therapy directly addresses the cause of HMD, surfactant deficiency, and is now a mainstay in the early management of HMD. Multiple controlled trials have shown that surfactant replacement markedly decreases the mortality and morbidity of babies with HMD, especially small, premature babies. Surfactant replacement increases compliance and decreases resistance in surfactant-deficient lung units, thereby reducing both the distending pressures needed to inflate the lung and the work of breathing in the spontaneously breathing infant. In addition, surfactant replacement improves ventilation to open, poorly ventilated lung units and increases their alveolar Po_2. As a result, hypoxic vasoconstriction is relieved, the right-to-left shunt decreases, and overall arterial oxygenation improves.

Four types of surfactant preparations are available:
- *Survanta®* (beractant), a surfactant derived from minced calf lung with added synthetic disaturated phosphatidylcholine
- *Infasurf®* (calfactant), a surfactant derived from alveolar washes from the airways of newborn calves
- *Curosurf®* (poractant alfa), a surfactant derived from minced porcine lung
- *Exosurf®* (colfosceril), a synthetic surfactant consisting primarily of disaturated phosphatidylcholine plus the alcohol of palmitic acid (hexadecanol)

Meta-analysis of clinical trials comparing a natural surfactant (Survanta®, Infasurf®, or Curosurf®) and an artificial surfactant (Exosurf®) reveal natural surfactants to be associated with lower oxygen requirements, fewer pulmonary air leaks, and lower mortality.

A large multicenter trial has compared Infasurf® with Survanta® in prevention and treatment of HMD. In the prevention arm, 86% of the Infasurf®-treated infants and 92% of the Survanta®-treated infants survived to discharge ($P = 0.06$). The subset of patients less than 600 g birth weight treated with Survanta® had an extraordinarily low mortality rate (26%) when compared to those treated with Infasurf® (63%). There were also fewer RDS deaths in the Survanta®-treated infants than in the Infasurf®-treated patients ($P = 0.01$). The Survanta®-treated infants had a longer duration of mechanical ventilation and oxygen supplementation, probably due to the high rate of survival of these less than 600 g birth weight babies. The authors of this study comment that this rate of survival may not be reproducible because other published rates of survival for babies this size suggest that most die with or without surfactant treatment. Other than the difference in mortality of this subgroup, there were no differences in the incidence of air leaks, complications of administration, or complications associated with prematurity, such as chronic lung disease. In both arms of the study, the number of surfactant doses required was similar for both surfactants, while the interval between surfactant doses was greater for infants treated with Infasurf® after the second prevention dose.

In addition, there are now two clearly defined treatment strategies for administration of surfactant. *Prophylactic therapy* requires that the surfactant preparation be instilled in the infant's trachea soon after birth, often before a diagnosis of HMD can be established. Prophylactic therapy is frequently administered in the delivery room. The benefits of prophylactic surfactant can still be achieved if surfactant is given immediately after initial resuscitation and stabilization. *Rescue therapy* is designed to treat infants with established HMD.

Since the mid-1980s, a large number of controlled trials have shown that therapy with surfactant is safe, reduces mortality from HMD, decreases the incidence of pulmonary air leaks, and decreases the incidence of intracranial hemorrhage in small infants. Furthermore, these studies have shown that two to three doses of surfactant are superior to a single dose for prophylaxis and rescue modes of treatment and that for very immature infants <30 weeks' gestation, prophylactic therapy is superior to rescue therapy.

Administration. In some institutions, all infants <30 weeks' gestation are intubated and ventilated in the delivery room and then are given *prophylactic surfactant* (see *Surfactant Administration*, Chapter 10). They receive at least two doses; a third dose is optional.

Infants >30 weeks' gestation are treated with rescue therapy when they must be intubated or when they have an a/A ratio of <0.22. In some institutions, all infants who require FIO_2 >0.5 to maintain Pao_2 >50 torr are candidates for intubation and treatment with surfactant. Surfactant can be administered to infants who are being supported by CPAP.

Rescue therapy also consists of two doses of surfactant, and a third dose is optional.

General Support
Resuscitation

Because infants born prematurely are at high risk for developing HMD, they should be resuscitated immediately after birth. This should include expansion of the lungs with positive pressure if spontaneous respiratory efforts do not result in complete lung expansion.

Temperature control

These infants must remain in a neutral thermal environment, either on a radiant warmer or in an isolette.

IV fluids

Infants with HMD should be given glucose-containing IV fluids to provide some energy substrate and prevent hypoglycemia (typically 6 mg/kg/min of glucose). They are often oliguric during the first 24 to 48 hours after birth, so it is our practice to restrict fluids in infants with HMD to 60 mL/kg/d. This practice may need to be modified in very immature infants where insensible water losses may be very high.

Circulatory support

Many infants with HMD, especially infants <28 weeks' gestation, have systemic hypotension. Excessive administration of volume to treat the hypotension is usually ineffective and often worsens the lung disease. If necessary, judicious use of volume to rule out hypovolemia can be tried, but then administration of dopamine is appropriate to increase cardiac output and diminish peripheral vasodilatation.

Infection

Because distinguishing HMD from bacterial pneumonia is difficult, consider antibiotic treatment of infants with HMD. Monitor drug levels and continue antibiotics until cultures are negative. In the severely ill or preterm infant, the lumbar puncture is often deferred until the respiratory status improves.

Respiratory Therapy

Oxygen administration, CPAP, and positive pressure ventilation still represent the mainstay in the management of the infant with HMD. All of these therapies work by increasing the Po_2 in poorly ventilated lung units, relieving hypoxic vasoconstriction, and reducing the right-to-left shunt. Administration of oxygen increases the diffusion gradient for oxygen into poorly ventilated lung units (Figure 3), while CPAP and IMV increase ventilation and increase the rate of oxygen delivery to those units. Oxygen and mechanical ventilation do not cure the infant, they merely support the infant during the transient illness. These modes of support can also cause injury, so the lowest level of support should be chosen to provide adequate delivery of oxygen to tissue.

Oxygen

The first level of support is supplemental oxygen (see *Oxygen Use and Monitoring* section, Chapter 10). The infant must be large and vigorous enough to be able to sustain tachypnea and an expiratory grunt to preserve functional residual capacity. Also, the infant should not have, or be at high risk for, apnea. Therefore, the candidates for supplemental oxygen alone are large premature infants >1,500 g.

Continuous positive airway pressure

CPAP is reserved for larger premature infants who can maintain spontaneous ventilation without apnea (see *Continuous Positive Airway Pressure* section, Chapter 10). Typically, these infants are >1,500 g birth weight and ≥30 weeks' gestation. CPAP begins when infants require FIO_2 >0.5 to maintain PaO_2 >50 torr. While nasal CPAP is often effective in improving oxygenation in infants with HMD, exclusive use of endotracheal tube CPAP allows simultaneous administration of rescue doses of surfactant.

Positive pressure ventilation

Some institutions intubate and ventilate from birth all infants <30 weeks' gestation. Older infants become eligible for positive pressure ventilation if they develop apnea or if they cannot maintain adequate oxygenation with an FIO_2 of 1.00 and maximum CPAP (8 to 10 cm H_2O). These institutions do not routinely ventilate infants with increasing $PaCO_2$ in the absence of apnea or hypoxemia. (For more information, see *Positive Pressure Ventilatory Support* section, Chapter 10.)

High-frequency ventilation

During high-frequency oscillatory ventilation, the infant is ventilated at very rapid rates (3,000 breaths/min) at tidal volumes less than dead-space volume. Theoretically, ventilation with low tidal volumes decreases barotrauma to the lung and results in fewer complications. Controlled trials of oscillatory ventilation for infants with HMD have not shown any consistent benefit over conventional ventilation. Moreover, three of the trials found an increased incidence of severe IVH in infants who received oscillatory ventilation. This therapy for HMD must still be considered experimental.

Extracorporeal membrane oxygenation

Large infants with HMD who fail to respond to surfactant therapy and to mechanical ventilation may be candidates for extracorporeal membrane oxygenation (ECMO; see *Extracorporeal Membrane Oxygenation* section, Chapter 10). Typically, these infants must be greater than 34 weeks' gestation and weigh more than 2,000 g.

Failure to Improve

Occasionally, infants will fail to improve with surfactant replacement therapy. These infants should be carefully evaluated for the presence of a PDA or other congenital heart disease. On the other hand, some infants will improve transiently and then deteriorate on the second or third day of therapy. This is a classic presentation for a PDA or for nosocomial pneumonia.

Outcome

HMD is a transient disease and most infants who have it recover without sequelae. Although mortality increases with decreasing gestational age, administration of antenatal corticosteroids to the mother and surfactant to the newborn can significantly improve survival (Table 3). The incidence of chronic lung disease, defined as an oxygen requirement at 28 days of age, depends heavily on gestational age and ranges from less than 10% for infants weighing more than 1,000 g at birth to nearly 50% for those between 500 and 1,000 g at birth. Severe chronic lung disease requiring supplemental oxygen for weeks to years is now rare in many neonatal intensive care units. Neurologic sequelae such as IVH are clearly associated with HMD but are substantially reduced by the administration of antenatal corticosteroids.

By Alicia A. Moïse, MD, and Thomas N. Hansen, MD

Table 4: Risk Factors for TTN

- Premature delivery
- Maternal sedation
- Delivery by elective cesarean section
- Delayed clamping of the umbilical cord
- Maternal diabetes
- Fetal distress
- Maternal asthma

Transient Tachypnea of the Newborn

Epidemiology

TTN, also referred to as *respiratory distress syndrome type II* or as *delayed clearance of the fetal lung fluid*, is the most common cause of respiratory distress in newborns. Several factors have been identified as risks for TTN (Table 4), the most prominent being premature delivery and maternal sedation.

Pathophysiology

Lung fluid is contained in airways and air sacs and is secreted by the fetal lung. The volume of liquid within the potential air spaces of fetal lambs increases from 4 to 6 mL/kg body weight at midgestation to more than 20 mL/kg near term. Transepithelial chloride secretion is the chief driving force responsible for the production of this liquid in the fetal lung. As a result, fetal lung fluid has a much higher chloride concentration than does plasma, interstitial fluid, or amniotic fluid (Table 5). Secretion of fetal lung fluid appears to be hormone controlled and can be inhibited by β-adrenergic agents.

Approximately two thirds of fetal lung fluid is removed from the lung before birth, during labor. Late in gestation, the lung epithelium (columnar epithelial cells and type II alveolar cells) converts from chloride and fluid secretion to

Table 5: Composition of Fetal Lung Liquid

	Lung Liquid	Interstitial Fluid	Plasma	Amniotic Fluid
Sodium mEq/L	150	147	150	113
Potassium mEq/L	6.3	4.8	4.8	7.6
Chloride mEq/L	157	107	107	87
Bicarbonate mEq/L	3	25	24	19
pH	6.27	7.31	7.34	7.02
Protein g/dL	0.03	3.27	4.09	0.10

(Bland RD: *Acta Paediatr Scand* 1983;305:12)

sodium and fluid absorption by the combined action of epithelial sodium channels and sodium, potassium-ATPase. This process increases before term and is enhanced by the presence of a large protein osmotic pressure gradient (Table 5) into the interstitium of the lung. This absorbed lung water is then cleared by the microcirculation and lymphatics. At delivery, with expansion of the lungs, the increase in pulmonary blood flow accelerates this process. Abnormal epithelial sodium transport may be partly responsible for the delayed absorption of lung water.

Infants born prematurely or without labor have not had sufficient time to reabsorb fetal lung fluid and, consequently, are born with excess water in their lungs. Clearance of fetal lung fluid after birth will also be delayed if the infant's lung inflation is impaired because of prematurity or the impact of maternal sedation. Any condition, such as asphyxia, that increases the rate of transvascular fluid filtration in the lung will further delay clearance of fetal lung liquid (see *Pulmonary Edema* section, this chapter).

Finally, increases in central venous pressure can impair lymphatic drainage and reabsorption of fetal lung fluid. In

Figure 5: Chest radiograph of an infant with TTN. The lung volume is increased, and there are lacelike densities emanating from the hilum. Areas of consolidation probably represent alveolar flooding.

the newborn, venous pressure may be increased by perinatal hypoxia or by an excessive placental transfusion at delivery. Respiratory symptoms result from airway compression by fluid accumulating in the interstitium. Airway obstruction results in gas trapping, maldistribution of ventilation, and hypoxia from ventilation-perfusion mismatch.

Presentation

History

Infants with TTN usually have one or more of the risk factors listed in Table 4.

Physical examination

Tachypnea is the hallmark of the disease, with respiratory rates ranging from 60 to 120 breaths/min. In addition, expiratory grunting, chest wall retractions, nasal flaring, a barrel chest, and cyanosis in room air are frequent.

Chest radiograph

Typically, hyperinflation is seen with a sunburst pattern of linear densities emanating from the hilum. These densities represent fluid in the interstitium surrounding airways and pulmonary arteries. Occasionally, fluffy densities compatible with alveolar flooding or even pleural effusions are present (Figure 5).

Laboratory

Arterial blood gas measurements reveal hypoxemia in room air that is usually corrected by an FIO_2 <0.50. In the first hours after birth, these infants frequently have hypercarbia and a mild to moderate respiratory acidosis.

Differential Diagnosis

Bacterial pneumonia

Bacterial pneumonia is difficult to distinguish from TTN. Antibiotic treatment of infants with abnormal chest radiographs and persistent or worsening oxygen requirements may be warranted until cultures are negative.

Aspiration pneumonia

Aspiration pneumonia, from either meconium or amniotic fluid, may present like TTN but will have a much longer and more complicated course.

Hyaline membrane disease

HMD, also known as RDS, may initially present with TTN but worsens over time with loss of lung volume and progressive increases in oxygen requirement.

Pulmonary edema

Pulmonary edema from primary cardiovascular anomalies or from congenital abnormalities of the lymphatic system (pulmonary lymphangiectasia) can mimic TTN initially. These disorders can be distinguished by typical

Table 6: Risk Factors for PPHN

- Post-term delivery
- Placental insufficiency
- Meconium staining
- Postnatal hypoxia
- Hypoglycemia
- Hypothermia
- Polycythemia
- Maternal prostaglandin inhibitors
- Bacterial pneumonia/sepsis
- Diaphragmatic hernia

findings of heart disease and by their failure to improve over time.

Management

TTN is a self-limited disease that usually resolves completely within 48 to 72 hours. Modest fluid restriction of 60 mL/kg/d IV is appropriate while assessing the need for supplemental oxygen. Oxygen requirements are usually highest at the onset of the disease and then decrease progressively. Infants with TTN do not usually require FIO_2 >0.5 or positive pressure ventilatory support. Diuretics do not alter the clinical course.

Failure to Improve

TTN is a diagnosis of exclusion. Infants with increasing oxygen requirements, infants who require FIO_2 >0.5, or infants with any circulatory insufficiency probably do not have TTN, and the diagnosis should be reconsidered. The most common disorder confused with TTN is mild HMD. However, the possibility that the infant has pneumonia or pulmonary edema from other causes should be considered.

Outcome

Almost all infants with TTN recover completely without residual pulmonary disability.

By Michael E. Speer, MD, and Thomas N. Hansen, MD

Persistent Pulmonary Hypertension of the Newborn

In infants with persistent pulmonary hypertension of the newborn (PPHN), hypoxemia results from left-to-right shunting of blood secondary to elevated pulmonary vascular resistance (PVR). Numerous underlying disease processes can present with a clinical picture of PPHN.

Epidemiology

In a large, multicenter observational study, the incidence of PPHN was 1.9 per 1,000 live births, and 58% of the infants were male. Several risk factors for PPHN have been identified (Table 6).

Pathophysiology

Transition from intrauterine to extrauterine life requires the PVR of the fetus to decrease abruptly at birth. In infants with PPHN, this decrease does not occur. The elevated PVR diverts blood flow away from the pulmonary circulation through the foramen ovale and ductus arteriosus into the systemic circulation. These right-to-left shunts result in severe hypoxemia refractory to administration of oxygen (Figure 6).

The two categories of disorders of the pulmonary vascular bed that result in PPHN are *maladaptation* and *maldevelopment*.

With *maladaptation*, the pulmonary vascular bed is structurally normal but PVR remains high. PPHN from maladaptation implies active vasoconstriction, which may be transient or persistent (Table 7).

Transient constriction usually occurs in infants who have some perinatal complication that interferes with the normal transition from intrauterine to extrauterine life. Treatment of the complication results in prompt resolution of pulmo-

Figure 6: Circulatory pathways in an infant with PPHN. In infants with PPHN, pulmonary vascular resistance remains high after birth and pressures remain elevated in the pulmonary artery (PA), right ventricle (RV), and right atrium (RA). Poorly oxygenated blood returning from the superior vena cava (SVC) and inferior vena cava (IVC) returns to the right atrium. Because right atrial pressure is increased, much of this poorly oxygenated blood is shunted across the foramen ovale (FO) to the left atrium (LA) where it mixes with oxygenated blood returning via the pulmonary veins (PV). This atrial-level right-to-left shunt reduces oxygen content of arterial blood throughout the systemic arterial circulation. In addition, since pulmonary artery pressure is greater than systemic arterial pressure, poorly oxygenated blood from the pulmonary artery is shunted right-to-left through the ductus arteriosus (DA) to the descending aorta. As a result, the oxygen content, and hence the Pao_2 and Sao_2 of blood obtained from below the DA, is often less than that of blood obtained from above the DA.

nary hypertension. Although polycythemia is not associated with active constriction, it is included in the category of maladaptation because it is rapidly reversible with reduction of the hematocrit.

114

Table 7: Causes of PPHN From Pulmonary Maladaptation

Transient	Persistent
• Hypoxia	• Meconium aspiration pneumonia
• Hypothermia	• Amniotic fluid aspiration
• Hypoglycemia	• Bacterial pneumonia
• Polycythemia	• Bacterial sepsis

Persistent vasoconstriction is associated with more severe complications of the transition. Conditions such as bacterial pneumonia result in release of mediators, like thromboxane, that result in intense pulmonary vasoconstriction. This persistent vasoconstriction is often accompanied by evidence of plugs of platelets in the pulmonary microcirculation.

With *maldevelopment*, the pulmonary vessels are abnormal. The medial musculature is hypertrophied and extends into normally nonmuscularized arteries down to the level of the alveolus. Excessive muscularization impinges on the vessel lumen, increasing vascular resistance. A common thread linking most cases of maldevelopment is chronically increased pulmonary blood flow in utero. Because the pulmonary and systemic circulations of the fetus are connected, conditions such as intrauterine hypoxia or asphyxia that increase systemic arterial blood pressure in the fetus will divert more blood to the lung, resulting in pulmonary vessel maldevelopment.

Presumably, fetal hypoxia and asphyxia also play a role in the vessel maldevelopment that complicates intrauterine aspiration of meconium. In experimental animals, closure of the ductus arteriosus in utero forces all of the right ventricular output through the lungs and also results in maldevelopment of pulmonary vessels. Because ductal patency in late

Table 8: Causes of PPHN From Pulmonary Maldevelopment

Maldevelopment	*Underdevelopment*
• Intrauterine asphyxia	• Diaphragmatic hernia
• Meconium aspiration	• Potter's syndrome
• Fetal ductal closure	• Other causes of pulmonary hypoplasia
• Congenital heart disease	

gestation is maintained by prostaglandins, intrauterine ductal closure may occur in human pregnancies if the mother is exposed to prostaglandin synthetase inhibitors such as aspirin or indomethacin.

Finally, infants with certain types of congenital heart disease, especially those with obstructed anomalous venous drainage, may have abnormal pulmonary vessels, and pulmonary hypertension often complicates their postoperative course.

Infants with hypoplastic or underdeveloped lungs will have persistently elevated PVR because of the reduction in the number of blood vessels per cross-sectional area of lung. In these infants, pulmonary vessels are also maldeveloped (Table 8).

A recently described rare cause of PPHN is alveolar capillary dysplasia or misalignment of lung vessels.

Presentation
History

The typical infant with PPHN is term or post-term with a history of one or more of the risk factors in Table 6.

Figure 7: Chest radiograph of an infant with idiopathic PPHN. The lung fields are black, reflecting the reduced pulmonary blood flow. The heart is moderately enlarged. (Adapted from Hansen TN, Corbet AJ. In: Taeusch HW, et al, eds. *Schaffer and Avery's Diseases of the Newborn.* 6th ed. Philadelphia, WB Saunders, 1991.)

Physical examination

The infant is cyanotic and usually tachypneic. Other signs of respiratory distress are related to the underlying lung disease. There may be a heart murmur characteristic of tricuspid insufficiency or a single S_2.

Chest radiograph

In PPHN after asphyxia or ductal closure, the lung fields are black, and the heart size is normal or increased. For other causes, the chest x-ray reflects the underlying lung disease (Figure 7).

Laboratory

Arterial blood gases reveal hypoxemia with normal Pa_{CO_2}. Right-to-left shunting of blood across the ductus may cause the measured Sa_{O_2} to be higher in preductal blood compared with postductal blood. Blood obtained from the right radial artery usually has a higher Sao_2 than blood from the umbilical artery, or the pulse oximeter demonstrates a differential Sao_2 between the right arm and the rest of the body. This differential Sao_2 strongly supports a diagnosis of PPHN. However, if the right-to-left shunt is primarily at the atrial level or if the ductus was closed in utero by exposure to prostaglandin synthesis inhibitors, there will be no Sao_2 gradient. Increasing the Fio_2 to 1.00 (the hyperoxia test) may increase Pao_2 in infants with PPHN, especially early in their course. When Pao_2 can never be increased, even transiently with hyperoxia or hyperventilation, the infant should be carefully evaluated for cyanotic heart disease.

Cardiac evaluation

The electrocardiogram may reveal ST segment changes compatible with subendocardial ischemia. The echocardiogram reveals normal cardiac anatomy, while Doppler studies reveal right-to-left shunting across the ductus arteriosus and foramen ovale. In addition, a jet of tricuspid insufficiency can often be detected, confirming the elevated right ventricular pressures.

Differential Diagnosis

Infection is a common cause of PPHN. We treat all infants with PPHN with antibiotics until cultures are negative.

Cyanotic congenital heart disease, especially total anomalous venous return, is difficult to distinguish from PPHN. Almost all patients with PPHN will have an adequate Pao_2 at some point in their course. If they never achieve adequate oxygenation, even transiently, then the clinician should consider heart disease as a cause.

Management

PPHN is a self-limited disease, and treatment is generally supportive. The goal of therapy is to lower oxygen demands and maintain oxygen delivery to the tissues until the PVR decreases. There have been limited randomized trials of therapies for PPHN. Only inhaled nitric oxide (iNO) and extracorporeal membrane oxygenation (ECMO) have been rigorously studied.

Decrease oxygen demand

These infants must be in a neutral thermal environment to minimize oxygen consumption. If they are receiving assisted ventilation, they should be sedated with morphine sulfate (0.1 mg/kg per dose) or fentanyl (bolus of 2 to 10 µg/kg per dose). Sedation also limits additional pulmonary vasoconstriction in response to stimuli such as suctioning. Neuromuscular blockade with pancuronium bromide, 0.1 mg/kg per dose, is reserved for infants requiring extremely high ventilator pressures.

Increase oxygen delivery

Oxygen delivery is determined by the cardiac output, the arterial blood oxygen content, hemoglobin concentration, and Sao_2.

Cardiac output should be supported with volume replacement and dopamine at rates of infusion up to 20 µg/kg/min.

Hemoglobin concentration should be maintained at approximately 15 g/dL by transfusion with packed red cells. Higher hemoglobin concentrations may result in hyperviscosity and exacerbate right-to-left shunting.

Oxygen saturation and Pao_2 should be increased by first improving the distribution of ventilation and then by directly attempting to lower the PVR.

Improve distribution of ventilation

In infants with PPHN and parenchymal lung disease, open, underventilated lung units contribute to hypoxemia, as in HMD. Therefore, management should be similar to that of the infant with HMD (see *Hyaline Membrane Disease* section, this chapter).

Because of the presence of open, poorly ventilated lungs, positive end-expiratory pressure (PEEP) is often useful in improving oxygenation in infants with PPHN and parenchymal lung disease.

Ventilation

Alkalinization, hyperventilation, and the avoidance of hypoxemia using conventional ventilation techniques may reduce pulmonary artery pressures. This was first proposed as a therapy for infants with pulmonary hypertension with no associated lung disease and was based on animal studies that demonstrated sensitivity of the pulmonary vasculature to hypoxia and acidosis. Subsequently, two separate investigators reported a small number of infants with high pulmonary artery pressures who responded to a brief period of hyperventilation. Since these initial reports, the intensity of ventilation has increased, and this strategy has been applied to infants with parenchymal lung disease with associated pulmonary hypertension, both of which may contribute to the increased incidence of chronic lung disease.

Gentle ventilation. The concept of gentle ventilation was originally reported in a retrospective study of infants with PPHN treated with a regimen using minimal ventilator settings to maintain Pao_2 between 50 and 70 mm Hg and $Paco_2$ between 40 and 60 mm Hg. Sedation and paralysis were avoided. All infants survived, and only one developed chronic lung disease. This study's findings were supported by a second case report. Although not conclusive, the lack of randomized trials demonstrating the benefit of hyperventilation and the potential concerns of respiratory alkalosis resulting in hearing loss or development delay bring into question the role of hyperventilation for all but the most severely affected infants with PPHN.

High-frequency oscillatory ventilation. The use of high-frequency oscillatory or jet ventilation has been suggested as therapy for infants with PPHN from a variety of causes. There has been a single, controlled trial and several uncontrolled observational trials of the effect of high-frequency ventilation on this disease. This technique decreases $Paco_2$ and, in the case of the oscillator, is an effective tool to increase oxygenation by increasing mean airway pressure and preventing atelectasis. The use of high-frequency ventilation may prevent the need for ECMO in selected patients; however, it is not known if there is a difference in long-term outcome in these patients.

Surfactant replacement

In many centers, infants with PPHN and parenchymal lung disease receive surfactant replacement (see *Surfactant Administration* section, Chapter 10).

Lower PVR

If improving distribution of ventilation fails to improve oxygenation, attempts should be made to lower the PVR.

Induced alkalosis

Raising the pH to between 7.55 and 7.65 by inducing respiratory or metabolic alkalosis will often lower PVR and improve oxygenation. To prevent lung injury from hyperventilation, a combination of mild hyperventilation with infusion of sodium bicarbonate is preferred.

Drug therapy

The ideal drug for PPHN would lower PVR and increase oxygenation with no direct effect on the systemic circulation. Since there is no intravenous vasodilator specifically for the pulmonary circulation, use of intravenous vasodilators has become limited with the advent of iNO therapy.

Inhaled nitric oxide. A meta-analysis of the results of 12 randomized trials of iNO therapy in hypoxemic term and near-term infants demonstrated that iNO improved oxygenation and reduced the need for ECMO. No improvement is seen with the use of iNO in infants with congenital diaphragmatic hernia. These studies used iNO in doses of 10 to 80 ppm in infants with an oxygen index >25 or a Pao_2 <100 in an Fio_2 = 1. Trials to determine the lowest effective dose are ongoing. In the meantime, iNO should be weaned to the lowest effective dose. Nitrogen dioxide and methemoglobin levels should be monitored during nitric oxide administration (see *Inhaled Nitric Oxide* section, Chapter 10).

Intravenous vasodilators. Nitroprusside is a pulmonary and systemic vasodilator that is given by an infusion of 1 to 5 mg/kg/min. It is rapidly cleared from the circulation if hypotension occurs. Because cyanide and thiocyanate are metabolic by-products of nitroprusside, their levels should be monitored. Prostacyclin has been used in patients with primary pulmonary hypertension, but there are no studies of its use in PPHN. There are also several case reports of the use of magnesium sulfate for treatment of PPHN.

Monitoring. Optimally, the Pao_2 should be maintained between 80 and 100 torr. There is no physiologic reason to maintain a higher Pao_2, and hyperoxia increases the risks of oxygen toxicity to the lungs and other organs. In severe forms of PPHN, it may be safer to maintain the Pao_2 at a lower value, 35 to 45 torr, rather than risk lung injury from excessive mechanical ventilation. Clinicians must pay strict attention to ensuring adequate oxygen delivery by supporting the circulation and maintaining an adequate hemoglobin concentration. Monitoring should include arterial lactate concentrations and acid base status. A rising arterial lactate or a progressive metabolic acidosis suggests that oxygen delivery is not adequate. After 3 to 5 days of a high concentration of oxygen ($Fio_2 > 0.50$), the PVR is no longer labile and oxygen should be weaned empirically to prevent pulmonary oxygen toxicity.

ECMO
When all other modes of therapy have failed to improve oxygenation, ECMO may be used to sustain oxygenation until the PVR falls (see *Extracorporeal Membrane Oxygenation* section, Chapter 10).

Failure to Improve
Infants with PPHN should begin to improve after 3 to 5 days, even on ECMO. Any infant who fails to improve should be evaluated for cyanotic congenital heart disease or some form of irreversible PPHN, such as alveolar capillary dysplasia.

Outcome
Data on outcome of these infants are limited. It is difficult to determine whether abnormalities in developmental outcome are related to the underlying disease process or to the therapy. Mortality and need for ECMO range from 20% to 40%, and the incidence of abnormal neurologic outcome ranges from 12% to 25%. High incidences of hearing impairment, cerebral infarction, and

Figure 8: Blood flows from the right atrium (RA), to the right ventricle (RV), through the pulmonary artery (PA), into the capillaries in the alveolar septum. Blood returns to the heart through the pulmonary veins (PV), to the left atrium (LA), and then to the left ventricle (LV). Fluid filtration into the pulmonary interstitium occurs primarily from the capillaries in the alveolar septum (inset). Filtered fluid is transported by the pulmonary lymphatics to the thoracic duct and then returned to the central venous circulation. The rate of transvascular fluid filtration is governed by a balance between capillary and interstitial hydrostatic pressures (Pmv and Ppmv, respectively) and capillary and interstitial oncotic pressures (πmv and πpmv, respectively) and by the relative permeability of the capillary wall to fluid. Pmv tends to drive fluid out of the capillary into the interstitium, while Ppmv tends to force fluid back into the capillary. On the other hand, πmv pulls fluid into the capillary from the interstitium, while πpmv pulls fluid from the interstitium into the capillary. The net balance of these forces favors filtration of fluid from the capillary into the interstitium. However, the capillary permeability to fluid and protein is low, so that the rate of fluid filtration (<10 mL/h) is small compared to the large amount of blood circulated through the lung (>40,000 mL/h).

intracranial hemorrhage have been reported in several studies.
By Mary E. Wearden, MD, and Thomas N. Hansen, MD

Pulmonary Edema

Epidemiology

Pulmonary edema, defined as an increase in water content of the lung parenchyma, is a major component of many neonatal lung diseases.

Pathophysiology

In the lung, fluid filters continuously from capillaries in the alveolar septum into the alveolar interstitium (Figure 8). This filtered fluid is returned to the circulation by the pulmonary lymphatics. Pulmonary edema occurs when the rate of fluid filtration from the microcirculation into lung tissue exceeds the rate of its removal by lymphatics.

Fluid filtration

The rate of transvascular fluid filtration (Table 9) is governed by (1) the balance between hydrostatic and oncotic pressures and (2) the permeability of the capillary wall to fluid. Interstitial hydrostatic pressure (Ppmv) is similar to alveolar pressure, which is nearly equal to atmospheric pressure, and has little effect on net fluid filtration. Changes in intravascular oncotic pressures are balanced by similar changes in interstitial oncotic pressure, so the net effect of oncotic pressure on fluid filtration is also small. Therefore, the capillary hydrostatic pressure is the dominant pressure governing fluid filtration. This means that there are two basic causes of increased fluid filtration in the lung: increased capillary hydrostatic pressure and increased capillary permeability.

There are two main determinants of capillary hydrostatic pressure: left atrial pressure and pulmonary blood flow. Capillary hydrostatic pressure is always less than pulmonary artery pressure and greater than left atrial pressure. As a result, increases in left atrial pressure always increase capillary hydrostatic pressure. In addition, the pulmonary vascular bed of the neonate is fully recruited at rest, so resistance to blood

Table 9: Causes of Increased Transvascular Fluid Filtration

⇑ Left Atrial Pressure	⇑ Blood Flow	⇑ Permeability
• Fluid overload • Heart disease - Left-sided obstruction - Left-to-right shunt • Cardiomyopathy • Asphyxia	• Heart disease - Left-to-right shunt • ⇓ Lung vascular bed - Lung hypoplasia - Broncho-pulmonary dysplasia - Hyaline membrane disease	• Oxygen toxicity • Aspiration • Sepsis • Pneumonia • Alveolar over-distention

flow through capillaries is fixed. Since pressure is the product of blood flow and resistance, any increase in pulmonary blood flow will directly increase capillary pressure. Similarly, any further decrease in the size of the vascular bed secondary to lung hypoplasia or loss of blood vessels, such as in bronchopulmonary dysplasia (BPD) or HMD, will result in a relative increase in blood flow to the remaining blood vessels and increased capillary pressure.

Capillary permeability is related to the size and number of channels available for filtration of fluid across the capillary wall. Increased capillary permeability or 'capillary leak' typically occurs secondary to conditions that injure the capillary endothelium. This injury may occur directly, by inhaled toxins such as oxygen, or indirectly, by activation of neutrophils with sepsis or pneumonia. Recently, alveolar overdistention has been shown to cause increased capillary permeability.

Lymphatic clearance

The lymphatics transport interstitial fluid through the thoracic duct into the systemic venous circulation. Recent studies found that neonate lymphatics transport fluid less efficiently than do adult lymphatics. Any impairment in lymphatic function will result in accumulation of edema fluid in the pulmonary interstitium. Impaired lymphatic function may result from primary abnormality of the lymphatics, such as in pulmonary lymphangiectasia (Chapter 6), or secondary to functional obstruction by disorders that increase systemic venous pressure, such as BPD with cor pulmonale and superior vena cava syndrome.

Sequence of edema accumulation

Fluid filters out of capillaries in the alveolar septum into the alveolar interstitium. The hydrostatic pressure in the alveolar interstitium is close to alveolar pressure (zero to slightly positive), while the pressure in the extra-alveolar interstitium is negative relative to atmospheric pressure (see *Lung and Heart Interaction* section, Chapter 2). Since these two interstitial compartments are connected, fluid in the alveolar interstitium moves along this pressure gradient into the extra-alveolar interstitium, where it can be stored in the loose connective tissue surrounding pulmonary arteries, lymphatics, and airways. Fluid entry into the alveolar spaces (alveolar flooding) occurs in the later stages of edema formation. Its presence infers that the capability of the extra-alveolar interstitium to store fluid has been exceeded or that the alveolar epithelial barrier has been damaged.

Presentation

History

There is usually a history compatible with one of the disorders listed in Table 9.

Physical examination

Physical examination reflects that interstitial edema compresses airways and thus increases airway resistance, resulting in an obstructive lung disease. With alveolar flooding, plasma proteins inactivate surfactant and reduce lung compliance. Both phenomena result in the creation of a population of severely underventilated lung units. Infants are often cyanotic in room air, with nasal flaring, tachypnea, and an expiratory grunt. They have barrel chests and retractions. Auscultation of the chest reveals fine rales, rhonchi, and occasional wheezes. Infants with pulmonary edema secondary to heart failure usually have an enlarged heart, gallop rhythm, and murmurs compatible with the underlying cardiac disease.

Chest radiograph

On the chest radiograph, lung volume is usually increased. Fluid within the perivascular cuffs in the extra-alveolar interstitium appears as linear densities radiating from the hilum, while alveolar flooding results in diffuse, fluffy infiltrates. In severe cases, especially with lymphatic obstruction, pleural effusions may be present. In cases secondary to heart failure, chest radiography shows the heart is enlarged.

Laboratory

The $Paco_2$ is often increased early in infants with pulmonary edema. The Pao_2 is usually reduced in room air but increases with administration of supplemental oxygen.

Differential Diagnosis

Infants with pulmonary edema secondary to elevated left atrial pressure typically have signs and symptoms of heart failure, including gallop rhythms, murmurs, and cardiomegaly. Infants with asphyxia may also present with pulmonary edema secondary to elevated left atrial pressure. These infants usually have signs and symptoms of ischemic insult to other organs. However, cases of severe pulmonary edema secondary to transient cardiac dysfunction in the absence of other symptoms of a hypoxic-ischemic insult have been reported. The exception to patients presenting with elevated left atrial pressure and cardiomegaly is found in infants with obstructed anomalous pulmonary venous drainage, in whom the heart size is often small. Pulmonary venous obstruction should be considered in any infant with the combination of severe progressive pulmonary edema and circulatory insufficiency. Preterm infants with left-to-right shunts through a PDA may develop pulmonary edema secondary to increased pulmonary blood flow in the absence of significant left ventricular failure. Any premature infant who fails to improve after surfactant therapy or who deteriorates after an initial improvement should be evaluated for a PDA even in the absence of cardiomegaly. Pulmonary edema should be expected to complicate the course of any infant with a reduced pulmonary vascular bed (eg, pulmonary hypoplasia secondary to diaphragmatic hernia or loss of blood vessels secondary to BPD). Infants who are ventilated with high concentrations of oxygen for more than 2 to 3 days may develop pulmonary edema secondary to increased capillary permeability to protein. This may account for some of the later deterioration in pulmonary function that occurs in infants treated for PPHN. Pulmonary edema secondary to increased capillary permeability to protein often occurs in infants with sepsis or pneumonia and may complicate episodes of massive aspiration of gastric contents. Infants with pulmonary edema secondary to lymphatic dysfunction will often have pleural effusions and may have other lymphatic anomalies such as cystic hygroma. Pulmonary lymphangiectasia is a primary abnormality of pulmonary lymphatics that presents as progressive pulmonary edema with no evidence for cardiac dysfunction.

Management

Treatment of pulmonary edema should be directed at correcting the etiology. For patients with PDA, this means either medical or surgical closure. For patients with self-limited diseases such as asphyxia, sepsis, or HMD, care is directed at maintaining oxygenation, decreasing fluid filtration, and waiting for spontaneous resolution. For patients with chronic pulmonary edema from BPD, heart disease that cannot be corrected immediately, or lymphatic abnormalities, prolonged supportive care may be required. Patients with alveolar flooding are usually the most challenging to treat. Therapies directed at enhancing removal of edema fluid from the alveolar space are being studied and may turn out to be important in these patients.

Maintaining oxygenation

Oxygenation is supported by a combination of supplemental oxygen and positive airway pressure: either CPAP or IMV with PEEP (see Chapter 10). Positive airway pressure improves ventilation to open, poorly ventilated lung units and is effective in increasing Pao_2 in patients with pulmonary edema. However, positive airway pressure does not reduce the rate of fluid filtration in the lung, nor does it reduce the rate of edema accumulation.

Decreasing fluid filtration

Regardless of the cause of pulmonary edema, the only way to reduce the rate of fluid filtration and accumulation is to lower capillary hydrostatic pressure. Typically, this requires fluid restriction, but long-term severe fluid restriction may result in substantial growth impairment in infants. Therefore, diuretics are also used to lower circulating blood volume and hence capillary pressure. The most common diuretic used in infants with persistent pulmonary edema is furosemide (starting dose: 1 mg/kg/dose q 12 h). Aggressive diuretic therapy reduces cardiac output and renal perfusion, may result in severe metabolic disturbances such as hypokalemia and hypochloremic metabolic alkalosis, and should be used with caution. For infants with persistent pulmonary edema complicating BPD, administration of furosemide on an every-other-day regimen or substitution of a thiazide may reduce metabolic complications. The use of vasodilators to reduce capillary pressure and reduce fluid filtration in the neonate is untested. In infants with heart failure, digitalis may improve cardiac function and lower vascular pressures.

Improving lymphatic function

The only way to improve lymphatic function at the present time is to lower right atrial pressure, primarily through the use of diuretic therapy. In patients with BPD, it may also be possible to lower right atrial pressure by improving alveolar oxygenation and lowering PVR (see *Bronchopulmonary Dysplasia* section, Chapter 5).

Outcome

The outcome of patients with pulmonary edema is generally not dependent on the edema itself but rather on the disease process leading to the development of pulmonary edema. Prolonged medical management of pulmonary edema in infants is complicated by malnutrition from chronic fluid restriction and bouts of circulatory insufficiency from chronic diuretic use.

By Stephen E. Welty, MD, and Thomas N. Hansen, MD

Pulmonary Hemorrhage

Epidemiology

Pulmonary hemorrhage occurs in conjunction with several disorders in the neonatal period, including prematurity, erythroblastosis, intracranial bleeding, asphyxia, massive aspiration, congenital heart disease, sepsis, hypothermia, PDA, and, more recently, surfactant replacement. However, almost all pulmonary hemorrhages in neonates occur in very-low-birth-weight infants, and most of these premature infants also have a PDA with significant left-to-right flow.

Pathophysiology

Pulmonary hemorrhage is most often hemorrhagic pulmonary edema. Actual blood loss is not severe. Pulmonary hemorrhage results from a sudden, large increase in capillary hydrostatic pressure that causes rupture of some capillaries and massive fluid transudation from others. The sudden increase in pressure may result from a large left-to-right shunt such as a PDA or from massive arterial and venous constriction following intracranial injury from asphyxia or IVH.

Presentation

Infants present with a history of bloody fluid in the trachea. Lung compliance decreases suddenly, and the patient usually becomes intensely cyanotic, often with signs of cardiovascular collapse. Chest radiography shows that lung fields have bilateral opacifications. The hematocrit on edema fluid is significantly lower than whole blood. Most infants have severe hypoxemia and hypercarbia.

Management

Treatment of pulmonary hemorrhage should be directed at correcting the etiology whenever possible. For patients with a PDA, medical or surgical closure is indicated. Pulmonary hemorrhage rarely represents a disorder of coagulation, so treatment with coagulation factors is not indicated. Therapy directed at the hemorrhage itself is supportive. Suctioning should be performed judiciously to keep the airway clear. Positive pressure ventilation with PEEP will improve oxygenation until edema fluid clears. A pulmonary hemorrhage in premature infants increases morbidity and mortality significantly; thus, preventive therapy is desirable. Prophylactic indomethacin administration to premature infants on the first days of life appears to reduce the incidence of clinically significant PDAs and pulmonary hemorrhages. Based on these results, some centers administer indomethacin to premature infants on the first days of life to prevent the development of a clinically significant PDA.

Outcome

Outcome depends predominately on the cause of the pulmonary hemorrhage. A pulmonary hemorrhage in extremely-low-birth-weight infants is devastating, substantially increasing morbidity and mortality.

By Stephen E. Welty, MD, and Thomas N. Hansen, MD

Pleural Effusions

Epidemiology

Pleural effusions in the newborn typically accompany conditions that increase right atrial pressure or otherwise impair lymphatic function. These are congestive heart failure, chylothorax, hydrops fetalis, central venous catheter accidents, superior vena cava syndrome, and infection.

Table 10: Composition of Pleural Liquid in Various Disorders

Condition	Color*	Protein Concentration[†]
Heart failure Hydrops fetalis SVC syndrome	Straw, clear	< Serum
Central venous catheter accident	Straw, clear or milky	< Serum
Chylothorax	Straw, clear or milky	< Serum
Infection	Turbid	> Serum

* Color of the effusion secondary to a catheter accident is milky if lipids are being infused; otherwise, it is straw-colored and clear. Color of the effusion secondary to a chylothorax is milky if the infant is being fed milk; otherwise, it is straw-colored and clear.

Pathophysiology

Fluid accumulates in the pleural space when the rate of fluid filtration across the pleural surfaces exceeds the rate of removal by pleural lymphatics. Filtration pressure in the parietal pleura is governed by systemic venous pressure, while filtration pressure in the visceral pleura is governed by both systemic and pulmonary venous pressures. In patients with heart failure, hydrops fetalis, or superior vena cava syndrome, elevated venous pressures increase the rate of filtration of fluid while simultaneously impairing the ability of the lymphatic system to clear this fluid. Congenital chylothorax results from intrauterine obstruction of the thoracic duct, with subsequent formation of fistulas between the intrathoracic

Lipid Concentration[‡]	White Cells[§]
Low	Few
Low or high	Few
Low or high	High, mostly lymphocytes
Low	High, mostly PMNs

[†] The protein concentration when < serum is usually 2 to 4 g/dL.
[‡] High lipid concentrations may be as much as 1,000 mg/dL.
[§] White cell counts may be as high as 10,000/mL.

portion of the duct and the pleural space. Acquired chylothorax occurs secondary to direct injury to the thoracic duct, usually at surgery.

Presentation

Congenital pleural effusions from hydrops fetalis or chylothorax will sometimes be detected in utero by ultrasound. A history of a central catheter (eg, for total parenteral nutrition [TPN], ECMO) is found in effusions secondary to superior vena cava syndrome or perforation of the catheter into the pleural space.

Signs and symptoms of respiratory distress are caused by compression of lung tissue by the pleural liquid and are therefore directly related to the size of the effusion. Infants with large or bilateral effusions often present with respiratory failure. The affected side of the chest may bulge, while the breath sounds over that side are decreased. Congenital bilateral effusions may be difficult to detect but should be suspected in any infant with hydrops or congenital anomalies of the lymphatic system, such as cystic hygroma. Chest radiography shows that the affected side of the chest is often opacified and the heart shifted to the contralateral side. Small effusions may only be detectable by decubitus views. Laboratory examination of fluid obtained by pleurocentesis can often determine the etiology of the pleural effusion (Table 10).

Differential Diagnosis

Pleural effusions should be suspected in any infant with hydrops fetalis and respiratory failure in the delivery room. In these infants, emergency thoracentesis may be lifesaving. Similarly, congenital chylothorax should be suspected in infants with anomalies related to the lymphatic system, such as webbed neck or cystic hygroma. Pleural effusions after cardiac surgery are usually secondary to injury to the thoracic duct. Infants who experience sudden respiratory deterioration while receiving parenteral nutrition through a central venous catheter may well have an acquired effusion secondary to intrapleural leakage of the IV fluids.

Management

Thoracentesis will relieve symptoms related to pleural effusion and provide fluid to assist in differential diagnosis. Further management is related to the underlying cause. Pleural effusion secondary to leak of parenteral alimentation fluid requires removal of the central catheter. Effusions secondary to infection are rare but usually resolve with appropriate antibiotic therapy. Chylous effusions are particularly problematic and may require repeated thoracenteses and even chronic drainage via a thoracostomy tube. Chronic drainage causes substantial protein loss and may also result in lymphopenia. Once drainage is established, these infants are placed on diets containing medium-chain triglycerides rather than long-chain fats to try to reduce thoracic duct flow. Unfortunately, oral feedings of protein and water also stimulate thoracic duct flow, so this regimen has limited utility. A variety of other techniques have been used to treat persistent chylothorax with varying degrees of success. These include direct repair of the thoracic duct, obliteration of the pleural space with sclerosing agents, pleural peritoneal shunts, and ligation of the thoracic duct below the diaphragm.

Outcome

The outcome for infants with pleural effusions is usually good. Most will resolve with treatment of the underlying disorder. While two thirds of infants with chylothorax will respond to repeated thoracenteses alone, the mortality is still significant (approaching 15%).

By Stephen E. Welty, MD, and Thomas N. Hansen, MD

Meconium Aspiration Syndrome

Meconium staining of the amniotic fluid (MSAF) is a common problem, occurring in 9% to 20% of all deliveries. MSAF is rare before 37 weeks' gestation and common after 42 weeks' gestation (Figure 9). MSAF is not diagnostic of fetal distress and does not appear to be an independent predictor of subsequent neurologic morbidity in the infant. However, some of these infants subsequently develop meconium aspiration syndrome (MAS), which is associated with increased perinatal morbidity and mortality and, therefore, is a problem of particular importance in the newborn period.

Pathophysiology

Meconium is a viscous, greenish liquid that fills the fetal gastrointestinal tract. It is composed of gastrointestinal secretions, cellular debris, bile, pancreatic juice, mucus, blood, swallowed lanugo, and vernix. In utero, meconium passage may occur either in response to fetal hypoxia, with a transient period of hyperperistalsis and relaxation of anal sphinc-

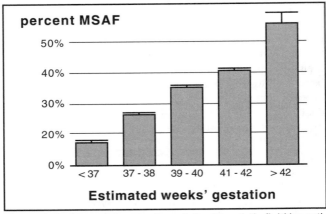

Figure 9: Incidence of meconium-stained amniotic fluid by estimated gestational age, ± 95% CI. (Used with permission, Dysart M, Graves BW, Sharp ES, et al: The incidence of meconium-stained amniotic fluid from 1980 through 1986, by year and gestational age. *J Perinatol* 1991;11:245-248).

ter tone, or as a normal, physiologic event in fetal gut maturation. Aspiration of meconium may occur in utero as the compromised, hypoxic, and acidotic fetus passes meconium and begins to gasp. More frequently, aspiration occurs with the initial breaths after delivery.

Acute large airway obstruction may occur as meconium is aspirated into the trachea. Subsequently, chemical pneumonitis and interstitial edema may obstruct smaller airways. Completely obstructed airways result in distal atelectasis. Airways with partial obstruction may allow more air to enter than to exit the distal airspace, producing air trapping. This stage of meconium aspiration is characterized by infiltration of leukocytes into the interstitial and alveolar spaces, alveolar edema, necrosis of alveolar and airway epithelia, and accumulation of proteinaceous debris in the alveoli. Alveolar injury results in surfactant inactivation and decreased lung compliance. Hypoxemia results from decreased alveolar ventilation, continued perfusion of poorly ventilated lung units, and right-to-left shunt secondary to increased PVR. PVR is increased by:

- local constriction of pulmonary vessels perfusing poorly ventilated lung units;
- global constriction of pulmonary vessels by vasoactive substances present in the aspirated meconium;
- platelet aggregation in pulmonary vessels in response to vasoactive substances in aspirated meconium; and
- maldevelopment of pulmonary vessels secondary to chronic intrauterine hypoxia.

Presentation
History

Infants with MAS are often postmature with an antenatal course frequently complicated by fetal distress. The amniotic fluid is meconium stained.

Physical examination

Tachypnea, grunting, nasal flaring, retractions, and cyanosis develop shortly after birth and progress over 12 to 24 hours. Gas trapping results in a barrel-chested appearance. These infants often have diffuse rales and rhonchi.

Chest radiograph

Initially, the chest radiograph may demonstrate streaky, linear densities similar to those seen in the infant with TTN. Later, the chest radiograph reveals large-volume lungs with diffuse, patchy, parenchymal infiltrates alternating with areas of overexpansion (Figure 10). Pneumomediastinum and pneumothorax are common. Occasionally, in infants with severe alveolar damage and surfactant inactivation, the chest radiograph may reveal low-volume lungs with homogeneous densities similar to those seen in infants with HMD.

Laboratory

Measurements of arterial blood gas tensions reveal arterial hypoxemia and hypercarbia. Infants with significant PPHN will often have a higher arterial oxygen saturation in

Figure 10: Radiograph of infant with MAS. The lungs are hyperinflated and dark (due to air trapping) with areas of haziness representing consolidation and alveolar edema.

preductal blood than in postductal blood. Spectrophotometric analysis of urine reveals an absorption at 405 nm characteristic of bile pigments present in meconium.

Differential Diagnosis

The major differential diagnoses include TTN, HMD, and bacterial pneumonia. Infants with TTN show steady improvement after birth, while those with meconium aspiration will continue to deteriorate. Infants with HMD are almost always premature, while those with meconium aspiration are term or post-term. MAS may be difficult to distinguish from bacterial pneumonia, and we often treat these infants with antibiotics, pending negative blood cultures. Aspiration of amniotic fluid with vernix caseosa may have a presentation like MAS, and the management of the two conditions is similar.

Prevention

Current recommendations for prevention of MAS call for a combined obstetric and pediatric approach to the infant born through thick or 'pea soup' meconium. This approach includes:

- Immediate suctioning of the infant's nasopharynx/oropharynx by the obstetrician as the head appears on the perineum or abdomen and before delivery of the thorax;
- Postdelivery visualization of the vocal cords by laryngoscopy and direct suctioning of the trachea with an endotracheal tube for those infants with meconium-stained amniotic fluid who are depressed at birth but not for vigorous infants.

Studies have shown that there is no evidence that endotracheal intubation and aspiration of the airways in nonasphyxiated meconium-stained babies is beneficial. However, it is likely that routine aspiration of the upper airways is beneficial and should not be discarded. Therefore, until additional research is completed, the depressed or nonvigorous newborn delivered through meconium-stained amniotic fluid probably still should be suctioned and undergo endotracheal intubation at birth.

Unfortunately, some infants born through thick meconium-stained fluids will develop MAS despite adequate delivery room management. It is thought that in utero aspiration may occur and that, despite aggressive suctioning at birth, MAS may not be preventable.

In addition to early clearing of the trachea, recent data suggest that intrapartum amnioinfusion may benefit infants with MSAF, possibly by diluting the meconium, by reducing its toxicity, and by correcting the oligohydramnios often associated with MSAF. It is possible that some of the benefit of amnioinfusion is that it may reduce the risk of cord compression and acidemia, both of which could ultimately result in antepartum aspiration. Studies suggest a potential benefit of amnioinfusion in decreasing the incidence of meconium below the vocal cords, but more studies are needed to determine if this technique will enhance a favorable outcome in labors complicated by MSAF.

Management

Symptomatic infants with meconium suctioned from their trachea should be given chest physiotherapy and warmed, humidified oxygen to breathe.

There is no clear evidence that infection contributes to the pathogenesis of MAS, and the role of antibiotics is controversial. However, meconium is known to enhance bacterial growth by reducing host resistance, and there is an increased risk of intra-amniotic infection when MSAF is present. Therefore, treatment of those infants with antibiotics should be considered pending negative blood cultures.

Tracheal lavage may result in deterioration in lung function and is not recommended.

General supportive care and treatments to lower PVR are described in the *Persistent Pulmonary Hypertension of the Newborn* section in this chapter.

There is evidence that infants with MAS have surfactant inactivation in that meconium in the alveoli can injure type II alveolar epithelial cells and interfere with surfactant production. Surfactant replacement therapy, if started within 6 hours after birth, has been shown to improve oxygenation and reduce the severity of pulmonary morbidity in some cases. Recent studies conclude that in infants with MAS, surfactant administration may reduce the severity of the respiratory illness and decrease the number of infants with progressive respiratory failure requiring support with ECMO.

Oxygen and ventilation

The approach to oxygen administration and ventilation is similar to that used for HMD (see *Oxygen Use and Monitoring*, Chapter 10). Because of the presence of open, poorly ventilated lung units, judicious application of PEEP (4 to 7 cm H_2O) is often useful in improving oxygenation in infants with MAS. Mechanical ventilation should be reserved for infants with apnea from birth asphyxia or for those who cannot maintain their Po_2 >50 mm Hg in 100% oxygen. Again, judicious use of PEEP (4 to 7 cm H_2O) may improve oxygenation. For aggressive mechanical ventilation in the large, vigorous newborn, neuromuscular blockade may optimize ventilatory support and decrease the chance of air leak. Because MAS is characterized by airway obstruction, particular attention must be paid to inspiratory time and ventilator rate to prevent unintentional PEEP that would exacerbate gas trapping and alveolar rupture.

Failure to Improve

Infants with MAS may deteriorate for 12 to 24 hours after birth but should begin to improve after 3 to 5 days—even when on ECMO. Any infant who fails to improve should be evaluated for cyanotic congenital heart disease or for a form of irreversible PPHN such as alveolar capillary dysplasia. Because meconium must ultimately be cleared from the lung by phagocytes, respiratory symptoms may persist for weeks after birth.

For those infants with MAS with profound hypoxia and PPHN, ECMO may be appropriate when conventional strategies fail.

Outcome

Symptoms related to MAS may persist for days to weeks. In the past, mortality for infants with MAS was as high as 30%. However, with the advent of a gentler approach to ventilation and, for severe cases, the availability of ECMO, mortality is now less than 10% and in some centers approaches zero. Infants with MAS are at increased risk for complications of mechanical ventilation, including air block and bronchopulmonary dysplasia.

By Karen E. Johnson, MD, Timothy R. Cooper, MD, and Thomas N. Hansen, MD

Pneumonia

Epidemiology

Pneumonia can be caused by bacterial, viral, spirochetal, protozoan, and fungal pathogens. The pneumonic process may begin before, during, or after delivery. The infant may be infected transplacentally, via infected amniotic fluid, after colonization at delivery, and nosocomially. Nosocomial infections,

Table 11: Common Organisms Associated With Neonatal Pneumonia

Transplacental
- Rubella
- Cytomegalovirus
- Herpes simplex virus
- Adenovirus
- Mumps virus
- *Toxoplasma gondii*
- *Listeria monocytogenes*
- *Mycobacterium tuberculosis*
- *Treponema pallidum*

Amniotic Fluid
- Cytomegalovirus
- Herpes simplex virus
- Enteroviruses
- Genital mycoplasma
- *L monocytogenes*
- *Chlamydia trachomatis*
- *M tuberculosis*
- Group B streptococci (GBS)
- *Escherichia coli*
- *Haemophilus influenzae* (nontypeable)
- *Ureaplasma urealyticum*

At Delivery
- GBS
- *E coli*
- *Staphylococcus aureus*
- *Klebsiella* sp
- Other streptococci
- *H influenzae* (nontypable)
- *Candida* sp
- *C trachomatis*
- *Ureaplasma urealyticum*

Nosocomial
- *S aureus*
- *S epidermidis*
- GBS
- *Klebsiella* sp
- *Enterobacter*
- *Pseudomonas*
- Influenza virus
- Respiratory syncytial virus
- Enteroviruses

in many instances, can be traced to poor handwashing and over-crowding. The most common organisms associated with each route of infection are listed in Table 11.

The preterm infant is much more prone to infection than the term infant. The reasons relate to an immature immune system coupled with a lack of protective maternal antibodies.

Pathophysiology

Congenital pneumonia is not an infrequent finding at autopsy; 15% to 38% of stillborn infants have evidence of pulmonary inflammation. In most of these pneumonias, infiltration of alveoli or destruction of bronchopulmonary tissue is rare, bacteria are seen infrequently, and cultures are often negative. Aspiration or ingestion of infected amniotic fluid appears to be the most frequent cause of bacterial pneumonia. Those infections occurring during and after the birth process have findings similar to pneumonias seen in older children. The lungs contain areas of cellular exudate with vascular congestion, hemorrhage, and necrosis.

Presentation

History

Infants who have congenital pneumonia are often critically ill at delivery or may be stillborn. The mother may give a history of an infectious process preceding delivery or may exhibit signs and symptoms of chorioamnionitis.

Physical examination

In infants who acquire their disease after birth, the signs and symptoms are frequently those of systemic infection: lethargy, poor feeding, fever, and respiratory distress or apnea. Rales and changes in the quality of the breath sounds may or may not be present.

Chest radiograph

Changes may mimic those of HMD in instances of early bacterial pneumonia, particularly those caused by group B streptococci, or be nonspecific, streaky densities or confluent opacities. Abscess cavities can be seen in staphylococcal disease but can also be found in pneumonia caused by *Escherichia coli* and *Klebsiella pneumoniae*.

Laboratory

Cultures of the gastric contents, throat, and nasopharynx are unrevealing or inaccurate. Direct tracheal aspiration via laryngoscopy with Gram stain and culture of the resulting material can be helpful. Bacteremia and meningitis often are found in infants with pneumonia, and cultures of blood and cerebrospinal fluid are recommended. Direct (arterial blood gas) or indirect (pulse oximetry or transcutaneous oxygen) assessment of oxygenation should be undertaken.

Differential Diagnosis

HMD, TTN, meconium aspiration, lung hypoplasia, pulmonary edema and hemorrhage, and congenital heart disease are relatively common conditions to consider in patients with neonatal pneumonia.

Management and Outcome

Obviously, prompt institution of antimicrobials is crucial. For early-onset disease, a penicillin and an aminoglycoside are usually recommended. For infection acquired in the hospital, a penicillinase-resistant penicillin or vancomycin and an aminoglycoside or third-generation cephalosporin are appropriate. Many neonatal ICUs have infections caused by *Staphylococcus epidermidis* or methicillin-resistant *S aureus*, requiring vancomycin. If infection by *Ureaplasma urealyticum* or *Chlamydia trachomatis* is suspected, erythromycin is the preferred antibiotic. Other supportive measures include cardiopulmonary management, fluids, and nutritional support.

In the British Perinatal Mortality Study, pneumonia was considered the cause of death in 5.5% of stillborn and neonatal deaths. The use of prophylactic intrapartum antibiotics has recently been shown to decrease the incidence of early-onset infection caused by group B *Streptococcus* and other organisms. The overall mortality of sepsis ranges from 5% to 10% in the term infant to as high as 67% in the neonate <1,500 g. Infants born with fulminant group B streptococcal infection suffered a 50% mortality in the past. Modern neonatal ICU support may decrease this number. Pneumonia is still a fatal complicating factor in infants with underlying congenital heart disease, central nervous system malformations, and anomalies of the gastrointestinal tract.

By Michael E. Speer, MD, and Leonard E. Weisman, MD

Suggested Readings

Hyaline Membrane Disease

Antenatal corticosteroids revisited: repeat courses. *NIH Consens Statement* 2000;17(2):1-18.

Avery ME, Mead J: Surface properties in relation to atelectasis and hyaline membrane disease. *Am J Dis Child* 1959;97:517.

Ballard RA, Ballard PL, Boardman RC, et al: Antenatal thyrotropin releasing hormone for the prevention of chronic lung disease in the preterm infant. *Pediatr Res* 1997;41:1461A. Abstract.

Bloom BT, Kattwinkel J, Hall RT, et al: Comparison of Infasurf (calf lung surfactant extract) to Survanta (beractant) in the treatment and prevention of respiratory distress syndrome. *Pediatrics* 1997;100:31-38.

Chu J, Clements JA, Cotton EK, et al: Neonatal pulmonary ischemia: clinical and physiological studies. *Pediatrics* 1967;40:709.

Corbet AJ, et al: Ventilation-perfusion relationships as assessed by aADN$_2$ in hyaline membrane disease. *J Appl Physiol* 1974;36:74-81.

Fujiwara T, Chida S, Watabe Y, et al: Artificial surfactant therapy in hyaline membrane disease. *Lancet* 1980;12:55.

Gluck L, Kulovich MV: Lecithin-sphingomyelin ratios in amniotic fluid in normal and abnormal pregnancy. *Am J Obstet Gynecol* 1973;115:539.

Gregory GA, Kitterman JA, Phibbs RH, et al: Treatment of idiopathic respiratory distress syndrome with continuous airway pressure. *N Engl J Med* 1971;284:1333.

Gribetz I, Frank NR, Avery ME: Static volume pressure relations of excised lungs of infants with hyaline membrane disease: newborn and stillborn infants. *J Clin Invest* 1959;38:2168.

Halliday HL: Natural vs synthetic surfactants in neonatal respiratory distress syndrome. *Drugs* 1996;51:226-237.

Hallman M, Teramo K: Measurement of the lecithin-sphingomyelin ratio and phosphatidylglycerol in amniotic fluid: an accurate method for the assessment of fetal lung maturity. *Br J Obstet Gynecol* 1981;88:806.

Hansen TN, Corbet AJ, Kenny JD, et al: Effects of oxygen and constant positive pressure breathing on aADCO$_2$ in hyaline membrane disease. *Pediatr Res* 1979;13:1167-1171.

Hansen TN, Corbet AJ: Disorders of the transition. In: Ballard R, Taeusch W, eds. *Schaffer's Diseases of the Newborn*. Philadelphia, WB Saunders Co, 1991, pp 498-504.

Horbar JD, Soll RF, Sutherland JM, et al: A multicenter, randomized, placebo-controlled trial of surfactant therapy for respiratory distress syndrome. *N Engl J Med* 1989;320:959.

Horbar JD, Wright LL, Soll R, et al: A multicenter, randomized trial comparing two surfactants for the treatment of neonatal respiratory distress syndrome. *J Pediatr* 1993;123:757.

Jobe AH: Pulmonary surfactant therapy. *N Engl J Med* 1993;328:861.

Jobe AH, Mitchell BR, Gunkel JH: Beneficial effects of the combined use of prenatal corticosteroids and postnatal surfactant on preterm infants. *Am J Obstet Gynecol* 1993;168:508.

Kattwinkel J: Surfactant. Evolving issues [review]. *Clin Perinatol* 1998; 25:17-32.

Kattwinkel J, Bloom BT, Delmore P, et al: Prophylactic administration of calf lung surfactant extract is more effective than early treatment of respiratory distress syndrome in neonates of 29 through 32 weeks' gestation. *Pediatrics* 1993;92:90.

Kendig JW, Notter RH, Cox C, et al: A comparison of surfactant as immediate prophylaxis and as rescue therapy in newborns of less than 30 weeks' gestation. *N Engl J Med* 1991;324:865.

Kendig JW, Ryan RM, Sinkin RA, et al: Comparison of two strategies for surfactant prophylaxis in very premature infants: a multicenter randomized trial. *Pediatrics* 1998;101:1006-1012.

Liechty EA, Donovan E, Purohit D, et al: Reduction of neonatal mortality after multiple doses of bovine surfactant in low birth weight neonates with respiratory distress syndrome. *Pediatrics* 1991;88:19.

Liggins GC, Howie RN: A controlled trial of antepartum glucocorticoid treatment of prevention of the respiratory distress syndrome in premature infants. *Pediatrics* 1972;50:515.

Long W, Corbet A, Cotton R, et al: A controlled trial of synthetic surfactant in infants weighing 1250 g or more with respiratory distress syndrome. *N Engl J Med* 1991;325:1696.

Long W, Thompson T, Sundell H, et al: Effects of two rescue doses of a synthetic surfactant on mortality rate and survival without bronchopulmonary dysplasia in 700- to 1350-gram infants with respiratory distress syndrome. *J Pediatr* 1991;118:595.

NIH Consensus Development Panel Effect of Corticosteroids for Fetal Maturation on Perinatal Outcomes: Effect of corticosteroids for fetal maturation on perinatal outcomes. *JAMA* 1995;273:413-418.

Nilsson R, Grossmann G, Robertson B: Lung surfactant and the pathogenesis of neonatal bronchiolar lesions induced by artificial ventilation. *Pediatr Res* 1978;12:249.

OSIRIS Collaborative Group: Early versus delayed neonatal administration of a synthetic surfactant - the judgment of OSIRIS. *Lancet* 1992;340:1363.

Richardson P, Pace WR, Valdes E, et al: Time dependence of lung mechanics in preterm lambs. *Pediatr Res* 1992;31:276.

Shapiro DL, Notter RH, Morin III, et al: Double-blind, randomized trial of a calf lung surfactant extract administered at birth to very premature infants for prevention of respiratory distress syndrome. *Pediatrics* 1985;76:593.

Soll RF, Hoekstra RE, Fangman JJ, et al: Multicenter trial of single-dose modified bovine surfactant extract (Survanta®) for prevention of respiratory distress syndrome. *Pediatrics* 1990;85:1092.

Wright LL, Verter J, Stevenson DK, et al: Increased antenatal glucocorticoid use decreases mortality and morbidity in the NICHD Neonatal Research Network's very low birth weight infants. *Pediatr Res* 1997;41:1269A. Abstract.

Transient Tachypnea of the Newborn

Avery ME, Gatewood OB, Brumley G: Transient tachypnea of the newborn: possible delayed resorption of fluid at birth. *Am J Dis Child* 1966;111:380.

Bland RD: Formation of fetal lung liquid and its removal near birth. In: Polin RA, Fox WW, eds. *Fetal and Neonatal Physiology.* Philadelphia, WB Saunders Co, 1992, pp 782-789.

Demissie K, Marcella SW, Breckenridge MB, et al: Maternal asthma and transient tachypnea of the newborn. *Pediatrics* 1998;102:84-90.

Hansen T, Corbet A: Disorders of the transition. In: Taeusch HW, Ballard RA, eds. *Avery's Diseases of the Newborn,* 7th ed. Philadelphia, WB Saunders Co, 1998, pp 613-615.

Krauss AN, Auld PAM: Pulmonary gas trapping in premature infants. *Pediatr Res* 1971;5:10.

Sundell H, Garrott J, Blankenship WJ: Studies on infants with type II respiratory distress syndrome. *J Pediatr* 1971;78:754.

Persistent Pulmonary Hypertension of the Newborn

Auten RL, Notter RH, Kendig JW, et al: Surfactant treatment of full-term newborns with respiratory failure. *Pediatrics* 1991;87:101-107.

Ballard RA, Leonard CH: Developmental follow-up of infants with persistent pulmonary hypertension of the newborn. *Clin Perinatol* 1984;11:737.

Bartlett RH, Roloff DW, Cornell RG, et al: Extracorporeal circulation in neonatal respiratory failure: a prospective randomized study. *Pediatrics* 1985;76:479.

Clark RH, Yoder BA, Sell MS: Prospective, randomized comparison of high-frequency oscillation and conventional ventilation in candidates for extracorporeal membrane oxygenation. *J Pediatr* 1994;124:447-454.

Drummond WH, Gregory GA, Heymann MA, et al: The independent effects of hyperventilation, tolazoline and dopamine on infants with persistent pulmonary hypertension. *J Pediatr* 1981;98:603.

Dworetz AR, Moya FR, Sabo B, et al: Survival of infants with persistent pulmonary hypertension without extracorporeal membrane oxygenation. *Pediatrics* 1989;84:1-6.

Geggel RL, Reid LM: The structural basis of PPHN. *Clin Perinatol* 1984;11:525-549.

Gersony WM, Duc GV, Sinclair JC: "PFC" syndrome (persistence of the fetal circulation). *Circulation* 1969;39(suppl):III-87.

Hansen TN, Gest AL: Oxygen toxicity and other ventilatory complications of treatment of infants with persistent pulmonary hypertension. *Clin Perinatol* 1984;11:653.

Hansen TN, Corbet AJ: Disorders of the transition. In: Ballard R, Taeusch W, eds. *Schaffer's Diseases of the Newborn.* Philadelphia, WB Saunders Co, 1991, pp 506-509.

Hendricks-Munoz KD, Walton JP: Hearing loss in infants with persistent fetal circulation. *Pediatrics* 1988;81:650.

Hickey PR, Hansen DD, Wessel DL, et al: Blunting of stress responses in the pulmonary circulation of infants by fentanyl. *Anesth Analg* 1985;64:1137.

Kinsella JP, Neish SR, Shaffer E, et al: Low-dose inhalational nitric oxide in persistent pulmonary hypertension of the newborn. *Lancet* 1992;340:819-820.

Levin DL, Heymann MA, Kitterman JA, et al: Persistent pulmonary hypertension of the newborn infant. *J Pediatr* 1976;89:626.

Morin FC III: Ligating the ductus arteriosus before birth causes persistent pulmonary hypertension in the newborn lamb. *Pediatr Res* 1989;25:245.

Naeye RL, Schochat SJ, Whitman V, et al: Unsuspected pulmonary vascular abnormalities associated with diaphragmatic hernia. *Pediatrics* 1976;58:902.

O'Rourke PP, Crone RK, Vacanti JP, et al: Extracorporeal membrane oxygenation and conventional medical therapy in neonates with persistent pulmonary hypertension of the newborn: a prospective randomized study. *Pediatrics* 1989;84:957-963.

Roberts JD, Polaner DM, Lang P, et al: Inhaled nitric oxide in persistent pulmonary hypertension of the newborn. *Lancet* 1992;340:818-819.

Schreiber MD, Heymann MA, Soifer SJ: Increased arterial pH, not decreased $PaCO_2$, attenuates hypoxia-induced pulmonary vasoconstriction in newborn lambs. *Pediatr Res* 1986;20:113.

Wilcox DT, Glick PL, Karamanoukian H, et al: Pathophysiology of congenital diaphragmatic hernia. V. Effect of exogenous surfactant therapy on gas exchange and lung mechanics in the lamb congenital diaphragmatic hernia model. *J Pediatr* 1994;124:289-292.

Wung JT, James LS, Kilchevsky E, et al: Management of infants with severe respiratory failure and persistance of the fetal circulation, without hyperventilation. *Pediatrics* 1985;76:488.

Pulmonary Edema

Albertine KH: Ultrastructural abnormalities in increased-permeability pulmonary edema. *Clin Chest Med* 1985;6:345.

Bland RD, Hansen TN: Neonatal lung edema. In: Said SI, ed. *The Pulmonary Circulation and Acute Lung Injury*. Mount Kisco, NY, Futura Publishing Co, p 225, 1985.

Brigham KL, Woolverton W, Blake L, et al: Increased sheep lung vascular permeability caused by *Pseudomonas* bacteremia. *J Clin Invest* 1974;54:792.

Carlton DP, Cummings JJ, Scheerer RG, et al: Lung overexpansion increases pulmonary microvascular protein permeability in young lambs. *J Appl Physiol* 1990;69:577-583.

Drake R, Giesler M, Laine G, et al: Effect of outflow pressure on lung lymph flow in unanesthetized sheep. *J Appl Physiol* 1985;58:70.

Fein A, Grossman RF, Jones JG, et al: The value of edema fluid protein measurement in patients with pulmonary edema. *Am J Med* 1979;67:32.

Feltes TF, Hansen TN: Pulmonary edema. In: Garson AJ, Bricker JT, McNamara DG, eds. *The Science and Practice of Pediatric Cardiology*. Philadelphia, Lea and Febiger, 1990, pp 386-400.

Johnson, SA, Vander Straten MC, Parallada JA, et al: Thoracic duct function in fetal, newborn, and adult sheep. *Lymphology* 1996;29:50-56.

Stastny B, Kind C: Acute pulmonary oedema due to transient myocardial dysfunction: an uncommon cause of respiratory distress in the term neonate. *Eur J Pediatr* 1998;157:59-62.

Staub NC, Nagano H, Pearce ML: The sequence of events during fluid accumulation in acute pulmonary edema. *Jap Heart J* 1967;8:683-689.

Staub NC: The pathogenesis of pulmonary edema. *Prog Cardiovasc Dis* 1980;33:53-80.

Verghese GM, Ware LB, Matthay BA, et al: Alveolar epithelial fluid transport and the resolution of clinically severe hydrostatic pulmonary edema. *J Appl Physiol* 1999;87:1301-1312.

Pulmonary Hemorrhage

Cole VA, Normand CS, Reynolds EO, et al: Pathogenesis of hemorrhagic pulmonary edema and massive pulmonary hemorrhage in the newborn. *Pediatrics* 1973;51:175-187.

Kluckow M, Evans N: Ductal shunting, high pulmonary blood flow, and pulmonary hemorrhage. *J Pediatr* 2000;137:68-72.

Malik AB: Mechanisms of neurogenic pulmonary edema. *Circ Res* 1985;57:1.

Pandit PB, O'Brien K, Asztalos E, et al: Outcome following pulmonary haemorrhage in very low birthweight neonates with surfactant. *Arch Dis Child Fetal Neonatal Ed* 1999;81:F40-F44.

Rowe S, Avery ME: Massive pulmonary hemorrhage in the newborn. II. Clinical considerations. *J Pediatr* 1966;69:12.

Pleural Effusions

Chernick V, Reed MH: Pneumothorax and chylothorax in the neonatal period. *J Pediatr* 1970;76:624.

Chervenak FA, Isaacson G, Blacemore KJ, et al: Fetal cystic hygroma: cause and natural history. *N Engl J Med* 1983;309:822.

Miserocchi G: Pleural pressures and fluid transport. In: Crystal RG, West JB, Barnes PJ, et al, eds. *The Lung.* New York, Raven Press Ltd, 1991, p 885.

Rodeck CH, Fisk NM, Fraser DI, et al: Long-term in utero drainage of fetal hydrothorax. *N Engl J Med* 1988;319:1135.

Smeltzer DM, Stickler GB, Fleming RE: Primary lymphatic dysplasia in children: chylothorax, chylous ascites, and generalized lymphatic dysplasia. *Eur J Pediatr* 1986;145:286.

Stringel G, Mercer S, Bass J: Surgical management of persistent postoperative chylothorax in children. *Can J Surg* 1984;27:543.

Wiener-Kronish JP, Berthiaume Y, Albertine KH: Pleural effusions and pulmonary edema. *Clin Chest Med* 1985;6:509.

Meconium Aspiration Syndrome

Al-Mateen KB, Dailey K, Grimes MM, et al: Improved oxygenation with exogenous surfactant administration in experimental meconium aspiration syndrome. *Pediatr Pulmonol* 1994;17:75-80.

Carson BS, Losey RW, Bowes WA, et al: Combined obstetric and pediatric approach to prevent meconium aspiration syndrome. *Am J Obstet Gynecol* 1976;126:712.

Davis RO, Philips JB, Haris BA, et al: Fatal meconium aspiration syndrome occurring despite airway management considered appropriate. *Am J Obstet Gynecol* 1985;151:731.

Desmond MM, Moore J, Lindley JE, et al: Meconium staining of the amniotic fluid: a marker of fetal hypoxia. *Obstet Gynecol* 1957;9:91.

Findlay, RD, Taeusch HW, Walther FJ: Surfactant replacement therapy for meconium aspiration syndrome. *Pediatrics* 1996;97:48-52.

Fox WW, Berman LS, Downes JJ, et al: The therapeutic application of end-expiratory pressure in the meconium aspiration syndrome. *Pediatrics* 1975;56:214.

Fox WW, Gewitz MH, Dinwiddie R, et al: Pulmonary hypertension in the perinatal aspiration syndromes. *Pediatrics* 1977;59:205.

Gregory GA, Gooding CA, Phibbs RH, et al: Meconium aspiration in infants - a prospective study. *J Pediatr* 1974;85:848.

Khammash H, Perlman M, Wojtulewicz J, et al: Surfactant therapy in full term neonates with severe respiratory failure. *Pediatrics* 1993;92:135-139.

Linder N, Aranda JV, Tsur M, et al: Need for endotracheal intubation and suction in meconium-stained neonates. *J Pediatr* 1988;112:613-615.

Liu WF: Delivery room intubation of thin meconium in the low risk newborn: a clinical trial. *Pediatr Res* 1998;43:182A. Abstract 1058.

Lotze A, Mitchell BR, Bulas DI, et al: Multicenter study of surfactant (beractant) use in the treatment of term infants with severe respiratory failure. Survanta in Term Infants Study Group. *J Pediatr* 1998;132:40-47.

Wiswell TE, Gannon CM, Jacob J, et al: Delivery room management of the apparently vigorous meconium-stained neonate: results of the multicenter, international collaborative trial. *Pediatrics* 2000;105(1 pt 1):1-7.

Matthews TG, Warshaw JB: Relevance of the gestational age distribution of meconium passage in utero. *Pediatrics* 1979;64:30.

Park KH, Bae CW, Chung SJ: In vitro effect of meconium on the physical surface properties and morphology of exogenous pulmonary surfactant. *J Korean Med Science* 1996;11:429-436.

Rubin BK, Tomkiewicz RP, Patrinos ME, et al: The surface and transport properties of meconium and reconstituted meconium solutions. *Pediatr Res* 1996;40:834-838.

Tran N, Lowe C, Sivieri EM, et al: Sequential effects of acute meconium obstruction on pulmonary function. *Pediatr Res* 1980;14:34.

Usta IM, Mercer BM, Aswad NK, et al: The impact of a policy of amnioinfusion for meconium-stained amniotic fluid. *Obstet Gynecol* 1995;85:237-241.

Wiswell TE, Henley MA: Intratracheal suctioning, systemic infection, and the meconium aspiration syndrome. *Pediatrics* 1992;89:203-206.

Pneumonia

Hansen TN, Corbet AJ: Neonatal pneumonias. In: Ballard R, Taeusch W, eds. *Schaffer's Diseases of the Newborn*. Philadelphia, WB Saunders Co, 1991, p 527.

Isaacs D, Royle JA: Intrapartum antibiotics and early onset neonatal sepsis caused by group B *Streptococcus* and by other organisms in Australia.

Australasian Study Group for Neonatal Infections. *Pediatr Infect Dis J* 1999;18:524-528.

Marks MI, Klein JO: Bacterial infections of the respiratory tract. In: Remington JS, Klein JO, eds. *Infectious Diseases of the Fetus and Newborn Infant*. 4th ed. Philadelphia, WB Saunders Co, 1995, pp 891-908.

Stoll BA, Weisman LE, eds. Infections in perinatology. *Clinics in Perinatology* 1997;24:1-283.

Chapter 5

Subacute and Chronic Acquired Parenchymal Lung Diseases

Air Block

Epidemiology

Air block is far more common in the newborn period than at any other period of life. Although the observed frequency appears to be decreasing, reports of air block vary with the underlying lung disease as well as with methods of resuscitation and ventilation (Table 1). Besides those with acute lung disease, infants with hypoplastic lungs, diaphragmatic hernias, and renal anomalies have a high incidence of air block.

In mature infants, air block is usually manifested by a *pneumomediastinum* or a *pneumothorax*. In small, less than 1,500-g, premature infants, *pulmonary interstitial emphysema (PIE)* is more common.

Pathophysiology

PIE and pneumothoraces occur less as a consequence of high transalveolar pressures than because of abnormal distribution of gas and subsequent alveolar overdistention. Therefore, the normal lung, evenly ventilated and constrained by the thorax, will rarely develop air block. However, with disease (eg, hyaline membrane disease [HMD] with microatelectasis, meconium aspiration syndrome [MAS] with 'ball valve effect'), or in healthy newborns breathing their first breaths, underventilated areas allow the overdistention of ventilated alveoli when high ventilation pressures or long inspiratory times are used. The alveoli tethered by adjacent

Table 1: Reported Frequencies of Pneumothorax

Normal term infants	0.5%–2%
TTN	5%–10%
Hyaline membrane disease (HMD)	up to 20%
HMD and CPAP	up to 20%
HMD and mechanical ventilation	20%–50%
Meconium aspiration syndrome	up to 50%

TTN = Transient tachypnea of the newborn
CPAP = Continuous positive air pressure

bronchi and blood vessels are less free to expand in all directions and are the most likely to rupture into the adjacent, perivascular, loose connective tissue.

Loculated air at this stage produces PIE. The perivascular connective tissue in the extremely premature infant is more abundant and less dissectable. Air frequently remains trapped at this site, finding its way into the lymphatics. In the mature infant, air usually dissects along this connective tissue plane toward the mediastinum, creating a pneumomediastinum or, with rupture into the pleural space, a pneumothorax. Although the air present in a pneumomediastinum is seldom under tension, very high pleural pressure can result from a pneumothorax. This high pressure may decrease the gradient for blood flow to the right atrium (whose pressure reflects pleural pressure) or cause mediastinal compression. This may then decrease venous return and cardiac output. Occasionally, air dissects from the mediastinum up into subcutaneous tissues of the neck (*subcutaneous emphysema*) or into the abdomen (*pneumoperitoneum*).

Mechanical ventilation increases the risk of air block, especially with ventilatory strategies that favor maldistributed ventilation. Long inspiratory times compromise exhalation times and may cause air trapping. In addition, slower rates require higher tidal volumes to achieve normal minute ventilation, and with abnormal distribution of ventilation, overdistention can occur. Hand bagging, especially by the inexperienced, may result in high pressures and long inspiratory times. Bronchial intubation may create overexpansion of the ventilated lung and atelectasis of the contralateral lung, especially with volume ventilators. Finally, agitated babies, who cry and fight the ventilator, may have unexpected patterns of ventilation resulting in alveolar overdistention.

Presentation
History and physical examination
While some pneumothoraces are asymptomatic, the presentation may be precipitous with an acute onset of hypoxemia and even cardiovascular collapse. If symptomatic, a rapid increase in respiratory rate and symptoms of respiratory distress are almost always found. An increasing anteroposterior diameter on the affected side is a dependable sign, although uncommon. Decreased breath sounds and chest excursion, while suggestive, are nonspecific. Heart sounds may become muffled, and the point of maximum impulse may shift. If venous return is obstructed, diastolic blood pressure may be increased and cardiac output decreased. If cardiac output is affected, tachycardia, bradycardia, or evidence of systolic hypotension and decreased pulses may be found.

Even with large collections of air, a pneumomediastinum is usually asymptomatic or associated with only mild tachypnea. In some babies, heart sounds may be muffled. Subcutaneous emphysema is recognizable by the palpable crepitant mass in the neck, upper thorax, or scalp. The clinical manifestations of a pneumoperitoneum vary with the volume of air and the presence or absence of tension. Many are asymptomatic. If there is sufficient tension, the functional residual capacity of the lung may be compromised and venous return to the heart may decrease secondary to compression of the inferior vena cava.

Symptoms of PIE are more insidious than those of a pneumothorax; frequently, onset is first found on chest radiograph. PIE is primarily manifested by an increasingly noncompliant lung and worsening oxygenation. With sufficient overdistention, venous return and cardiac output are diminished.

Transillumination

A strong presumptive diagnosis of pneumothorax can be made without a radiograph to avoid postponing treatment in an emergency. Transillumination with a high-intensity, fiberoptic probe in a darkened room has been shown to have high sensitivity and specificity. False negatives may be caused by large infants with increased skin thickness, small collections of air, or situations where the thymus is elevated against the chest wall. False positives are seen with subcutaneous edema, pneumomediastinum, lobar emphysema, or PIE. The transilluminator is applied directly to the skin of the chest wall and gradually moved over alternate sides of the chest. Normally, the ring of light surrounding the probe will extend about 1 cm. A larger or asymmetric ring of light suggests a pneumothorax. When the air leak is large, the entire chest may light up. Transillumination is least helpful to diagnose PIE.

Chest radiograph

If large, a pneumothorax can be easily identified by chest radiograph. Identification of smaller collections can be difficult. Air may be visible only in scattered areas or only along the medial or basilar aspect of the lung. Anterior air may present as a large, hyperlucent hemithorax with increased sharpness at the edge of the mediastinum. When doubt exists, a cross-table lateral or a decubitus radiograph can help.

The appearance of a pneumomediastinum can take on a wide variety of configurations, some of which can be bizarre. Most typically, air collects around the heart, elevating the lobes of the thymus. This finding can resemble a billowing spinnaker sail of a racing yacht and is referred to as the 'spinnaker sail' sign. When both lobes of the thymus are elevated, an 'angel wing' configuration has been described. When a

Figure 1: Pneumomediastinum and right-sided pneumothorax. This radiograph shows the right lobe of the thymus as lifted up and away from the cardiac silhouette in the typical 'spinnaker sail' configuration. The left lobe of the thymus also appears in the superior left hemithorax and might be confused with a mass or area of consolidation. A moderately large pneumothorax is seen on the right as a dark area without pulmonary parenchymal markings.

large volume of mediastinal air is present, the thymic lobes can be elevated far into the apex of the chest and can be mistaken for atelectasis or an intrapulmonary mass.

Differentiating a pneumomediastinum from a medial pneumothorax can be a challenge. Medial pneumothoraces, which normally lie lateral to the lobes of the thymus, are usually observed when the volume is small to moderate (Figure 1). Differentiation can be aided by a lateral view. With a pneumomediastinum, an area of extreme hyperlucency in the superior retrosternal space is almost always seen. An anterior pneumothorax more often occupies the entire superior surface of the heart. Rarely, air from a pneumomediastinum may lie be-

Figure 2: Pneumopericardium. This infant, who previously had a right pneumothorax, now presents with an air-filled pericardial sac. This is distinguishable from a pneumomediastinum or medial pneumothorax by the air found beneath the cardiac silhouette and the outline of the pericardial sac.

low the heart and may be confused with a pneumopericardium. Generally, air from a pneumopericardium not only lies below the heart, but also totally encircles it (Figure 2).

In infants with PIE, the chest radiograph (Figure 3) is most remarkable for tortuous 2- to 3-mm-diameter bubbles of air that follow the perivascular sheaths from the hilum and do not empty with expiratory films. With progression of PIE (and often over just a few hours), the bubbles become less tortuous and develop into larger cysts. As a result of the air trapping, the lung volume is large and depression of the diaphragm can become profound. Decreased

Figure 3: Pulmonary interstitial emphysema (PIE). In this premature infant, the bubbly changes are seen throughout both lungs. In many infants, they are more prominent toward the hilum and may appear to be air bronchograms. The bubbles in PIE are larger and less uniform in outline than those seen in hyaline membrane disease. The lungs have a large volume, flattening the diaphragm and squeezing the heart (which is only about 40% of the thoracic diameter).

venous return and hypoxic vasoconstriction may result in a general darkening of the lung fields. PIE is frequently associated with other forms of extrapleural air (eg, pneumothorax, pneumopericardium).

Laboratory

Pneumothoraces and PIE are both manifested by decreased blood oxygen levels and carbon dioxide retention. There may be a mixed respiratory and metabolic acidosis.

Management of Pneumothorax

A small-volume, asymptomatic pneumothorax may only require observation. Although a nitrogen washout in a 100% oxygen hood for 24 to 48 hours has been used to manage mildly symptomatic term infants, there are significant potential morbidities that should be considered, and unmonitored oxygen should not be used. The risk of administering high oxygen concentrations for a disease with such little morbidity seems excessive. Nitrogen washout can only occur in the total absence of nitrogen (see *Ventilation-Perfusion Relationships* section, Chapter 2). Consequently, less than 100% oxygen will not wash out nitrogen.

In an emergency, air may be aspirated with a 22- to 25-g scalp vein needle placed over the superior aspect of the rib in the midclavicular line. The clinician should place the end in a sterile water bottle or apply a syringe and aspirate just enough to relieve symptoms. This should prevent damage to the lung and allow for subsequent chest tube placement.

Symptomatic infants or those requiring mechanical ventilation most likely will require chest tube placement. The goal is to place the tip of the chest tube between the lung and the anterior chest wall. After appropriate analgesia and sterile preparation, incise the skin at the first to third intercostal space at the midclavicular line or the sixth to seventh intercostal space at the midaxillary line. Avoid the tissue of the areola or breast. Then bluntly dissect with a curved hemostat. Tunnel one to two interspaces to the second intercostal space at the midclavicular line or the fourth or fifth space at the midaxillary line. Insert an 8- to 12-F chest tube without trocar. Direct the tube anteriorly to optimize drainage of air, and connect to 10- to 15-cm H_2O continuous suction. Secure with a suture, and cover with antibiotic ointment and an occlusive dressing. Verify placement and effectiveness with a chest radiograph. Determine anterior-vs-posterior positioning with a lateral radiograph. Complications of chest tube insertion include inadvertent placement in the subcutaneous tissue, as well as perforations of the pulmonary parenchyma that occur up to 35% of the time and usually heal uneventfully without developing a bronchopleural fistula. Chest tubes may bruise the diaphragm or mediastinal structures, producing paralysis or erosion.

Generally, an air leak resolves after several days. Continued bubbling suggests that a hole of the chest tube is lying outside the chest or that loose connections in the drainage equipment, an air leak at the incision site, or a pleural fistula is present. Consider removal of the tube when there has been no bubbling for 24 hours and no air is seen on the chest radiograph. Before removal of the tube, place the tube to underwater seal for 24 hours, clamp the tube for a time, then remove rapidly. Apply an occlusive dressing to the wound. Follow up with chest radiograph and observe for recurrence.

Pneumomediastinum

Mediastinal air seldom achieves sufficient pressure to compromise circulation, and specific treatment is not required. Clinical observation is important because these babies can deteriorate if a pneumothorax develops.

Pulmonary interstitial edema

The keys to successful management of PIE are early recognition, minimization of further air leak, and adjustment of ventilatory goals. Serial chest radiographs and a high index of suspicion in infants at risk for PIE are critical.

PIE produces extrinsic pressure on airways leading to adjacent alveoli and can result in gas trapping in these units. Interruption of this cycle is achieved by maneuvers that decrease ventilation to these poorly ventilated areas. Because of increased airway resistance, the time constant (see *Lung Mechanics* section, Chapter 2) to these areas is longer than in the normally ventilated unit. Shortening the inspiratory time to 0.1 to 0.15 second will selectively decrease ventilation to the PIE-affected alveoli. Compensation with higher peak inspiratory pressure (PIP) may then be required to maintain oxygenation and ventilation. Minimize these changes and provide positive end-expiratory pressure (PEEP) just sufficient to prevent airway collapse. Higher PIP and PEEP each exacerbate air trapping.

To avoid excessive ventilation settings, the clinician may need to modify the desired Pao_2, $Paco_2$, and pH. Accept Pao_2 of 35 to 45 while minimizing oxygen consumption, optimizing hemoglobin and circulatory status, and monitoring for worsening lactic acidosis. Elevations in the $Paco_2$ are acceptable, as long as the pH remains greater than 7.15 to 7.20. Occasionally, PIE will be unilateral; it then may be helpful to selectively intubate the less affected side or position the baby with that side up. Some institutions have had success using high-frequency ventilation (see *High-Frequency Jet Ventilation* and *High-Frequency Oscillatory Ventilation* sections, Chapter 10).

Pneumopericardium

In the presence of life-threatening tamponade, a pericardial drain can be inserted using the following steps. Prepare an 18- to 20-gauge IV cannula by attaching an IV extension tube, open stopcock, and syringe. Cover the transilluminator tip with a sterile glove to allow use within the sterile field. After appropriate analgesia and skin preparation, make a small stab wound in the left xiphosternal angle and insert the IV cannula, directing it toward the tip of the left scapula, using the transilluminator as a guide to outline the pneumopericardium. While applying constant suction on the syringe, advance the cannula until air is evacuated. If air reaccumulates, secure the cannula, place it to continuous suction, and confirm its position by chest radiograph. Frequently, the small internal diameter of the IV cannula does not provide sufficient drainage. In this case, consider a more permanent tube placed by cutdown.

Outcome

While most infants with pneumothoraces will have an uneventful recovery, they may have higher mortality and morbidity. In very-low-birth-weight (VLBW) infants, mortality can increase by threefold to fourfold with air block. Air embolization is rare but fatal when it occurs. Pleural fistulas may require open thoracotomy. Subsequent bronchopulmonary dysplasia (BPD) appears to be more frequent. The incidence of intraventricular hemorrhage increases. This may be associated with impaired venous return and hypercarbia-induced increase in cerebral blood flow or with sudden improvement in cerebral perfusion after chest tube placement. Symptoms of syndrome of inappropriate antidiuretic hormone secretion (SIADH) have been reported.

Infants with PIE have a much more guarded prognosis. They have a higher incidence of pneumopericardium. Their mortality is significantly higher, as is their incidence of subsequent BPD; it may be as high as 50%.

By Timothy R. Cooper, MD

Chronic Pulmonary Insufficiency of Prematurity

Chronic pulmonary insufficiency of prematurity (CPIP), or late-onset respiratory distress, is less a disease than a physiologic consequence of prematurity. As described in Chapter 2, resting lung volume is determined by the balance of forces favoring collapse (spontaneous atelectasis of the lung) and the forces favoring expansion (the spring outward of the chest wall). The extremely premature infant weighing less than 1,200 g has a soft, flexible chest wall, with poorly ossified ribs and diminished muscle mass. In addition, the predominant sleep activity is rapid eye movement (REM), a time when tonic intercostal muscle activity is diminished and phasic activity is curtailed. Furthermore, the ribs lie more nearly horizontal, further decreasing the efficiency of the accessory respiratory muscles.

Finally, the flatter configuration and narrower zone of apposition of the diaphragm make this organ of respiration less effective as well. All these forces taken together favor alveolar collapse.

CPIP is characterized by the development of apnea, respiratory difficulty, and increasing oxygen requirements during the first weeks of life. Blood gases and pulmonary function testing show modest hypercapnia and an increased transalveolar gradient for O_2, CO_2, and N_2 (increased $AaDo_2$, $aADco_2$, and $aADn_2$). Poorly defined, diffuse, hazy-appearing parenchyma are seen on the chest radiograph.

Nasal continuous positive airway pressure (N-CPAP) administered until the baby is greater than 1,200 to 1,300 g, or about 30 weeks' gestation, can produce a good response. Caffeine helps by decreasing apnea, decreasing REM sleep, and increasing diaphragmatic and accessory muscle tone. If on weaning or discontinuing N-CPAP, the baby has an increase in oxygen requirement or apnea, the previous level of support should be resumed. This suggests a loss of lung volume resulting in hypoventilation and an elevated alveolar Pco_2 and, hence, lower alveolar Po_2. These signs may take 24 to 48 hours to develop as the infant gradually loses lung volume. Because continued growth will improve chest wall stability, the weaning attempts may be periodically repeated until successful.

By Timothy R. Cooper, MD

Bronchopulmonary Dysplasia

BPD is the clinical evolution of a sequence of injuries involving the interface of mechanical ventilation and the lung of the vulnerable host.

The classic definition of BPD has been a continued need for oxygen beyond 28 days of life. It has been suggested, however, that the definition be narrowed to those infants requiring oxygen supplementation or mechanical ventilation beyond 36 weeks' gestational age. Approximately 20% of babies <1,500 g at birth continue to require oxygen at 36 weeks. Because risk of death and major morbidity are closely related to chronic ventilator course, management of the ventilator-dependent infant is the focus of this section.

Etiology and Pathogenesis

Suggested etiologies of BPD have included pulmonary immaturity, oxygen toxicity, barotrauma, vitamin deficiency, failed antioxidant protection, excess fluid administration, patent ductus arteriosus (PDA), and chronic infection (eg, from *Ureaplasma*, *Chlamydia*, or cytomegalovirus). Although oxidant injury remains an important area of investigation, recent work has led to a comprehensive concept of a lung injury sequence that evolves following interaction of the immature lung and mechanical ventilation. Three pathways of injury occur in the clinical evolution of BPD:

(1) Structural injury to airways and alveoli in conjunction with inhibition of maturational processes.

(2) Stimulation of elastic tissue production and accelerated fibrosis.

(3) Activation of an intense inflammatory response. This contributes to ongoing airway injury, mucosal damage, and interstitial edema within the lungs.

In survivors, this is followed by a prolonged and disordered process of repair and resolution.

Genetic predisposition is suggested by an increased family history of asthma among BPD patients, as well as by evidence of early airway injury in certain VLBW subgroups. Goldman demonstrated that mean pulmonary resistance among ventilated premature infants in the first 5 days of life was about 90% higher in those who subsequently developed BPD. The surfactant-deficient or structurally immature lung is particularly vulnerable to bronchiolar lesions induced by mechanical ventilation, and disruption of airways occurs very early in the course of mechanical ventilation.

A unifying concept that explains induction of this airway injury is that of 'volutrauma.' Relative risk of BPD increases with decreasing PCO_2 below 40 mm Hg, an effect particularly striking with PCO_2 values below 29 mm Hg. Experimentally, if the chest is bound to prevent lung expansion, transpulmonary pressures above 50 cm H_2O may be applied without air leak or lung injury. Chest binding can also prevent pulmonary edema induced by high tidal volume ventilation. Such data suggest that acute lung injury is determined by the relationship between delivered tidal volume and maximum lung volume (Vmax). As tidal volume approaches the Vmax of an individual lung, airways become overdistended and geometrically distorted. Thus, volume-induced injury may occur in immature lungs with a low Vmax even at low ventilator pressures because the delivered tidal volume plus any PEEP applied may be near the Vmax for those lungs. Shearing and disruption are associated with necrosis of bronchial mucosa and activation of an intense inflammatory response, leading to further lung damage and progressive clinical symptoms.

Clinical Course

The clinical course of BPD in the surfactant era is more insidious than that originally described by Northway (Table 2). Most patients are surfactant-treated infants, <1,250 g at birth, without HMD but requiring mechanical ventilation during the first week of life because of apnea or structural immaturity of the lungs. The course of those who become chronically ventilator dependent can be divided into three clinical phases.

Phase I—Acute course and diagnosis

This evolves during the first month of life and most closely corresponds to Northway stages 1 and 2. A relatively benign course during the first 2 weeks gives way to continued ventilator dependency with progressive deterioration in pulmonary function, rising oxygen requirements, and opacification of previously clear lung fields on chest radiograph. Wide swings in Po_2 and oxygen saturation values are characteristic. Despite treatment of PDA, effective use of xanthines for apnea, and lack of evidence of infection, the infant remains ventilator dependent. Marked increases in microvascular permeability occur, and there is widespread necrosis of bronchial mucosa. Numerous inflammatory markers are found in the tracheal fluid of these ba-

Table 2: Northway's Stages of Bronchopulmonary Dysplasia	
Stage	**Chest Radiograph Findings**
1	Consistent with hyaline membrane disease.
2	Opaque lung fields with air bronchograms. Interstitial air is common.
3	Cystic lung fields with areas of hyperinflation and areas of atelectasis.
4	Massive lung fibrosis and edema; areas of consolidation and areas of overinflation.

bies compared with those with no signs of chronic pulmonary disease. Airways are obstructed with necrotic debris, and atelectasis may alternate with early cyst formation. Within 3 to 4 weeks, a process of exclusion has established BPD as the cause of persistent ventilator dependency.

Phase II—Course of chronic ventilator dependency

This phase includes features of Northway stages 3 and 4. Bronchiolar metaplasia, hypertrophy of smooth muscle, and interstitial edema produce uneven airway obstruction with worsening hyperinflation of the lung. Obliteration and abnormal muscularization of the pulmonary vascular bed progresses. Active inflammation slowly subsides to be replaced by a disordered process of structural repair. The early weeks of this phase remain unstable, with frequent changes in oxygen requirement and characteristic episodes of acute deterioration requiring increases in ventilator support. After 4 to 6 weeks, the clinical course becomes more static as fibrosis, hyperinflation, and pulmonary edema come to dominate the clinical picture. Increased airway smooth muscle is present, and tracheobronchomalacia is common. Chronic elevation of pulmonary vascular resistance (PVR) increases right ventricular afterload, impairs pulmonary lymphatic drainage, and leaves the infant vulnerable to episodes of acute cor pulmonale.

The course of phase II evolves over 3 to 9 months. During this time, growth and remodeling of lung parenchyma and the pulmonary vascular bed are associated with gradual improvement in pulmonary function and heart-lung interaction. Oxygen requirements fall to 40% or less, and the patient can be weaned from intermittent positive pressure ventilation (IPPV) to breathe spontaneously on continuous positive airway pressure (CPAP) or a pressure support mode of ventilation. After extubation, supplemental oxygen alone becomes sufficient.

Phase III—Discharge planning and transition to home care

This phase covers the transition from mechanical ventilation to the home care environment. Active, inflammatory lung damage has ceased, and the process of repair has become more orderly. Lung growth and remodeling of parenchyma and vasculature have progressed sufficiently to allow more stable pulmonary function without the need for positive pressure support. Lung mechanics, especially airway resistance, remain abnormal, however, and hyperinflation, fibrosis, and cysts often remain visible radiographically. Many more months of lung growth will be required to overcome these derangements.

The most important aspect of this phase is the recognition that, although the lung has improved, structure and function remain abnormal. Close monitoring of adequacy of oxygenation is essential for several weeks after extubation to be sure a subtle rise in PVR will not lead to insidious development of cor pulmonale. During this period, discharge planning can begin. Screening of hearing and development can proceed, along with increased attention to play therapy and any required physical therapy. Many infants will have problems with oral motor function and feeding. Effects of feeding on oxygenation must be evaluated closely. Special home care needs should be identified and a home dietary plan chosen and implemented. Most of these infants can be discharged with low-flow oxygen by nasal cannula, an oral diuretic, and modest fluid restriction (150 mL/kg/d) using a standard 24 kcal/oz formula that is readily available commercially. Continuation of inhaled medications by mask may be necessary. As long as the infant requires oxygen, both fluid restriction and diuretics will make lung function more efficient and help minimize PVR.

Cardiopulmonary Physiology

In advanced BPD, there is a marked increase in airway resistance and a decrease in dynamic compliance, which becomes frequency dependent. Tidal volume is reduced, and respiratory rate is increased. The uneven airway obstruction leads to gas trapping and hyperinflation with severe pulmonary clearance delay. In severe cases, only 36% of the functional residual capacity (FRC) is composed of well-ventilated lung units. If bronchomalacia is present, forced airway collapse may occur during active expiratory efforts associated with agitation. Little improvement in pulmonary function occurs before 6 months of age. By 3 years of age, compliance is near normal, and airway resistance is only about 30% higher than that of controls.

The fragile heart-lung interaction in these patients can be depicted as a three-compartment model. In one compartment, airways, gas exchange units, and blood vessels have been obliterated, producing a reduction in cross-sectional area of the pulmonary vascular bed and gas exchange surface. In the second compartment, uneven airway obstruction produces a population of underventilated (though often hyperinflated) lung units in which alveolar hypoxia induces hypoxic pulmonary vasoconstriction. This produces a further increase in resting PVR. The third compartment, with well-ventilated lung units and intact vasculature, must accept a disproportionate amount of pulmonary blood flow. These vessels, already maximally dilated, can accept additional flow only at the expense of high right ventricular afterload, high microvascular pressures, and increased fluid filtration into the perivascular interstitium. Chronically elevated right-sided cardiac pressures also inhibit pulmonary lymphatic drainage. Any further reduction in ventilation or fall in Pa_{O_2} in the underventilated compartment (such as that accompanying mucous plugging, bronchospasm, or reduction in F_{IO_2}) induces additional regional hypoxic vasoconstriction and forces yet more blood through the well-ventilated compartment, with further increase in pulmonary edema.

Understanding this fragile heart-lung interaction is essential to management of BPD. Pulmonary care is designed to minimize PVR, especially in the underventilated compartment, to avoid the vicious cycle of pulmonary edema causing deterioration in pulmonary function, which in turn causes more pulmonary edema, a course eventually terminating in acute right ventricular failure.

Management
Primary goals of management
- Provide complete, balanced nutrition together with enough time to allow growth of new lung and remodeling of the pulmonary vascular bed.
- Avoid cor pulmonale, a major cause of death, by providing comprehensive care and monitoring to minimize PVR.

Ventilator-dependent infants require months to recover. During this period, care is largely supportive and primarily improves short-term oxygenation and reduces work of breathing, without changing the underlying repair process. Attempting to wean supplemental oxygen too quickly risks increases in PVR, which may precipitate acute cardiopulmonary failure.

Supportive care and nutrition
Growth and development of new airways, gas exchange units, and pulmonary vasculature require 1 to 3 years and the provision of all primary and trace nutrients. A balanced nutrient intake must be provided in conjunction with fluid restriction, increased mineral wasting from diuretic therapy, and, at times, the catabolic effects of corticosteroids. Long-term dietary intake should meet all guidelines

of the American Academy of Pediatrics for term and preterm infants. A pediatric nutritionist should regularly assess the nutritional status and plan of care of all infants with chronic lung disease.

Infants with BPD benefit from fluid restriction to control pulmonary edema. In preterm infants, modest fluid restriction (150 mL/kg/day) is compatible with proper long-term nutrition using one of the commercial 24 kcal/oz, mineral-enhanced premature formulas or fortified human milk. These provide good-quality protein intake, trace nutrients, and increased calcium and phosphorus supplementation to optimize bone mineralization. When the infant reaches term, a standard 24 kcal/oz formula or mineral- and protein-enriched formula may be substituted. If necessary, additional calories may be added as corn oil (separate, individually dosed). These infants require close monitoring of growth and bone mineral status. If an infant remains fluid restricted at discharge, an enriched formula should be selected for care at home.

Severe impairment of lung mechanics may require restriction of fluids to 110 to 130 mL/kg/day. Adding caloric supplements alone to a 24 kcal/oz formula will not support growth at this low intake. Protein and trace nutrients will be deficient. A commercial 27 to 30 kcal/oz formula will provide a protein intake of 3 to 3.5 g/kg/day. Enriched formulas that can be mixed with premature formulas or human milk to increase nutrient content are available. However, all such efforts to increase nutrient density will raise osmolality. In babies 5 to 6 months of age or older, full nutrition can be maintained using 120 mL/kg/day of a protein-mineral-enriched formula, which can be prepared to achieve up to 30 kcal/oz. Infants receiving a special formula in restricted amounts may require iron and vitamin supplements.

Diuretics

Diuretics improve short-term lung mechanics and may promote a reduction in oxygen requirements or ventilator support. Two reported regimens have facilitated improvement in lung function and enhanced weaning from IPPV while minimizing effects of hypochloremic metabolic alkalosis:

(1) Furosemide (1 mg/kg/dose, b.i.d., IV, or 2 mg/kg/dose, b.i.d., enterally) given every other day is as effective as daily dosing and results in much less chloride depletion and urinary calcium loss.

(2) Hydrochlorothiazide (2 mg/kg/dose, b.i.d.) or chlorothiazide (20 mg/kg/dose, b.i.d.) combined with spironolactone (1.5 mg/kg/dose, b.i.d.) may be given daily. This regimen has improved lung mechanics and reduced urinary calcium excretion in some studies, but it may be associated with increased potassium and phosphorus loss.

Chronic diuretic therapy usually requires chloride supplementation of 2 to 4 mEq/kg/day above usual nutritional needs. At least one third should be provided as KCl.

Oxygen

Persistent pulmonary hypertension is a predictor of mortality in BPD. Oxygen is the primary tool to minimize PVR and avoid death from cor pulmonale. Fio_2 should be adjusted to maintain arterial Pao_2 above 55 mm Hg. Insidious hypoxemia is particularly common during feedings and sleep, when additional oxygen supplements may be necessary. Need for supplemental oxygen extends well beyond the period of positive pressure support. The impact of oxygen on outcome cannot be overemphasized because overzealous attempts to wean supplemental oxygen may precipitate acute cardiopulmonary failure and even death.

Bronchodilators

Increased resting airway tone has been demonstrated in infants with BPD, and numerous studies have reported improved lung mechanics after administration of β_2-agonists to ventilator-dependent infants.

Although a sound basis exists for bronchodilator therapy in BPD, clinical use is largely based on models for asthma. Bedside pulmonary function testing in small infants lacks adequate sensitivity to select specific responders to different treatment regimens and to guide the course of daily management. Cumulative cost is high. The National Heart, Lung and Blood Institute has published consensus panel guidelines for bronchodilator and anti-inflammatory therapy in young children with asthma. A few short-term studies in neonates have provided guidelines for use of certain inhaled medications in infants with BPD.

(1) Albuterol: Denjean described a dose-response relationship for ventilator-dependent premature infants using a metered-dose inhaler (MDI) to administer 1 or 2 puffs of 90 or 180 µg albuterol via a commercial spacer device placed between the ventilator circuit connector and the endotracheal tube. This method is cheaper than nebulizer administration. The dose may be given every 3 to 4 hours. For older, larger infants, 2 to 4 puffs per treatment may be required. Little information exists regarding the long-term safety or efficacy of chronic albuterol therapy in small infants. In children with asthma, prolonged use has been associated with diminution of effect and deterioration in pulmonary function. Routine daily use in patients with asthma is no longer recommended. Therefore, it is advisable to limit use of this agent to the early phases of management of BPD. When lung function has become more stable, a long-acting compound, such as salmeterol (1 to 2 puffs every 12 hours), may be used for maintenance therapy if continued bronchodilator use is necessary. Subsequent use of albuterol can then be reserved for rescue treatment of acute episodes of airway reactivity.

(2) Ipratropium bromide: Limited data suggest that this agent, at inhaled doses of 25 µg/kg, lowers respiratory system resistance in some preterm infants with BPD in a manner similar to albuterol. A dose-dependent effect has been demonstrated in older children with asthma at doses of 75 to 250 µg per treatment.

In asthmatic infants less than 1 year of age, clinical improvement has been reported with this dosage range. No specific side effects were reported in these limited studies. Administration to intubated patients (1 to 2 puffs given 2 to 3 times daily) can be accomplished using an MDI and spacer device connected to the endotracheal tube. Although the idea of synergy with β_2-agonists is appealing, a definitive role for cholinergic blockade in these patients has not been established, and long-term effects are unknown.

(3) Inhaled corticosteroids: LaForce reported improved airway resistance and lung compliance in a group of ventilator-dependent preterm infants after nebulization of beclomethasone for more than 2 weeks (50 µg/2 mL normal saline [NS], nebulized into the ventilator circuit t.i.d.). The incidence of infection was not increased in the small group studied. Alternatively, this drug may be given by MDI (42 µg/puff, 1 to 2 puffs twice daily) using a commercial spacer device connected to the endotracheal tube. This route represents an attractive alternative to systemic steroid therapy, but to date, no long-term benefits for inhaled steroids have been established. Likewise, evidence is lacking regarding long-term risks or side effects.

(4) Management of acute bronchospasm: Acute episodes of bronchospasm do occur in some infants with BPD. For severe episodes of airway reactivity, albuterol is the agent of choice. It may be given by MDI and spacer or by nebulization (0.15 mg/kg in 2.0 mL NS) into the ventilator circuit every 20 minutes for 3 doses. Alternatively, continuous nebulization of 0.5 mg/kg/h may be given for 1 to 2 hours. Either regimen can be followed by administration every 1 to 4 hours, with frequency decreasing as airflow improves. During acute episodes, the dose of inhaled corticosteroid can be doubled for 7 to 10 days. If frequent albuterol and inhaled steroid

therapy fails to reestablish stable pulmonary function in older infants, a short (5-day) tapering course of systemic steroids may be necessary.

Systemic corticosteroids

Initial animal research suggested that corticosteroids might enhance oxygen toxicity, interfere with lung growth, and accelerate pulmonary fibrosis. Early clinical studies, however, suggested an important role for these agents in management of BPD. Recently, the number of reports of serious side effects of systemic steroid therapy has increased. Three strategies for clinical use of systemic steroids have been reported, but each is accompanied by a risk of potential side effects in VLBW infants.

Late intervention (>3 weeks of age). Controlled trials have demonstrated a reduction in duration of assisted ventilation and need for oxygen after discharge among infants with established BPD treated with steroids after 3 weeks of age. Incidence of chronic lung disease or death at 36 weeks' gestation is reduced, but there is no increase in long-term survival. In this setting, short-term lung mechanics are improved in part by a brisk diuresis and decrease in lung water. Adrenal suppression can be avoided if course of treatment does not exceed 1 week. To optimize response to a pulse course of treatment, the patient should be receiving adequate ventilator support and oxygen, fluid restriction (150 mL/kg/day or less), and an effective regimen of diuretics. Dexamethasone (0.25 mg/kg/dose b.i.d.) can be given for 48 to 72 hours, then tapered by 50% per day over the next 3 to 5 days. Therapy is completed in 1 week. Because response occurs early in the course of steroid therapy, babies who fail to wean from IPPV after 1 week of treatment are unlikely to do so subsequently. However, some infants who initially respond require continued steroid therapy. Risk of glucose intolerance and hypertension is increased. A recent large meta-analysis found an increased rate of abnormal neurologic exam overall, but risk of moderate to severe impairment or cerebral palsy was not increased. A single-center controlled trial reported a significant increase in cerebral palsy and neurologic impairment, but its results were confounded by higher survival among treated infants. Thus, the potential short-term pulmonary benefits of this strategy must be weighed carefully against the possible serious long-term side effects.

Moderately early treatment (7 to 14 days). More recent studies have focused on early treatment to interrupt the lung injury cycle. Dexamethasone given during the first 2 weeks of life has been reported to reduce oxygen requirements, reduce duration of ventilator support, and decrease need for supplemental oxygen at 36 weeks' postconceptional age. However, many of these infants required either repeated courses of treatment or continued daily therapy for as long as 42 days. The incidence of hypertension, gastrointestinal bleeding, and infection is increased. Data regarding long-term neurologic outcome are limited. In the absence of data on developmental outcome, use of this strategy must be considered carefully.

Preventive therapy (<96 hours of age). A preventive role for steroid therapy has been investigated. Recent reports suggest that dexamethasone 0.5 to 1.0 mg/kg/day, initiated in the first 12 hours of postnatal life, results in earlier extubation and less oxygen dependency at 36 weeks postconception. Effects were particularly notable in surfactant-treated premature infants <1,250 g at birth. The duration of treatment in these reports varied between 1 day and 12 days. Again, hypertension and glucose intolerance were common side effects, but the rate of infection was not increased. However, a recent large, multicenter trial demonstrated significant increases in neurologic disabilities, gastrointestinal bleeding, and intestinal perforation among infants receiving this early steroid strategy. Because of the high risk of serious side effects, this strategy is not recommended.

The potential side effects and long-term risks of systemic steroid therapy must be weighed carefully against the impact of chronic ventilation in small premature infants. Routine use of dexamethasone for prevention or treatment of chronic lung disease in preterm infants is not currently recommended by the American Academy of Pediatrics. It is suggested that such use be limited to exceptional circumstances, such as an infant on maximum ventilator and oxygen support. In such circumstances, parents should be informed about the short- and long-term risks and should participate in the decision-making process.

Preventive care

Use of antioxidant therapy to prevent or ameliorate BPD remains an area of active research. Use of vitamin E has been ineffective; however, preliminary data suggest some benefit associated with early administration of superoxide dismutase. Although premature infants with BPD have been found to have lower serum vitamin A concentrations than others with respiratory distress syndrome, clinical trials involving supplementation have yielded equivocal results.

Early use of N-CPAP represents an attempt to avoid ventilator-induced injury altogether. Association of early hypocarbia and subsequent BPD has strengthened the concept of volutrauma and fostered several strategies for 'gentle ventilation' that combine low pressures, low tidal volumes, and short inspiratory times with permissive hypercarbia. However, a recent controlled trial using these techniques failed to demonstrate a reduction in occurrence of chronic lung disease. A reduction in incidence of BPD has been cited in select clinical trials of high-frequency oscillatory ventilation.

Infection, particularly respiratory syncytial virus (RSV), is a significant cause of postdischarge hospitalization and death in infants with BPD. Palivizumab (Synagis®) significantly reduces the risk of hospitalization due to RSV infection among these infants. The American Academy of Pediatrics recommends administration of palivizumab to infants and children <2 years of age who have BPD and have required medical therapy within 6 months of the anticipated RSV season.

Monitoring of Course and Coordination of Care

A comprehensive program of monitoring is necessary to achieve adequate growth and avoid cor pulmonale.

Nutritional monitoring

Patients should be weighed every 1 to 3 days, and length and frontal-occipital circumference measurements should be obtained weekly. Nutritional monitoring should include periodic determination of blood urea nitrogen (BUN), serum albumin, prealbumin, calcium, phosphorus, and alkaline phosphatase. A dietitian or physician skilled in infant nutrition should be actively involved in the care of these patients.

Oxygen monitoring

Long-term maintenance of adequate oxygenation is the key to preventing death from cor pulmonale. Adequacy of oxygenation can be evaluated by obtaining a 6- to 8-hour strip recording of transcutaneous oxygen tension ($TcPo_2$) or pulse oximetry (Spo_2) every 1 to 2 weeks. Attempts should be made to keep $TcPo_2$ above 55 mm Hg and Spo_2 above 94% in term and older infants (90% to 95% range in small premature infants). Arterial blood gas samples must be obtained periodically but may be difficult to interpret because of agitation or sampling difficulties.

Echocardiograms

Several studies have described the value of echocardiography in screening for pulmonary hypertension and assessing response of the pulmonary vascular bed to oxygen. Tricuspid regurgitation is common, and flow velocity can be determined by Doppler. A modified Bernoulli equation can be used to calculate the pressure gradient across this valve [pressure gradient = $4(Vmax)^2$]. This value plus assumed right atrial pressure provides an estimate of right ventricular systolic pressure. Increased mortality risk has been associated with pre-ejection period/right ventricular ejection fraction time ratios >0.30, and it is recommended that sufficient oxygen be given to avoid ratios >0.34. These two echocardiographic parameters can be measured every 4 to 6 weeks to estimate right ventricular afterload and assess adequacy of pulmonary care. If either parameter is abnormal, an increase in supplemental oxygen, as well as other components of pulmonary care, should be considered.

Developmental screening

Hearing screening should be done before discharge or before 6 months of age to allow early intervention by an audiologist, if needed. Developmental assessment may begin during the hospital stay as part of comprehensive long-term follow-up after discharge. Specific attention to oral motor dysfunction and feeding disorders may be necessary.

Planned, multidisciplinary care

Primary goals of care can best be achieved by a multidisciplinary care team directed by an experienced neonatologist or pediatric pulmonologist complemented by other physicians skilled in developmental assessment and nutrition. Team members include nurses, social workers, respiratory therapists, child life specialists, physical and occupational therapists, a dietitian, and an audiologist. The team should have regularly scheduled meetings and rounds to evaluate the progress of each patient with regard to goals of care. Such a team can maintain long-term, consistent, goal-directed care for each patient and is particularly adept at establishing a social environment that minimizes adverse aspects of chronic ventilator care and the intensive care unit environment. Early in the course of ventilator dependency, premature infants benefit from environmental modifications that reduce noise and discomfort and minimize the stress response. As infants become older, parents and caregivers must work together to provide a friendly, play-oriented environment. Some infants with BPD have associated neurologic dysfunction or hearing deficits. Feeding disorders are common. Resources to manage such disorders must be assembled and integrated into a regular schedule of play therapy against a backdrop of ongoing medical care. Maintenance of an appropriate social environment for these chronically hospitalized infants presents a considerable challenge and has significant impact on the medical course.

178

Because prognosis for long-term recovery in BPD is good, the psychology of BPD care is particularly important. It is essential that caregivers maintain an involved, optimistic attitude toward these infants.

Outcome

Outcome varies widely among different centers, with overall mortality ranging from 25% to 40%. Mortality rates have fallen in recent years, but survival to discharge is strongly related to duration of ventilation. Death rates of 21% to 57% are reported for infants requiring more than 1 month of IPPV. Many deaths are related to infection or cardiopulmonary failure associated with persistent pulmonary hypertension and cor pulmonale, but some result from associated problems of prematurity, such as bowel surgery and progressive liver failure.

Significant increases in growth failure, hearing loss, retinopathy of prematurity (ROP), and neurodevelopmental handicaps have been reported. However, Sauve found only a slight increase in the rate of hearing and developmental abnormalities in a population compared to matched controls, although growth failure and ROP occurred with increased frequency. In an 8-year follow-up study by Robertson, growth of BPD patients born <32 weeks' gestation was similar to that of matched controls. Multivariate analysis suggested that developmental disabilities found among groups of BPD patients were primarily related to complications of prematurity and adverse social factors.

As previously stated, improvement in pulmonary function occurs slowly in these patients over a period of 1 to 3 years in association with repair and regrowth of the lung. Day-to-day care is largely supportive and does little to hasten this process. Care providers are faced with many frustrations in management of these infants and must constantly remain focused on a long-term view. It is necessary to avoid constant changes in care or interventions that, at best, are costly and without long-term benefit and, at worst, may introduce a significant risk of side effects or long-term complications.

By James M. Adams, MD

Wilson-Mikity Syndrome

Epidemiology

Only rarely described since the use of CPAP, this syndrome was said to affect premature infants weighing less than 1,500 g. Although the etiology is unknown, male infants appear to be affected more often.

Pathophysiology

Although autopsy changes have rarely been reported, they include cystic emphysematous areas interspersed with areas of collapse, cellular thickening of the alveolar septa, increase in fibroelastic tissue, and patchy emphysema. Hypersecretion, aspiration, or immature structure may result in localized pulmonary collapse and air trapping, decreased lung compliance, and increased airway resistance. Higher mean airway pressure from CPAP may prevent this process.

Presentation

Infants with no history of respiratory distress but with symptoms of tachypnea, cyanosis, hypercapnia, retractions, or apnea develop Wilson-Mikity syndrome between 1 and 4 weeks of age. These symptoms may progress for about 2 months. The infants usually become oxygen dependent, with slow recovery and resolution during the ensuing 1 to 2 years.

The chest radiographic findings are indistinguishable from those of BPD. They progress from initial coarse, nodular infiltrates to development of hyperexpansion, with cystlike changes in the lung. These classic 'bubbly' changes appear to result from areas of alveolar overexpansion surrounded by areas of atelectasis.

Differential Diagnosis

The condition must be distinguished from BPD and other causes of cystic lung disease. In contrast to BPD, the findings of pulmonary hypertension, right ventricular hypertrophy, and pulmonary fibrosis are uncommon.

Management

Wilson-Mikity syndrome should respond well to N-CPAP.

Outcome

The reported mortality of 30% to 50% from more than two decades ago is difficult to extrapolate to more recent times. It is expected that the outcome should be better than that observed with BPD. In survivors, there usually is complete radiographic resolution by 2 years.

By Timothy R. Cooper, MD

Suggested Readings

Air Block

Allen RW, Jung AL, Lester PD: Effectiveness of chest tube evacuation of pneumothorax in neonates. *J Pediatr* 1981;99:629.

Brooks JG, Bustamante SA, Koops BL, et al: Selective bronchial intubation for the treatment of severe localized pulmonary interstitial emphysema in newborn infants. *Pediatrics* 1977;91:648.

Chernick V, Avery ME: Spontaneous alveolar rupture at birth. *Pediatrics* 1963;32:816.

Meadow WL, Cheromcha D: Successful therapy of unilateral pulmonary emphysema: mechanical ventilation with extremely short inspiratory time. *Am J Perinatol* 1985;2:194.

Ogata E, Gregory GA, Kitterman JA, et al: Pneumothorax in respiratory distress syndrome: incidence and effect on vital signs, blood gases and pH. *Pediatrics* 1976;58:177.

Plenat F, Vert P, Didier F, et al: Pulmonary interstitial emphysema. *Clin Perinatol* 1978;5:351.

Reppert SM, Ment LR, Todres ID: The treatment of pneumopericardium in the newborn infant. *J Pediatr* 1977;905:115.

Varano LA, Maisels MJ: Pneumopericardium in the newborn: diagnosis and pathogenesis. *Pediatrics* 1974;53:941.

Chronic Pulmonary Insufficiency of Prematurity

Krauss AN, Klain DB, Auld PA: Chronic pulmonary insufficiency of prematurity (CPIP). *Pediatrics* 1975;55:55-58.

Bronchopulmonary Dysplasia

Abman SH, Wolfe RR, Accurso FJ, et al: Pulmonary vascular response to oxygen in infants with severe bronchopulmonary dysplasia. *Pediatrics* 1985;75:80-84.

Avery GB, Fletcher AB, Kaplan M, et al: Controlled trial of dexamethasone in respirator-dependent infants with bronchopulmonary dysplasia. *Pediatrics* 1985;7:106-111.

Bancalari E, Gerhardt T: Bronchopulmonary dysplasia. *Pediatr Clin North Am* 1996;33:1-23.

Benatar A, Clarke J, Silverman M: Pulmonary hypertension in infants with chronic lung disease: noninvasive evaluation and short-term effect of oxygen treatment. *Arch Dis Child Fetal Neonatal Ed* 1995;72:F14-F19.

Bolivar JM, Gerhardt T, Gonzalez A, et al: Mechanisms for episodes of hypoxemia in preterm infants undergoing mechanical ventilation. *J Pediatr* 1995;127:767-773.

Brozanski BS, Jones JG, Gilmour CH, et al: Effect of pulse dexamethasone therapy on the incidence and severity of chronic lung disease in the very low birth weight infant. *J Pediatr* 1995;126:769-776.

Carlton DP, Cummings JJ, Scheerer RG, et al: Lung overexpansion increases pulmonary microvascular protein permeability in young lambs. *J Appl Physiol* 1990;69:577-583.

Collaborative Dexamethasone Trial Group: Dexamethasone therapy in neonatal chronic lung disease: an international placebo-controlled trial. *Pediatrics* 1991;88:421-427.

Davis A, Vickerson F, Worsley G, et al: Determination of dose response relationship for nebulized ipratropium in asthmatic children. *J Pediatr* 1984;105:1002-1005.

Denjean A, Guimaraes H, Migdal M, et al: Dose-related bronchodilator response to aerosolized salbutamol (albuterol) in ventilator-dependent premature infants. *J Pediatr* 1992;120:974-979.

Dreyfuss D, Saumon G: Role of tidal volume, FRC and end-expiratory volume in the development of pulmonary edema following mechanical ventilation. *Am Rev Respir Dis* 1993;148:1194-1203.

Durand M, Sardesai S, McEvoy C: Effects of early dexamethasone therapy on pulmonary mechanics and chronic lung disease in very low birth weight infants: a randomized, controlled trial. *Pediatrics* 1995;95:584-590.

Everard ML, Stammers J, Hardy JG, et al: New aerosol delivery system for neonatal ventilator circuits. *Arch Dis Child* 1992;67(7 Spec No):826-830.

Fouron J, Le Guennec J, Villemant D, et al: Value of echocardiography in assessing the outcome of bronchopulmonary dysplasia in the newborn. *Pediatrics* 1980;65:529-535.

Garg M, Kurzner SI, Bautista DB, et al: Clinically unsuspected hypoxia during sleep and feeding in infants with bronchopulmonary dysplasia. *Pediatrics* 1988;81:635-642.

Garland JS, Buck RK, Allred EN, et al: Hypocarbia before surfactant therapy appears to increase bronchopulmonary dysplasia risk in infants with respiratory distress syndrome. *Arch Pediatr Adolesc Med* 1995;149:617-623.

Gladstone IM, Jacobs HC, Ehrenkranz RA: Pulmonary function tests and fluid balance in neonates with chronic lung disease during dexamethasone treatment. *Pediatr Res* 1989;25A, Abstract 1277.

Goldman SL, Gerhardt T, Sonni S, et al: Early prediction of chronic lung disease by pulmonary function testing. *J Pediatr* 1983;102:613-616.

Goodman G, Perkin RM, Anas NG, et al: Pulmonary hypertension in infants with bronchopulmonary dysplasia. *J Pediatr* 1988;112:67-72.

Groneck P, Gotze-Speer B, Oppermann M, et al: Association of pulmonary inflammation and increased microvascular permeability during the development of bronchopulmonary dysplasia: a sequential analysis of inflammatory mediators in respiratory fluids of high-risk preterm neonates. *Pediatrics* 1994;93:712-718.

Halliday HL, Dumpit FM, Brady JP: Effects of inspired oxygen on echocardiographic assessments of pulmonary vascular resistance and myocardial contractility in bronchopulmonary dysplasia. *Pediatrics* 1980;65:536-540.

Henry RL, Hiller EJ, Milner AD, et al: Nebulised ipratropium bromide and sodium cromoglycate in the first two years of life. *Arch Dis Child* 1984;59:54-57.

Hernandez LA, Peevy KJ, Moise AA, et al: Chest wall restriction limits high airway pressure-induced lung injury in young rabbits. *J Appl Physiol* 1989;66:2364-2368.

Jobe AJ: The new BPD: an arrest of lung development. *Pediatr Res* 1999;46:641-643.

Jobe AH, Bancalari E: Bronchopulmonary dysplasia. *Am J Respir Crit Care Med* 2001;163:1723-1729.

Kleinman RE, ed. *Pediatric Nutrition Handbook*. 4th ed. Elk Grove, IL: American Academy of Pediatrics, 1998.

Kao LC, Warburton D, Cheng MH: Effect of oral diuretics on pulmonary mechanics in infants with chronic bronchopulmonary dysplasia: results of a double-blind crossover sequential trial. *Pediatrics* 1984;74:37-44.

Kao LC, Warburton D, Platzker AC, et al: Effect of isoproterenol inhalation on airway resistance in chronic bronchopulmonary dysplasia. *Pediatrics* 1984;73:509-513.

Kramer R, Birrer P, Modelska K, et al: A new baby-spacer device for aerosolized bronchodilator administration in infants with bronchopulmonary disease. *Eur J Pediatr* 1992;151:57-60.

Kraybill EN, Runyan DK, Bose CL, et al: Risk factors for chronic lung disease in infants with birth weights of 751 to 1000 grams. *J Pediatr* 1989;115:115-120.

LaForce WR, Brudno S: Controlled trial of beclomethasone dipropionate by nebulization in oxygen and ventilator dependent infants. *J Pediatr* 1993;122:285-288.

McCubbin M, Frey EE, Wagener JS, et al: Large airway collapse in bronchopulmonary dysplasia. *J Pediatr* 1989;114:304-307.

Miller RW, Woo P, Kellman RK, et al: Tracheobronchial abnormalities in infants with bronchopulmonary dysplasia. *J Pediatr* 1987;111:779-782.

National Asthma Education and Prevention Program: *Expert Panel Report. Guidelines for Diagnosis and Management of Asthma.* Bethesda, MD: National Institutes of Health, 1991. NIH Publication No. 91-3042.

National Asthma Education and Prevention Program: *Expert Panel Report 2. Guidelines for the Diagnosis and Management of Asthma.* Bethesda, MD: National Institutes of Health and National Heart, Lung and Blood Institute, 1997. NIH Publication 97-4051.

Nilsson R, Grossmann G, Robertson B: Lung surfactant and the pathogenesis of neonatal bronchiolar lesions induced by artificial ventilation. *Pediatr Res* 1978;12:249-255.

Northway WH, Rosan RC, Porter DY: Pulmonary disease following respirator therapy of hyaline membrane disease. *N Engl J Med* 1967;276:357-368.

Overstreet DW, Jackson JC, van Belle G, et al: Estimation of mortality risk in chronically ventilated infants with bronchopulmonary dysplasia. *Pediatrics* 1991;88:1153-1160.

Ozdemir A, Brown MA, Morgan WJ: Markers and mediators of inflammation in neonatal lung disease. *Pediatr Pulmonol* 1997;23(4):292-306.

Pearson E, Bose C, Snidlow T, et al: Trial of vitamin A supplementation in very low birth weight infants at risk for bronchopulmonary dysplasia. *J Pediatr* 1992;121:420-427.

Postnatal corticosteroids to treat or prevent chronic lung disease in preterm infants. *Pediatrics* 2002;109:330-338.

Prevention of respiratory syncytial virus infections: indications for use of palivizumab and update on the use of RSV-IGIV. American Academy of Pediatrics Committee on Infectious Diseases and Committee on Fetus and Newborn. *Pediatrics* 1998;102:1211-1216.

Rastogi A, Akintorin SM, Betz ML, et al: A controlled trial of dexamethasone to prevent bronchopulmonary dysplasia in surfactant treated infants. *Pediatrics* 1996;98:204-210.

Robertson B: The evolution of neonatal respiratory distress syndrome into chronic lung disease. *Eur Respir J* 1989;2:33s-37s.

Robertson CM, Etches PC, Goldson E, et al: Eight-year school performance, neurodevelopmental, and growth outcome of neonates with bronchopulmonary dysplasia: a comparative study. *Pediatrics* 1992;89:365-372.

Rush MG, Englehardt B, Parker RA, et al: Double-blind, placebo-controlled trial of alternate-day furosemide therapy in infants with chronic bronchopulmonary dysplasia. *J Pediatr* 1990;117:112-118.

Sauve RS, Singhal N: Long-term morbidity of infants with bronchopulmonary dysplasia. *Pediatrics* 1985;76:725-733.

Schuh S, Parkin P, Rajan A, et al: High- versus low-dose, frequently administered, nebulized albuterol in children with severe, acute asthma. *Pediatrics* 1989;83:513-518.

Shenai JP, Kennedy KA, Chytil F, et al: Clinical trial of vitamin A supplementation in infants susceptible to bronchopulmonary dysplasia. *J Pediatr* 1987;111:269-277.

Sosullski R, Abbasi S, Fox WW: Therapeutic value of terbutaline in bronchopulmonary dysplasia. *Pediatr Res* 1982;16:309A.

Stark AR, Carlo WA, Tyson JE, et al: Adverse effects of early dexamethasone in extremely-low-birth-weight infants. National Institute of Child Health and Human Development Neonatal Research Network. *N Engl J Med* 2001;344:95-101.

Stephure DK, Singhal N, McMillian DD: Safety of dexamethasone for bronchopulmonary dysplasia. *Pediatr Res* 1989;25, Abstract 546.

Thibeault DW, Mabry SM, Ekekezie II, et al: Lung elastic tissue maturation and perturbations during the evolution of chronic lung disease. *Pediatrics* 2000;106:1452-1459.

Watts JL, Ariagno RL, Brady JP: Chronic pulmonary disease in neonates after artificial ventilation: distribution of ventilation and pulmonary interstitial emphysema. *Pediatrics* 1977;60:273-281.

Wheater M, Rennie JM: Poor prognosis after prolonged ventilation for bronchopulmonary dysplasia. *Arch Dis Child Fetal Neonatal Ed* 1994;71:F210-F211.

Wilkie RA, Bryan MH: Effect of bronchodilators on airway resistance in ventilator dependent neonates with chronic lung disease. *J Pediatr* 1987;278-282.

Yeh TF, Torre JA, Rastogi A, et al: Early postnatal dexamethasone therapy in premature infants with severe respiratory distress syndrome: a double-blind, controlled study. *J Pediatr* 1990;117:273-282.

Wilson-Mikity Syndrome

Burnard ED: The pulmonary syndrome of Wilson and Mikity and respiratory function in very small premature infants. *Pediatr Clin North Am* 1966;13:999.

Hodgman JE, Mikity VG, Tatter D, et al: Chronic respiratory distress in the premature infant. Wilson-Mikity syndrome. *Pediatrics* 1969;44:179.

Krauss AN, Levin AR, Grossman H, et al: Physiologic studies on infants with Wilson-Mikity syndrome. *J Pediatr* 1970;77:27.

Chapter 6

Congenital Diseases Affecting the Lung Parenchyma

Cystic Malformations of the Lung

Cystic malformations are not common causes of respiratory distress. Most are incidental findings in asymptomatic infants. Others present with respiratory distress from recurrent infection, wheezing, or expiratory stridor caused by airway obstruction. On the chest radiograph, round radiolucent cysts may be seen within the pulmonary parenchyma. However, it is often not the cysts per se that draw attention but the surrounding consolidated or emphysematous parenchyma. With multiple cysts, a diaphragmatic hernia should be considered. Other causes of cystic parenchyma (eg, bronchopulmonary dysplasia, bacterial pneumonias with pneumatoceles) can usually be excluded by the timing of their onset. Cystic lesions of the lung may also be caused by barotrauma in mechanically ventilated newborns, and these lesions may be difficult to discern on radiographs from those that are congenitally acquired.

Today, many cystic malformations are diagnosed antenatally using fetal ultrasonography. It is often difficult to discern one cystic lesion from another without further evaluation. Recent diagnostic imaging reports have found that, occasionally, congenital masses of the lung found on prenatal ultrasound images performed late in gestation 'disappeared' on postnatal evaluation. Although there are cases of spontaneous regression of these lesions, studies suggest that children with 'disappearing' fetal lung masses have persistent abnormalities that are often subtle on radiographs but may be well demonstrated with computed tomography (CT) imaging after birth.

Congenital Lobar Emphysema

Epidemiology

Congenital lobar emphysema (CLE) is the most common cause of cystic malformation of the lung in neonates. It presents within the first 6 months of life, occurs more frequently in males (1.8:1), and occasionally occurs within families. CLE may affect the left upper lobe (50%), the right middle lobe (24%), or the right upper lobe (18%), and it is frequently associated with congenital heart disease (30%) such as tetralogy of Fallot, ventricular septal defect, total anomalous venous return, and patent ductus arteriosus.

Pathophysiology

Characteristically, multiple lobes of the lung contain alveoli distended 3 to 10 times normal size. This is not true emphysema—there is no destruction of lung tissue—but rather distal overinflation of otherwise normal tissue caused by partial airway obstruction (Table 1).

Presentation

Most affected infants present with mild symptoms of airway obstruction and respiratory distress without cyanosis. Chest radiography reveals hyperinflated lobes—often herniated across the midline—and compression of the adjacent lung (Figure 1). CLE can be distinguished from other cysts, pneumothoraces, or pneumatoceles by the presence of bronchovascular markings extending to the periphery of the involved lobe and by atelectasis of adjacent tissue. Infants with pulmonary interstitial emphysema will have a history of mechanical ventilation. Other diagnostic studies are rarely necessary.

Management

Some infants acutely need pulmonary toilet and continuous positive airway pressure (CPAP) to maintain patency and ad-

<table>
<tr><td colspan="2">Table 1: Causes of Partial Airway
Obstruction in Congenital
Lobar Emphysema</td></tr>
</table>

- Local bronchial cartilage deficiency resulting in redundant mucosa and bronchial wall collapse

- Hypoplasia of a segment of airway or a flap-valve formed by redundant mucosal folds

- Partial rotation of the lobe around its hilar pedicle

- External compression by blood vessels or by mediastinal or intrapulmonary masses

- Polyalveolar lobe containing an excess of alveoli and an inadequate blood supply

equate drainage. Some clinicians advocate bronchoscopy to identify and remove the source of airway obstruction. Most cases do not progress, and symptoms in mildly affected children usually resolve within a year as the severity of airway obstruction diminishes. With severe distress, lobectomy may be required.

Outcome

The long-term prognosis is excellent.

Bronchogenic Cyst
Epidemiology

The bronchogenic cyst is the most common cause of a cyst in the lung but rarely presents in the neonate.

Pathophysiology

During pulmonary development, abnormal budding of the respiratory tract at any point before the alveolus produces a cyst. These cysts are lined with columnar, cuboidal, or pseudostratified epithelium and contain walls with smooth muscle and cartilage. With no communication to the airway, lung liquid secretions are trapped. Bronchogenic cysts are found predominantly in the mediastinum near the carina and are seldom large.

Figure 1: Radiograph of an infant with congenital lobar emphysema. Both lungs are hyperinflated with multiple large cysts.

Presentation
This cyst produces symptoms by airway compression. Smaller cysts may be asymptomatic, incidental findings. On chest radiograph, most cysts are fluid-filled and appear as smooth, round, or oval masses. Lung distal to the compressed airway will be either atelectatic or emphysematous.

Management
Surgical excision may be necessary.

Outcome
Most cases are asymptomatic. Prognosis after resection should be good.

Neurenteric and Enteric Cyst
Epidemiology
Other intrathoracic, fluid-filled cysts (esophageal, gastrogenic, and enterogenous cysts) are extremely rare in the neonate.

Pathophysiology
These cysts are usually located in the posterior mediastinum and are lined with gastrointestinal epithelium and layers of smooth muscle. They are believed to be duplicated segments of the gastrointestinal tract that have become partially or completely detached from their parent viscera. The close association with vertebral anomalies is thought to result from common primary embryonic defects.

Presentation
Bronchial compression by the cyst may result in distal overdistention, atelectasis, or respiratory distress. Distinction between bronchogenic, neurenteric, and enteric cysts is difficult and may require CT or magnetic resonance imaging.

Management
Surgical resection may be indicated.

Outcome
The long-term prognosis for normal activity and lung function is extremely good.

Cystic Adenomatoid Malformation
Epidemiology
Cystic adenomatoid malformation (CAM) is a rare cystic lesion found more often in males (1.8:1).

Pathophysiology
CAM is a hamartomatous lesion consisting of numerous, intercommunicating, bronchiolus-like structures of variable size with many immature cells and surrounded by a rim of lung tissue. There are three types of CAM—I, II, and III—with distinct clinical, radiographic, and histologic features.

Presentation
Polyhydramnios, prematurity, and stillbirth are common in all three types of CAM. Antenatal ultrasound diagnosis is possible. Infants usually develop progressive respiratory dis-

tress at birth as the cysts, filling with air, cause mediastinal shift and compression of the remaining lung. A chest radiograph is usually diagnostic and demonstrates multiple, progressively enlarging cysts. Placement of a radiopaque, orogastric catheter may help to differentiate CAM from a diaphragmatic hernia. Occasionally, if the cysts grow large and thin-walled, CAM is difficult to distinguish from lobar emphysema or a large pneumothorax.

Management

Surgical resection is almost always required.

Outcome

When the symptoms progress rapidly, mortality is high.

Type I CAM is the most common (70% of cases) and presents as single or multiple large (3 to 10 cm) cysts. These cysts are confined to one lobe, filled with air or fluid, and usually communicate with the bronchi. Polyhydramnios resulting from mechanical obstruction of venous return occurs in 10% of cases. Only 11% have associated anomalies. About one third of affected children present after 1 year of age, usually with cough, fever, or mild dyspnea; 90% survive.

Type II CAM is found in 18% of cases and is composed of multiple, evenly distributed, medium-sized (0.5 to 2.0 cm) cysts that resemble terminal bronchioles. It occurs in young infants, 50% of whom have other anomalies. These anomalies are often severe and include sirenomelia, renal agenesis, and extralobar pulmonary sequestration. Because of the severe associated anomalies, only 56% of these infants survive.

Type III CAM, found in 10% of cases, is usually a large, bulky lesion with evenly distributed, small (less than 0.2 cm) cysts occupying an entire lobe or lung. This type resembles the early canalicular stage of fetal lung development and may be the result of an insult at the time of lung bud branching (26 to 28 days). Mediastinal displacement and polyhydramnios are extremely common. Associated anomalies are not described. Only 60% of infants with this condition survive.

By Karen E. Johnson, MD, and Timothy R. Cooper, MD

Other Lung Malformations
Pulmonary Sequestration
Epidemiology

Pulmonary sequestration is a rare cause of respiratory distress during the newborn period.

Pathophysiology

Pulmonary sequestration presents as a mass of lung tissue located within normal lung parenchyma but with an abnormal communication with the tracheobronchial tree. There are two types of pulmonary sequestration, intralobar and extralobar. Intralobar pulmonary sequestration occurs most commonly as a portion of lung within the lower lobe of a normal lung and results from chronic pulmonary infections that obliterate or obstruct the airway and normal blood supply. This sequestered lobe does not communicate with the major airways and derives its blood supply from the aorta. Recurrent infections are common.

Extralobar pulmonary sequestration (accessory lobe) consists of pulmonary tissue isolated from the lung and surrounded by its own pleura. It communicates with either the lung or gut. Occasionally familial, this sequestration has a 4:1 male predominance. More than 90% are left-sided and are located between the lower lobe and the diaphragm. About half of these children have other anomalies (Table 2), often of foregut derivation. The blood supply is from the aorta, although venous blood is occasionally provided from a branch of the pulmonary artery. Venous drainage through the azygos and hemiazygos veins results in a left-to-right shunt. Infections are less common than with intralobar sequestrations.

Presentation

Both types of sequestration are usually diagnosed in childhood after a history of recurrent pneumonia. Pulmonary sequestrations appear on a chest radiograph as a unilateral, triangular or oval posteriobasilar mass. They are usually located toward the midline. Cystic changes are common. A barium swallow may show gastrointestinal communication. Aortog-

Table 2: Anomalies Associated With Pulmonary Sequestration

Foregut anomalies
- Tracheoesophageal fistula
- Esophageal duplication
- Neurenteric cysts
- Esophageal diverticulum
- Esophageal cysts
- Bronchogenic cysts
- Megacolon

Skeletal deformities
- Funnel chest
- Vertebral anomalies
- Polydactyly

Diaphragmatic hernias

Congenital heart disease
- Atrial septal defect
- Ventricular septal defect
- Congenital absence of pericardium
- Truncus arteriosus
- Tricuspid atresia
- Transposition of the great arteries
- Subvalvular aortic stenosis

Renal anomalies

Cerebral anomalies
- Hydrocephalus

raphy demonstrates the abnormal blood supply. Pulmonary sequestrations must be distinguished from solid type III CAM, bronchogenic cysts, and mediastinal tumors (neural crest tumors, teratomas, and hamartomas).

Management

Surgical resection is often required.

Pulmonary Arteriovenous Fistula

Epidemiology

A rare cause of neonatal cyanosis is abnormal vascular communications between pulmonary arteries and veins.

Pathophysiology

Single or multiple, visible or microscopic, these fistulas most commonly involve the lower lobes. Frequently, pulmonary arteriovenous fistulas are associated with skin hemangiomas or hereditary telangiectasis. Although not usually symptomatic until adulthood, arteriovenous fistulas have been reported to present in the newborn period as refractory cyanosis with a harsh murmur. Chest radiography may show a small mass lesion, but radionuclide perfusion study or digital subtraction angiography are frequently needed. The electrocardiogram may demonstrate left ventricular hypertrophy. Contrast echocardiography may be more sensitive than arteriography in making the diagnosis.

Management

Treatment usually involves lobectomy.

Outcome

The prognosis depends on the extent of the lesion.

Congenital Pulmonary Lymphangiectasia

Epidemiology

A rare condition, congenital pulmonary lymphangiectasia is more common in males and is occasionally familial or associated with Noonan's syndrome.

Pathophysiology

Usually there is only dilatation of the pulmonary lymphatic vessels. The condition results either from a primary developmental defect or from lymphatic obstruction. It may also be associated with lymphatic disorders at other sites or with congenital heart diseases that have high pulmonary venous pressures (eg, hypoplastic left heart syndrome, total anomalous pulmonary venous return, pulmonary venous atresia or stenosis).

Presentation

Affected infants usually are full term and present with cyanotic respiratory distress shortly after birth. On chest radiograph, the lungs are hyperexpanded, with diffuse, coarse, granular densities representing dilated lymphatics. Pleural effusions are common. The diagnosis is often confused with pneumonia, pulmonary edema, or pulmonary interstitial emphysema. Confirmation of the condition is difficult and may require lung biopsy. On autopsy, the lungs are lobulated with marked dilatation of the subpleural lymphatic vessels and thick, fibrotic interlobular septa.

Management

Supportive therapy can be attempted (see *Pulmonary Edema* section, Chapter 4). There is no specific treatment for this disorder.

Outcome

In severe cases, survival of infants beyond the neonatal period is rare.

Pulmonary Agenesis

Epidemiology

Pulmonary agenesis may involve complete or partial absence of pulmonary tissue. Bilateral agenesis is extremely rare and fatal. Isolated lobar agenesis can also occur. Unilateral pulmonary agenesis is more common, may be hereditary, and is slightly more common in females.

Pathophysiology

Unilateral pulmonary agenesis usually affects the left lung and is frequently associated with other congenital anomalies (eg, VACTERL [vertebral, anal, cardiac, tracheal, esophageal, renal, and limb] association). A large variety of bronchial branching abnormalities are described, and vascular anomalies are frequent.

Presentation

Affected infants present with tracheal deviation and a nearly symmetric chest resulting from partial occupation of the contralateral chest by the remaining hypertrophied lung.

Table 3: Causes of Bilateral Neonatal Pulmonary Hypoplasia

Extrathoracic Compression

Oligohydramnios

Potter's syndrome

Bilateral cystic kidneys

Posterior urethral valves

Prune-belly syndrome

Neurogenic bladder

Bilateral ureteropelvic junction obstruction

Atresia of urethra

Prolonged amniotic fluid leakage

Chronically elevated diaphragm—no oligohydramnios

Large abdominal masses

Massive ascites

Membranous diaphragm

Thoracic Cage Compression

Thoracic dystrophies

Asphyxiating thoracic dystrophy

Achondroplasia

Achondrogenesis

Thanatophoric dwarfism

Osteogenesis imperfecta

Ellis-van Creveld syndrome

Short-limb polydactyly syndrome

Metatropic dwarfism

Hypophosphatasia

Thoracic Cage Compression
Thoracic dystrophies (continued)
Chondrodystrophia fetalis calcificans

Camptomelic dwarfism

Spondyloepiphyseal dysplasia

Neuromuscular disease with 'functional' compression
Werdnig-Hoffmann disease

Myotonic dystrophy

Amyotonia congenita

Myasthenia gravis

Decreased intrauterine breathing

Phrenic nerve agenesis or damage

Anencephaly

Intrathoracic Compression
Diaphragmatic hernia

Diaphragmatic agenesis

Chylous hydrothorax

Fetal hydrops

Large intrathoracic tumor, cyst, or heart

Idiopathic

Modified from Swischuk LE: *Imaging of the Newborn, Infant and Young Child.* 3rd ed. Baltimore, MD, Williams & Wilkins, 1988.

The presence of breath sounds is variable. Respiratory distress and cyanosis are not common. Chest radiograph reveals opacification and mediastinal shift into the affected hemithorax and, in the most severe cases, increased pulmonary vascular markings on the unaffected side. The chest radiograph findings can be confused with atelectasis.

Management

Bronchoscopy, bronchography, and arteriography can be helpful to outline the arterial and bronchial branches and to demonstrate the presence of associated cardiovascular anomalies.

Outcome

Prognosis depends on the presence of other congenital anomalies and on the capacity for sufficient pulmonary blood flow.

Pulmonary Hypoplasia

Epidemiology

Pulmonary hypoplasia, which can be unilateral or bilateral, is a developmental disorder resulting in decreased numbers of alveoli, bronchioles, and arterioles. Primary hypoplasia is uncommon, and its cause is unknown. It may be seen with other anomalies.

Pathophysiology

Most infants have secondary hypoplasia of lung tissue resulting from extrathoracic compression (oligohydramnios), intrathoracic compression (congenital diaphragmatic hernia), or thoracic compression (asphyxiating thoracic dystrophy and myotonic dystrophy) (Table 3).

Infants with oligohydramnios and renal agenesis are more often severely affected, and pulmonary histology indicates developmental arrest before 16 weeks' gestation. Factors other than amniotic fluid volume are involved because the contribution of fetal urine to production is most important later in gestation. In contrast, in infants with normal renal function, the association between prolonged oligohydramnios and hypoplasia is greater when oligohydramnios occurs before the pulmonary canalicular phase at 26 weeks' gestation.

Table 4: Features of Potter's Syndrome

- Breech presentation
- Wizened facies
- Limb malformations (flexion contractures, Potter's facies, and edematous, spade-shaped hands)
- Bell-shaped thorax
- Severe respiratory insufficiency
- Persistent pulmonary hypertension of the newborn
- Significant air leak
- Amnion nodosum—multiple nodules on the fetal surface of the placenta

Presentation

The neonate with extrathoracic compression usually presents with a constellation of findings similar to Potter's syndrome (Table 4). Infants with prolonged oligohydramnios from nonrenal causes almost always have associated skeletal deformities. The chest radiograph reveals small, relatively hyperlucent lung fields. Evidence of air block is common. Abdominal ultrasound is necessary to rule out a renal or urologic cause.

Management

Ventilatory management of these infants is difficult and involves judicious use of inspiratory pressures (during initial resuscitation and later) and shortened inspiratory times to attain acceptable oxygenation (see *Persistent Pulmonary Hypertension of the Newborn* section, Chapter 4). It is frequently wise to accept marginal arterial blood gas tensions and avoid additional trauma to the lungs. It is also important to augment ventilator therapy with chemical alkalinization and to maximize oxygen-carrying capacity and cardiac output. The use of surfactant in these infants may promote oxygenation and improve ventilation.

Outcome

Outcome depends on the severity of the lung disease and the underlying etiology. Infants with significant pulmonary hypoplasia will almost always have positional, often transient, limb deformities. Pulmonary hypoplasia associated with renal agenesis is uniformly fatal.

By Joyce M. Koenig, MD, and Timothy R. Cooper, MD

Suggested Readings

Congenital Lobar Emphysema

Campbell PE: Congenital lobar emphysema: etiological studies. *Aust Paediatr J* 1969;5:226.

McBride JT, Wohl MEB, Strieder DJ, et al: Lung growth and airway function after lobectomy in infancy for congenital lobar emphysema. *J Clin Invest* 1980;66:962.

Shannon DC, Todres ID, Moylan FMB: Infantile lobar hyperinflation: expectant treatment. *Pediatrics* 1977;59:1012.

Bronchogenic Cyst

Boyden EA: Bronchogenic cysts and the theory of intralobar sequestration: new embryologic data. *J Thorac Surg* 1958;35:604.

de Paredes CG, Pierce WS, Johnson DG, et al: Pulmonary sequestration in infants and children. A 20-year experience and review of the literature. *J Pediatr Surg* 1970;5:136.

Ramenofsky ML, Leape LL, McCauley RG: Bronchogenic cyst. *J Pediatr Surg* 1979;14:219.

Neurenteric and Enteric Cyst

Kugelman A, Weinger-Abend M, Miselevich I, et al: Acquired pulmonary cyst in the newborn infant. *Pediatr Pulmonol* 1997;24:298.

Superina RA, Ein SH, Humphreys RP: Cystic duplications of the esophagus and neuroenteric cysts. *J Pediatr Surg* 1984;19:527.

Cystic Adenomatoid Malformation

Bale PM: Congenital cystic malformation of the lung. A form of congenital bronchiolar ("adenomatoid") malformation. *Am J Clin Pathol* 1979;71:411.

Merenstein GB: Congenital cystic adenomatoid malformation of the lung: report of a case and review of the literature. *Am J Dis Child* 1969;118:772.

Stocker JT: Congenital and developmental diseases. In: Dail DH, Hammar SP, eds. *Pulmonary Pathology*. New York, Springer-Verlag, 1988, p 58.

Stocker JT, Madewell JE, Drake RM: Congenital cystic adenomatoid malformations of the lung: classification and morphologic spectrum. *Hum Pathol* 1977;8:155.

Winters WD, Effmann EL, Nghiem HV, et al: Disappearing fetal lung masses: importance of postnatal imaging studies. *Pediatr Radiol* 1997;27:535.

Pulmonary Sequestration

Coran AG, Drongowski R: Congenital cystic disease of the tracheobronchial tree in infants and children. Experience with 44 consecutive cases. *Arch Surg* 1994;129:521.

Landing BH, Dixon LG: Congenital malformations and genetic disorders of the respiratory tract. *Am Rev Respir Dis* 1979;120:151.

Laurin S, Hagerstrand I: Intralobar bronchopulmonary sequestration in the newborn—a congenital malformation. *Pediatr Radiol* 1999;29:174.

Nicolette LA, Kosloske AM, Bartow SA, et al: Intralobar pulmonary sequestration: a clinical and pathological spectrum. *J Pediatr Surg* 1993; 28:802.

Savic B, Birtel FJ, Tholen W, et al: Lung sequestration: report of seven cases and review of 540 published cases. *Thorax* 1979;34:96.

Stocker JT: Sequestration of the lung. *Semin Diagn Pathol* 1986;3:106.

Stocker JT, Kagan-Hallet K: Extralobar pulmonary sequestration: analysis of 15 cases. *Am J Clin Pathol* 1979;72:917.

Pulmonary Arteriovenous Fistula

Dines DE, Seward JB, Bernatz PE, et al: Pulmonary arteriovenous fistulas. *Mayo Clin Proc* 1983;58:176.

Fiane AE, Stake G, Lindberg HL: Congenital pulmonary arteriovenous fistula. *Eur J Cardiothorac Surg* 1995;9:166.

Hodgson CH, Burchell HB, Good CA, et al: Hereditary hemorrhagic telangiectasia and pulmonary arteriovenous fistula. *N Engl J Med* 1959; 261:625.

Marianeschi SM, McElhinney DB, Reddy VM: Pulmonary arteriovenous malformations in and out of the setting of congenital heart disease. *Ann Thorac Surg* 1998;66:688.

Congenital Pulmonary Lymphangiectasia

Bouchard S, Di Lorenzo M, Youssef S, et al: Pulmonary lymphangiectasia revisited. *J Pediatr Surg* 2000;35:796.

Felman AH, Rhatigan RM, Pierson KK, et al: Pulmonary lymphangiectasis: observation in 17 patients and proposed classification. *Am J Roentgenol Radium Ther Nucl Med* 1972;116:548.

Laurene KM: Congenital pulmonary cystic lymphangiectasia. *J Pathol Bacteriol* 1955;70:325.

Noonan JA, et al: Congenital pulmonary lymphangiectasia. *Am J Dis Child* 1970;120:314.

Pulmonary Agenesis

Cunningham ML, Mann N: Pulmonary agenesis: a predictor of ipsilateral malformations. *Am J Med Genet* 1997;70:391.

Maltz DL, Nadas AS: Agenesis of the lung. Presentation of eight new cases and review of the literature. *Pediatrics* 1960;42:175.

Schecter DC: Congenital absence or deficiency of lung tissue. The congenital subtractive bronchopneumonic malformations. *Ann Thorac Surg* 1968;6:286.

Pulmonary Hypoplasia

Hislop A, Hey E, Reid L: The lungs in congenital bilateral renal agenesis and dysplasia. *Arch Dis Child* 1979;54:32.

Langston C, Thurlbeck WM: Conditions altering normal lung growth and development. In: Thibeault DW, Gregory GS, eds. *Neonatal Pulmonary Care*, 2nd ed. Norwalk, Conn, Appleton-Century-Crofts, 1986, pp 1-32.

Lauria MR, Gonik B, Romero R: Pulmonary hypoplasia: pathogenesis, diagnosis, and antenatal prediction. *Obstet Gynecol* 1995;86:466.

Perlman M, Levin M: Fetal pulmonary hypoplasia, anuria and oligohydramnios: clinical pathologic observations and review of the literature. *Am J Obstet Gynecol* 1974;118:119.

Perlman M, Williams J, Hirsch M: Neonatal pulmonary hypoplasia after prolonged leakage of amniotic fluid. *Arch Dis Child* 1976;51:349.

Sun B: Use of surfactant in pulmonary disorders in full-term infants. *Curr Opin Pediatr* 1996;8:113.

Swischuk LE, Richardson CJ, Nichols MM, et al: Primary pulmonary hypoplasia in the neonate. *J Pediatr* 1979;95:573.

Thibeault DW, Beaty EC, Hall RT, et al: Neonatal pulmonary hypoplasia with premature rupture of fetal membranes and oligohydramnios. *J Pediatr* 1985;107:273-277.

Chapter 7

Diseases Affecting the Diaphragm and Chest Wall

Diseases of the Diaphragm

Congenital Diaphragmatic Hernia

Epidemiology

Congenital diaphragmatic hernia (CDH) is a relatively common neonatal disorder with an incidence of 1:2,000 to 1:5,000 live births. Despite progress in pre- and postnatal management, patients born with an isolated CDH suffer substantial morbidity and mortality. Previously reported survival rates were optimistically noted to be around 50%, but many institutions are now achieving improved survival rates. Most infants with CDH are mature; two thirds are male; and in 90% of cases, the hernia is left sided. While CDH is a predominantly sporadic disorder, a rare familial form with a much higher recurrence risk has also been reported. CDH is associated with a reported 36% incidence of other malformations or chromosomal anomalies.

Pathophysiology

Diaphragmatic hernias occur through a left posterolateral defect (foramen of Bochdalek—90%) or a right retrosternal defect (foramen of Morgagni—10%). The right side is believed to be protected by the liver during development.

The diaphragm develops anteriorly as a septum between the heart and liver. It grows posteriorly to close laterally at the foramen of Bochdalek at 8 to 10 weeks' gestation. The bowel migrates back from the yolk sac at about 10 weeks. If it arrives in the abdomen before the diaphragm has closed, a hernia results. Depending on the size of the diaphragmatic defect, the stomach as well as the small and large bowel, spleen, and liver can herniate into the chest. Pulmonary hypoplasia ensues from the resulting lung compression. Although the ipsilateral lung is most severely affected, the contralateral lung is also compressed as the mediastinum is shifted. Survival is closely related to the degree of pulmonary hypoplasia.

Pulmonary hypoplasia is manifested by a decrease in the number of bronchial generations and the number of alveoli per acinus. The number of pulmonary arterioles per square centimeter of pulmonary vascular bed is reduced. In addition, there is muscular hyperplasia of the pulmonary arterioles with abnormal extension of muscle into arterioles at the acinar level. Those vascular abnormalities place infants with CDH at high risk for severe persistent pulmonary hypertension of the newborn (PPHN; see *Persistent Pulmonary Hypertension of the Newborn* section, Chapter 4).

Presentation

Prenatal diagnosis of CDH is made by ultrasound demonstration of the stomach or bowel in the thorax as a fluid-filled retrocardiac mass. CDH is frequently associated with polyhydramnios. Once the diagnosis of CDH is established, it is necessary to look for other associated malformations that occur. The morbidity and mortality rates in fetuses with CDH may range from 10% to 50%. The principal advantage of prenatal detection of CDH is that it facilitates delivery at a tertiary center with immediate neonatal resuscitation, optimal ventilatory care, and surgical expertise. A multidisciplinary team approach should be used.

Studies in the literature have attempted to determine prenatal markers in fetuses with CDH that predict postnatal outcome. Indirect measures of severity have been proposed, such as age at diagnosis, degree of mediastinal shift, polyhydramnios, lung-to-head ratio, and the presence of intrathoracic stomach and liver. Liver herniation into the hemithorax has been shown to be present when there is a larger diaphragmatic defect with greater pulmonary compression af-

Figure 1: Radiograph of an infant with congenital diaphragmatic hernia. Multiple loops of air-filled bowel can be seen in the right chest, causing the mediastinum to shift to the left. Note there is no orogastric tube present; this should be routine. After placing the infant on intermittent gastric suction, the size of the herniated bowel was smaller, and the infant was easier to ventilate.

fecting lung size, thus lowering the lung-to-head ratio. Early prenatal diagnosis (before 25 weeks' gestation), liver herniation into the hemithorax, and a low lung-to-head ratio (less than 1.4) are reported as independent predictors of a poor postnatal outcome.

Postnatally, the diagnosis is made with a chest and abdomen radiograph (Figure 1), aided by a feeding tube placed in the stomach. This will demonstrate the hemithorax filled with a mass, usually incorporating air-filled bowel loops and the stomach within the chest. The heart is displaced to the contralateral side, and the abdomen is remarkably devoid of air. Symptoms are usually those of respiratory insufficiency and begin in the first hours or days of life, depending on the degree of compression of the lung by the herniated viscus. The infant with severe symptoms may present in the delivery room with deteriorating Apgar scores, scaphoid abdomen, increased anteroposterior diameter of the chest, displaced point of maximum impulse, and breath sounds that are decreased bilaterally or are absent on the affected side.

The differential diagnosis of CDH consists of cystic adenomatoid malformation of the lung, congenital lobar emphysema, lung cyst, pneumothorax, diaphragmatic paralysis, eventration of the diaphragm, and pleural effusion.

Management

The neonate with CDH and respiratory distress from birth must be treated as a medical emergency:

- Avoid bag-and-mask ventilation by immediate intubation and ventilation. Use low peak inspiratory pressure, a rapid rate, and minimal positive end-expiratory pressure (see *Persistent Pulmonary Hypertension of the Newborn* section, Chapter 4). Overdistention of the lungs in babies with CDH can increase pulmonary vascular resistance, causing pulmonary hypertension, and can result in lung injury caused by barotrauma. The use of high-frequency oscillatory ventilation (HFOV) as a primary modality of ventilation has been reported as a method of stabilization.

- Place a double-lumen orogastric tube to low, intermittent suction. This will reduce the amount of air in the hernia and further compression of the lung.

- Paralysis with pancuronium (0.05 to 0.1 mg/kg/dose IV p.r.n. movement) and sedation with morphine (0.1 mg/kg/dose IV) or fentanyl (2 to 10 µg/kg/dose IV) may be necessary to optimize ventilator support and decrease the danger of a pneumothorax. However, paralysis may lead to a loss in functional residual capacity and subsequently to a need for increased ventilatory support.
- Place an indwelling arterial catheter. Initiate noninvasive oxygen monitoring.
- If hypotension is present, provide colloid and continuous infusion of pressors, for example, dopamine (2.5 to 20 µg/kg/min IV drip).
- When respiratory acidosis is controlled, sodium bicarbonate may be used to correct metabolic acidosis.
- Evaluation for sepsis and administration of antibiotics should be considered.
- As in neonates with respiratory distress syndrome, there is a qualitative and a quantitative surfactant deficiency in CDH. Fetuses with CDH may benefit from antenatally administered maternal corticosteroids, but more studies are needed before this can be advocated. Postnatally, surfactant therapy should be considered, based on supportive evidence for surfactant deficiency in both the fetal lamb model and in human neonates with CDH. Surfactant must be used carefully, because the lungs are small relative to the infant's size. Our routine is to administer half the recommended dose of surfactant to infants with respiratory failure secondary to CDH.

The definitive treatment is surgical reduction of the hernia. There is no evidence that this is an emergency, however, and time should be spent adequately stabilizing the infant before surgery. The development of PPHN frequently complicates the postoperative clinical course. Frequently, the patient experiences a 'honeymoon' phase, during which the infant does quite well, but then deteriorates with severe hypoxemia secondary to PPHN. The management of these infants, including special therapies such as extracorporeal membrane oxygenation (ECMO) and inhaled nitric oxide (iNO), is identical to that detailed for infants with PPHN. There is echocardiographic evidence that after CDH repair, infants still have some degree of pulmonary hypertension up to 2 months of age.

Many clinicians consider ECMO for infants with CDH in whom maximal medical therapy has failed. However, ECMO is a treatment for pulmonary hypertension and not for pulmonary hypoplasia. It may succeed in improving survival by alleviating pulmonary hypertension only in those infants with an adequate amount of lung parenchyma. Patients with CDH may have pulmonary hypertension secondary to vasoconstriction or as a result of a dramatic decrease in lung parenchymal vessels. The timing of diaphragmatic repair as it relates to ECMO therapy is controversial. All proposed antenatal treatments are still experimental, and any benefits they may have over postnatal alternatives have yet to be proven.

Outcome

A multidisciplinary approach to the management of CDH—including antenatal assessment, planning, and treatment—may ensure access to state-of-the-art care for both the mother and fetus and may improve outcome.

Infants with severe respiratory distress presenting within 6 hours of birth have approximately a 50% chance of survival. In 1991, some centers suggested that ECMO might improve survival up to 60% to 65%. Various studies have suggested that a preoperative pH <7.00, Pco_2 >100, postductal Pao_2 <100, $AaDo_2$ >500, and mean airway pressure requirements >13 indicate a significant degree of pulmonary hypoplasia and very poor probability of survival.

Gastroesophageal reflux (GER) has become a significant postoperative and long-term problem after CDH repair, particularly in babies who require a large prosthetic diaphragmatic patch. This may be related to a weak diaphragmatic crus or a hiatal hernia. One study identified clinical GER in

89% of patients with CDH who underwent ECMO, and 44% of those with GER were discharged home on a regimen of nasogastric feedings. In addition, 50% of those infants treated with ECMO were at less than the 5th percentile for weight at both 1 and 2 years of age. In another study, 42% of survivors of ECMO required an antireflux operation to prevent recurrent episodes of aspiration. An aggressive multidisciplinary team approach to nutritional management in post-ECMO infants suggests improved results in adequate feeding and growth.

Fetal surgery is physiologically sound and technically feasible, but it does not improve outcome over standard postnatal treatment in fetuses with CDH without liver herniation. Advances in antenatal and postnatal management of CDH and their effects on long-term outcome are still under investigation.

Paralysis of the Diaphragm

Phrenic nerve injury with diaphragmatic paralysis is a rare cause of respiratory distress. It is most commonly found after birth trauma or thoracotomy. The injuries are usually observed in large-for-gestational-age infants after shoulder dystocia or in difficult breech extractions. The nerve roots of cervical nerves 3, 4, and 5 are stretched with lateral hyperextension and traction of the neck. The diagnosis is suggested in an infant with respiratory distress, signs of birth trauma, and an elevated hemidiaphragm on the affected side. During inspiration, the affected hemidiaphragm moves up into the chest, which represents paradoxical movement. As a result, the abdominal contents often shift toward the affected side. This can be seen on physical examination as a shift in the umbilicus toward the affected side during inspiration. This has been termed positive 'belly dancer's' sign. The involved diaphragm shows either limited or paradoxical movement on fluoroscopy or ultrasound examination. Treatment ranges from no intervention to continuous positive airway pressure by nasal prongs and intermittent mandatory ventilation. Most improve over a 2-month period. If the infant continues to require mechanical ventilation, surgical plication of the diaphragm should be performed.

Disorders of the Chest Wall

Skeletal and neuromuscular abnormalities may cause respiratory distress by restriction of thoracic volume. Although bony abnormalities are rare, they may be recognized immediately and are sometimes amenable to surgical correction. The severity of these disorders ranges from mild to incompatible with life.

Sternal Deformities

The most common sternal defect is pectus excavatum, an undue depression of the sternum. Rarely does this require correction unless it is progressive. Other defects of the sternum involve failure of fusion and include: (1) complete sternal separation, which allows protrusion of the cardiovascular structures (ie, ectopia cordis) and is commonly associated with lethal cardiac conditions; and (2) partial sternal separation, which leads to the development of upper sternal clefts. In both situations, early surgery is required to shield the underlying structures from injury.

Thoracic Deformities

Rare skeletal defects of the thoracic cage—involving broad, short ribs, a rigid thorax, and some degree of lung hypoplasia—are part of a disease group with generalized chondrodystrophy. Representatives of this group are asphyxiating thoracic dystrophy (Jeune syndrome), thanatophoric dwarfism, achondrogenesis, osteogenesis imperfecta, Ellis-van Creveld syndrome (chondroectodermal dysplasia), hypophosphatasia, spondylothoracic dysplasia, and rib-gap syndrome.

Respiratory distress can present at birth with severe retractions and a virtually immobile thorax. Diaphragmatic excursions are prominent, with respirations appearing entirely abdominal. Radiographically, the lungs appear airless with a diminished anteroposterior diameter. The chest has a squared-off appearance with short, clubbed ribs and a relatively large-appearing heart. A skeletal survey may help in differentiating the various syndromes. Treatment for pulmonary hypoplasia may be required (see *Pulmonary Hypoplasia* section, Chapter 6).

Muscles of the chest cage may be absent and may contribute to deformities. Deficiency of pectoral muscles on one side (Poland syndrome) may be associated with abnormal ribs and breast hypoplasia. Breathing may be paradoxical. Corrective surgery is usually done after puberty.

Muscle Weakness

Neuromuscular disorders may lead to thoracic dysfunction and respiratory failure. These primary neuromuscular disorders are usually associated with generalized muscular weakness or paralysis. These infants present with hypoventilation and a normal chest radiograph. Diseases in this group include myasthenia gravis, poliomyelitis, amyotonia congenita, muscular dystrophy, glycogen storage disease, and spinal cord injury or tumor.

By Charleta Guillory, MD, and Timothy R. Cooper, MD

Suggested Readings

Congenital Diaphragmatic Hernia

Adsick NS, Vacanti JP, Lillehei CW, et al: Fetal diaphragmatic hernia: ultrasound diagnosis and clinical outcome in 38 cases. *J Pediatr Surg* 1989; 24:654-657.

Albanese CT, Lopoo J, Goldstein RB, et al: Fetal liver position and perinatal outcome for congenital diaphragmatic hernia. *Prenat Diagn* 1998;18:1138-1142.

Bernbaum J, Schwartz IP, Gerdes M, et al: Survivors of extracorporeal membrane oxygenation at 1 year of age: the relationship of primary diagnosis with health and neurodevelopmental sequelae. *Pediatrics* 1995; 96:907-913.

Bloss RS, Aranda JV, Beardmore HE: Congenital diaphragmatic hernia: pathophysiology and pharmacologic support. *Surgery* 1981;89:518-524.

Breaux CW, Rouse TM, Cain WS, et al: Improvement in survival of patients with congenital diaphragmatic hernia utilizing a strategy of delayed repair after medical and/or extracorporeal membrane oxygenation stabilization. *J Pediatr Surg* 1991;26:333.

Crane JP: Familial congenital diaphragmatic hernia: prenatal diagnostic approach and analysis of twelve families. *Clin Genet* 1979;16:244.

Elbourne D, Field D, Mugford M: Extracorporeal membrane oxygenation for severe respiratory failure in newborn infants (Cochrane Review). *Cochrane Database Syst Rev* 2002;(1):CD001340.

Glick PL, Stannard VA, Leach CL, et al: Pathophysiology of congenital diaphragmatic hernia II: the fetal lamb CDH model is surfactant deficient. *J Pediatr Surg* 1992;27:382-388.

Glick PL, Leach CL, Besner GE, et al: Pathophysiology of congenital diaphragmatic hernia III: surfactant replacement for the high-risk neonate with congenital diaphragmatic hernia. *J Pediatr Surg* 1992;28:1-4.

Harrison MR, Adzick NS, Bullard KM, et al: Correction of congenital diaphragmatic hernia in utero VII: a prospective trial. *J Pediatr Surg* 1997;32:1637-1642.

Harrison MR, Bjordal RI, Langmark F, et al: Congenital diaphragmatic hernia: the hidden mortality. *J Pediatr Surg* 1978;13:227-230.

Ionoco JA, Cilley RE, Mauger DT, et al: Postnatal pulmonary hypertension after repair of congenital diaphragmatic hernia: predicting risk and outcome. *J Pediatr Surg* 1999;34:349-353.

Langer JC, Harrison MR, Adzich NS, et al: Perinatal management of the fetus with an abdominal wall defect. *Fetal Ther* 1987;2:216-221.

Levin DL: Morphologic analysis of the pulmonary vascular bed in congenital left-sided diaphragmatic hernia. *J Pediatr Surg* 1978;92:805.

Lipschutz GS, Albanese CT, Feldstein VA, et al: Prospective analysis of lung-to-head ratio predicts survival for patients with prenatally diagnosed congenital diaphragmatic hernia. *J Pediatr Surg* 1997;32:1634-1636.

Nakayama DK, Motoyama EK, Tagge EM: Effect of preoperative stabilization on respiratory system compliance and outcome in newborn infants with congenital diaphragmatic hernia. *J Pediatr Surg* 1991;118:793.

Somaschini M, Locatelli G, Salvoni L, et al: Impact of new treatments for respiratory failure on outcome of infants with congenital diaphragmatic hernia. *Eur J Pediatr* 1999;158:780-784.

Van Meurs KP, Newman KD, Anderson KD, et al: Effect of extracorporeal membrane oxygenation on survival of infants with congenital diaphragmatic hernia. *J Pediatr Surg* 1990;117:954.

Van Meurs KP, Robbins ST, Reed VL, et al: An early congenital diaphragmatic hernia: long-term outcome in neonates treated with extracorporeal membrane oxygenation. *J Pediatr* 1993;122:893-899.

Wilcox DT, Glick PL: Care of the fetus/newborn with congenital diaphragmatic hernia. *Fetal Maternal Med Rev* 1994;6:81-84.

Witters I, Legius E, Moerman P, et al: Associated malformations and chromosomal anomalies in 42 cases of prenatally diagnosed diaphragmatic hernia. *Am J Med Genet* 2001;103:278-282.

Paralysis of the Diaphragm

Haller JA, Pickard LR, Tepas JJ, et al: Management of diaphragmatic paralysis in infants with special emphasis on selection of patients for operative plication. *J Pediatr Surg* 1979;14:779.

Langer JC, Filler RM, Coles J, et al: Plication of the diaphragm for infants and young children with phrenic nerve palsy. *J Pediatr Surg* 1988;23:749.

Weisman LE, Woodall J, Merenstein G: Constant negative pressure in the treatment of diaphragmatic paralysis secondary to birth injury. In: *Birth Defects*: Original Article Series. XII, (6), pp 297-302, 1976. The National Foundation.

Chapter 8

Diseases of the Upper Airway

Disorders of the Nose, Mouth, and Pharynx

Upper airway obstruction from an intrinsic developmental defect or from secondary compression and distortion can cause severe respiratory insufficiency. The radiograph will show proximal pharyngeal distention with distal airway collapse (see *X-ray Patterns in Neonatal Lung Disease* section, Chapter 3). In contrast to lower airway disease, the lung volume is normal or subnormal.

Choanal Atresia

Epidemiology

Choanal atresia is reported to occur in 2 to 4 neonates in every 10,000 births. It has a familial tendency and a female-to-male ratio of 2:1. Two thirds of these atresias are unilateral, and 66% involve the right side. One half of affected children have associated anomalies, including Treacher Collins syndrome, tracheoesophageal fistula, palatal abnormalities, and the CHARGE association (coloboma, heart disease, choanal atresia, retarded growth and development, and genital and ear anomalies). Because 50% to 70% of children with choanal atresia have congenital heart disease, all children with choanal atresia should receive a cardiac evaluation.

Pathophysiology

Atresia occurs where the nasal cavity enters the nasopharynx. This obstruction may be bony (90%) or membranous. Some infants may have stenosis at the bony inlet or within the nasal passage, which can result in symptoms similar to unilateral choanal atresia.

Table 1: Syndromes Associated With Pierre Robin Sequence

- Stickler syndrome
- Camptomelic syndrome
- Cerebrocostomandibular syndrome
- Persistence of left superior vena cava syndrome
- Beckwith-Wiedemann syndrome
- Myotonic dystrophy
- Radiohumeral synostosis syndrome
- Spondyloepiphyseal dysplasia congenita
- Trisomy 11q
- Fetal alcohol syndrome
- Fetal hydantoin syndrome
- Fetal trimethadione syndrome

Presentation

Newborn infants are predominantly nasal breathers, so it is not surprising that nasal obstruction produces spells of cyanosis relieved by crying as well as by mouth breathing and severe retractions. Inability to pass a 3- to 5-French feeding tube through the nares may confirm suspicions. Contrast radiographs of the nasal passage will demonstrate the level of obstruction, but computed tomography (CT) of the nasopharynx defines the location and thickness of the obstruction and differentiates membranous from bony atresia. In the future, magnetic resonance imaging (MRI) may prove helpful.

Unilateral choanal atresia may escape detection for years. It should be suspected in infants presenting with unilateral, foul-smelling discharge on the affected side or respiratory distress associated with upper respiratory infections.

Management

Early transendonasal perforation of the atretic septum is recommended to prevent complications of intermittent hypoxia. While awaiting definitive treatment, an oral airway or endotracheal intubation may be required to maintain airway patency, and gavage feedings will be necessary. Postoperatively, nasal stents remain in place for about 6 weeks to maintain patency during wound healing.

Outcome

The prognosis may be poor when associated with multiple anomalies.

Pierre Robin Sequence

Epidemiology

Pierre Robin sequence (micrognathia, glossoptosis, and cleft palate) occurs once in every 2,000 live births. Inheritance may be dominant with variable expressivity. About 25% of affected children have manifestations of other syndromes (Table 1).

Pathophysiology

Mandibular hypoplasia at 9 weeks may force the tongue posteriorly, preventing closure of the palatal shelves. The cleft palate, found in 60% of infants with Pierre Robin sequence, is characteristically U-shaped in contrast to the typical inverted V-shape of most partial clefts. Because of the relative macroglossia, large negative pressures in the lower pharynx are created during inspiration and swallowing. This may further pull the tongue into the hypopharynx and produce pharyngeal obstruction. Recurrent episodes of hypoxia may eventually result in the development of cor pulmonale.

Presentation

The pharyngeal obstruction from this condition is usually less severe than that from choanal atresia. Cyanosis is usually intermittent, especially with feedings, supine positioning, or active sleep. Chronic obstruction causes CO_2 retention, failure to thrive, and cor pulmonale. Excessive air swallowing is frequent, resulting in gastric distention, vomiting, and aspiration.

Management

Placing the child in a prone position may clear the airway, but endotracheal intubation may be necessary to maintain the airway. A 3.5-mm endotracheal tube directed into the nasopharynx and left in place for weeks or months may be sufficient to prevent the negative pressures described above. Careful monitoring of the child (eg, multichannel tracing, home monitoring) is essential. Tracheostomy may be necessary if obstructive apnea persists.

Adequate nutrition and growth are also critical. Oral feedings may be accomplished with techniques similar to those used for infants with cleft palate. Orogastric tubes or gastrostomy may be necessary if the infant still has difficulty coordinating breathing and feeding. The palate is not usually repaired until 6 to 12 months of age.

Outcome

Generally, mandibular growth catches up with maxillary growth. In most cases, the airway obstruction resolves by 6 to 12 months, and the child develops a normal profile by 4 to 6 years of age.

Macroglossia

Airway obstruction from macroglossia may cause respiratory problems through mechanisms similar to that seen in the Pierre Robin sequence. There are many associated conditions, including trisomy 21, Beckwith-Wiedemann syndrome, congenital hypothyroidism, and large congenital tumors of the tongue (eg, hemangioma, teratoma, lymphangioma).

Partial glossectomy or excision of tumors or cysts may be indicated. Some hemangiomas may respond to corticosteroids.

Glossoptosis-Apnea Syndrome

Unilateral choanal atresia, choanal stenosis, or severe swelling of the nasal mucosa may generate a large negative oropharyngeal pressure. In the absence of adequate muscular control over the tongue, pharyngeal obstruction may develop.

Pharyngeal Incoordination

This condition has been observed in neonates with severe hypoxic-ischemic encephalopathy and pseudobulbar palsy, Arnold-Chiari malformation, and Möbius' syndrome. It usually produces choking and cyanosis during feedings. Aspiration pneumonia is a frequent complication. Orogastric or gastrostomy tube feedings are necessary.

Disorders of the Larynx

Laryngomalacia

Epidemiology

Laryngomalacia is relatively common, presenting at birth or within the first month of life.

Pathophysiology

This disease is characterized by easy collapse of the aryepiglottic folds, epiglottis, or larynx. The disorder occurs when poorly supported arytenoids, aryepiglottic folds, or epiglottis prolapse into the airway during inspiration.

Presentation

The condition usually presents as intermittent stridor that is influenced by position, crying, feeding, or sleeping. The stridor is inspiratory with significant chest retractions. Cyanosis, hypercarbia, abnormal cry, feeding problems, and failure to thrive are seldom present. Obstruction worsens with agitation. Radiographs of the neck may show prolapse of the aryepiglottic folds. Laryngoscopy provides the definitive diagnosis. Other conditions presenting as stridor are listed in Table 2.

Management

Conservative management is usually appropriate because spontaneous improvement is likely.

Vocal Cord Paralysis

Epidemiology

This condition is uncommon in the neonate.

Pathophysiology

Most often, unilateral paralysis occurs after injury to the recurrent laryngeal nerve. The usual causes are excessive stretching of the neck during delivery or trauma during surgical ligation of a patent ductus arteriosus. Bilateral paralysis is usually secondary to some severe central nervous system condition, including hypoxic-ischemic encephalopathy, Arnold-Chiari malformation, hydrocephalus, and brainstem dysgenesis.

Presentation

If the paralysis is unilateral, it usually involves the left side. The infant's cry is usually weak or hoarse, and stridor and retractions are not marked. Bilateral paralysis is more serious and may be associated with a characteristic high-pitched, crowing inspiratory stridor, pharyngeal incoordination, swallowing difficulties, recurrent apnea, or tracheal aspiration.

Vocal cord paralysis should be distinguished from other conditions that produce stridor (Table 2).

Management

Tracheostomy is usually needed for children with bilateral vocal cord paralysis.

Outcome

Unilateral paralysis usually improves in several weeks or months. However, bilateral paralysis has a poor prognosis that depends to a great extent on the underlying condition.

Subglottic Stenosis

Epidemiology

Acquired subglottic stenosis can be seen in 0.23% to 8% of surviving intubated babies.

Presentation

Glottic and subglottic stenosis usually result from prolonged or repeated intubation. Congenital subglottic stenosis can also occur and should be suspected if the diameter of the cricoid ring is less than 4 mm. Partial obstruction can also be caused by a laryngeal web or cyst. Supraglottic stenosis is rare. These children have inspiratory stridor with or without a hoarse cry. Soft tissue radiography, xeroradiography, and CT are helpful, but the definitive diagnosis is made by laryngoscopy.

Table 2: Differential Diagnosis of Stridor

Nose
Choanal atresia
Maternal reserpine
Syphilis

Mouth and Jaw
Pierre Robin
  sequence
Micrognathia
Macroglossia
Hypoplastic
  mandible
Thyroglossal cysts
Lingual thyroid

Larynx
Laryngomalacia
Bilateral vocal
  cord paralysis
Subglottic stenosis
Laryngeal tumor
Laryngotracheo-
  esophageal cleft
Laryngeal web
Reflex laryngospasm
Floppy epiglottis
Laryngeal stridor
  from hypopara-
  thyroidism (rare)
Calcified laryngeal
  and tracheal cartilage
Laryngitis (rare)
Laryngeal infection,
  bacterial or viral (rare)

Trachea and Bronchi
Tracheomalacia
Tracheal stenosis
Tracheal cyst
Bronchostenosis
Bronchomalacia
Lobar emphysema

Extrinsic
Neck or mediastinal
  mass
Goiter
Vascular ring
Hemangioma
Cystic hygroma
Teratoma
Tracheoesophageal
  fistula

Other
Neurogenic stridor
Stridor with apneic
  spells and cyanosis
Trisomy 21
Diphtheria
Neonatal tetanus

Iatrogenic
Obstruction of nares
  by tubes or tape
Postintubation
  laryngeal edema,
  stenosis, or vocal
  cord injury

Prevention

Acquired subglottic stenosis is associated with endotracheal tubes that fit too snugly, with prolonged intubation, and with numerous intubations. In some institutions, the policy is to always place endotracheal tubes small enough to result in an audible leak. In addition, clinicians may attempt to wean infants rapidly from mechanical ventilation to nasal continuous positive airway pressure.

Management

In mild cases, normal, spontaneous growth will often result in a sufficiently large cricoid for normal respiration. In more severe cases involving soft tissue stenosis, an anterior cricoid split may prove beneficial. In the most severe cases, tracheostomy may be necessary while waiting for growth of the cricoid. Stenosis that results from fibrous webs, cysts, or granulation tissue can be treated with endoscopic CO_2 laser ablation.

Outcome

In most cases, symptoms from subglottic stenosis will improve spontaneously. In cases requiring tracheostomy, 2 to 5 years may be required before removal of the tracheostomy. Laryngotracheal reconstruction may then be required.

Laryngeal Tumors

Laryngeal tumors are uncommon causes of airway obstruction and stridor in neonates. The most common benign tumor of the larynx is the laryngeal papilloma, which may be induced by human papillomaviruses 6 and 11. The clinical course is unpredictable, and airway obstruction may be fatal. Diagnosis is made by visual examination with a laryngeal mirror or a flexible fiberoptic laryngoscope. Treatment is surgical and involves ablation of the tumors with a CO_2 laser. The disease tends to recur and is difficult to cure.

Additional tumors include subglottic hemangioma (the second most frequent laryngeal mass), neurofibroma, lymphangioma, chondroma, fibroma, and rhabdomyoma. Malignant tumors are rare but include rhabdomyosarcoma, angiosarcoma, fibrosarcoma, chondrosarcoma, neurofibrosarcoma, and squamous cell carcinoma.

Laryngeal Webs

Laryngeal webs are uncommon congenital abnormalities. Their formation represents anomalous embryologic development of the larynx, but the mechanism of their development remains unknown. Diagnosis is endoscopic. Treatment is surgical open laryngeal reconstruction.

Disorders of the Trachea

Esophageal Atresia and Tracheoesophageal Fistula

Epidemiology

Esophageal atresia is a common anomaly seen in 1 in 3,000 live births. There is no sex preponderance, and 90% are associated with a tracheoesophageal fistula (TEF). Up to 80% of affected infants have multiple associated anomalies. These anomalies most often involve congenital heart disease (20%) and imperforate anus (10%) as part of the VACTERL association (which also includes vertebral, rib, renal, and limb anomalies). Many infants with Goldenhar's syndrome, CHARGE association, and trisomy 13, 18, and 21 also have esophageal atresia or TEF.

Pathophysiology

The esophagus and trachea first appear at the 21st day of gestation as a median ventral diverticulum of the primitive pharynx. By 34 to 36 days' gestation, lateral ridges divide the diverticulum to form the trachea and esophagus. Tracheoesophageal anomalies occur at this stage. Five major variants of tracheoesophageal abnormalities result from abnormal septation (Table 3).

Presentation

Esophageal atresia is occasionally suspected in a pregnancy complicated by polyhydramnios. At delivery, as many as 40% of affected infants are below the 10th percentile of weight for gestational age, and 36% weigh <2,500 g. The diagnosis

Table 3: Types of Tracheoesophageal Fistula (TEF)

Esophageal atresia with distal TEF	86%
Esophageal atresia without TEF	8%
H-type TEF without esophageal atresia	4%
Esophageal atresia with distal and proximal TEF	1%
Esophageal atresia with proximal TEF	0.05%

is most often made at the first feeding, when the baby has coughing, choking, and cyanotic episodes. Oral secretions are usually markedly increased. Atelectasis and pneumonia are common. The inability to pass a nasogastric tube into the stomach is diagnostic. This may be confirmed by a chest radiograph showing the tip of the tube in a wide, air-filled pouch in the upper mediastinum. Vertebral and rib anomalies may also be apparent. Contrast studies should be avoided because the aspiration of contrast medium from a blind esophageal pouch could produce pneumonia.

On occasion, esophageal atresia without a distal esophagus-to-trachea fistula is suspected in an unfed infant because of a persistent airless abdomen on the radiograph. In infants with a distal fistula, the bowel may be markedly distended. The child with an H-type fistula usually is older at diagnosis and often will have a history of recurrent pneumonia; confirmation of this variant is difficult and may require contrast radiography or esophagoscopy.

Esophageal atresia is generally not difficult to diagnose. However, H-type fistulas may be confused with other causes of chronic pneumonitis (eg, aspiration from gastroesophageal reflux, recurrent pneumonia, cystic fibrosis, pulmonary sequestration).

Management

Initially, continuous suctioning of the blind esophageal pouch with a double-lumen suction catheter is important. Maintain the child in a prone position, with the head of the bed elevated. In the larger newborn without respiratory distress, early primary surgical repair of the TEF without gastrostomy should be arranged. If surgery must be delayed, adequate nutritional support is essential.

In the newborn with respiratory distress, positive-pressure ventilation should be avoided, if possible; effective ventilator management is difficult in infants with a distal esophagus-to-trachea fistula because of loss of airway pressure across the fistula and subsequent abdominal distention. In these infants, emergency gastrostomy and ligation of the distal fistula may be needed.

Outcome

The survival rate is excellent. Death primarily results from associated anomalies, prematurity, or low birth weight. Postoperative complications include anastomotic leaks (21%), strictures (18%), and recurrent TEF (12%). The functional outcome after primary surgical repair is good, although a few survivors have reported dysphagia.

Laryngotracheoesophageal Cleft

This is the most complete manifestation of the abnormal embryogenesis that usually leads to esophageal atresia and TEF. In this case, incomplete fusion of the tracheoesophageal septum results in a longitudinal communication between the airway and the esophagus. Stridor, respiratory distress, and cyanosis are common. Surgical repair is difficult, and mortality is high.

Tracheal Agenesis

Tracheal agenesis is extremely rare, with fewer than 50 reported cases. Most cases are associated with severe genitourinary, vertebral, or cardiac anomalies. Displacement of the tracheoesophageal septum at 25 to 35 days' gestation causes failure of tracheal formation, with the bronchi arising from the esophagus. Usually, there is an associated TEF. The trachea is atretic below the vocal cords and absent to the carina. The condition should be suspected when respiratory efforts or manual ventilation fail to move air and when, on laryngoscopy, the trachea is not visualized below the larynx. Intragastric oxygen may prolong life until surgical repair can be attempted, but the prognosis is extremely poor.

Congenital Tracheal Stenosis

Congenital tracheal stenosis, which is very rare, involves a narrowed segment of the trachea or hypoplasia of the entire trachea, with or without involvement of the bronchi. Other associated anomalies include hypoplastic lungs, vascular rings, congenital heart defects, TEF, and hemivertebra. Tracheal stenosis produces inspiratory stridor, wheezing, and, often, cyanotic episodes. The diagnosis can be suggested by a chest radiograph with air as the contrast medium. Three-dimensional CT and flexible fiberoptic bronchoscopy are essential to confirm the diagnosis. Treatment varies, depending on the severity, and includes simple dilatation, segmental excision, or tracheoplasty. Mortality may be high, especially with more distal lesions.

Tracheobronchomalacia

Congenital tracheobronchomalacia is a rare disease caused by an inadequate cartilaginous framework. Secondary tracheobronchomalacia is also seen in the chronically ventilated preterm infant. Both types can result in airway closure at some point in the respiratory cycle and may present with symptoms of stridor or respiratory distress. The diagnosis is confirmed by bronchoscopy, which shows an approximation of the anterior and posterior walls of the trachea during expiration. In more severe cases, prolonged constant positive airway pressure may be required. The most severe cases may require prolonged tracheostomy. Fortunately, in most infants, spontaneous improvement can be expected by 6 to 12 months of life.

Table 4: Types of Vascular Rings

Lesion	Stridor	Swallowing dysfunction	Barium swallow
Double aortic arch	Yes	Yes	Bilateral indentation of esophagus
Right aortic arch and ligamentum/ductus	Yes	Yes	Bilateral indentation of esophagus right > left
Anomalous innominate artery	Yes	No	Normal
Anomalous left pulmonary artery	Yes	No	Anterior indentation between esophagus and trachea
Anomalous right subclavian artery	No	Occasional	Oblique indentation of posterior esophagus

Vascular Rings

Table 4 shows five common anomalies that are classified as vascular rings, the first four of which result in respiratory distress.

The double arch compresses the right and left sides of the trachea and esophagus; the right arch also compresses the posterior esophagus. A right aortic arch with a persistent ligamentum or ductus results in a similar pattern of compression. The anomalous innominate artery compresses the anterior trachea only. An anomalous left pulmonary artery arising from the right pulmonary artery passes between the trachea and esophagus and is the only lesion to compress the anterior esophagus.

Infants with tracheal compression have inspiratory stridor and wheezing. They usually develop symptoms late in the neonatal period and often lie with their head and neck hyperextended to stretch the trachea and make it less compressible. Chest radiograph may show mild overinflation, a right-sided aorta, and tracheal narrowing. A barium swallow may show indentation of the esophagus. MRI or bronchoscopy may be necessary to make an accurate diagnosis. The treatment is surgical reduction of the vascular ring.

By Gerardo Cabrera-Meza, MD, and Timothy R. Cooper, MD

Suggested Readings

Choanal Atresia

Duncan NO 3d, Miller RH, Catlin FI: Choanal atresia and associated anomalies: the CHARGE association. *Int J Pediatr Otorhinolaryngol* 1988;15:129-135.

Stahl RS, Jurkiewicz MJ: Congenital posterior choanal atresia. *Pediatrics* 1985;76:429-436.

Laryngeal Anomalies

Clements BS: Congenital malformations of the lungs and airways. In: Taussig LM, Landau LI, eds. *Pediatric Respiratory Medicine*. St. Louis, Mosby, 1998, pp 1106-1136.

Holzki J, Laschat M, Stratmann C: Stridor in the neonate and infant. Implications for the pediatric anesthetist. Prospective description of 155 patients with congenital and acquired stridor in early infancy. *Paediatr Anaesth* 1998;8:221-227.

Milczuk HA, Smith JD, Everts EC: Congenital laryngeal webs: surgical management and clinical embryology. *Int J Pediatr Otorhinolaryngol* 2000;52:1-9.

Samuel M, Burge DM, Griffiths DM: Prenatal diagnosis of laryngotracheoesophageal clefts. *Fetal Diagn Ther* 1997;12:260-265.

Smith RJH, Catlin FI: Congenital anomalies of the larynx. *Am J Dis Child* 1984;138:35-39.

Subglottic Stenosis

Marshak G, Grundfast KM: Subglottic stenosis. *Pediatr Clin North Am* 1981;28:941-948.

Ratner I, Whitfield J: Acquired subglottic stenosis in the very low-birthweight infant. *Am J Dis Child* 1983;137:40-43.

Triglia JM, Guys JM, Delarue A, et al: Management of pediatric laryngotracheal stenosis. *J Pediatr Surg* 1991;26:651-654.

Tracheoesophageal Fistula

Crisera CA, Connelly PR, Marmureanu AR, et al: Esophageal atresia with tracheoesophageal fistula: suggested mechanism in faulty organogenesis. *J Pediatr Surg* 1999;34:204-208.

Holder TM, Cloud DT, Lewis JE, et al: Esophageal atresia and tracheoesophageal fistula. *Pediatrics* 1964;34:542-549.

Montedonico S, Diez-Pardo JA, Lassaletta L, et al: Respiratory malformations associated with esophageal atresia (in Spanish). *Circ Pediatr* 1999;12:61-64.

Quan L, Smith DW: The VATER association. Vertebral defects, anal atresia, T-E fistula with esophageal atresia, radial and renal dysplasia: a spectrum of associated defects. *J Pediatr* 1973;82:104-107.

Spitz L, Kiely E, Brereton RJ: Esophageal atresia: five-year experience with 148 cases. *J Pediatr Surg* 1987;22:103-108.

Temtamy SA, Miller JD: Extending the scope of the VATER association: definition of the VATER syndrome. *J Pediatr* 1974;85:345-349.

Tsugawa C, Nishijima E, Muraj T: Recent advances in the treatment of esophageal atresia and congenital tracheal stenosis (in Japanese). *Nippon Geka Gakkai Zasshi* 1997;98:1008-1012.

Usui N, Kamata S, Ishikawa S, et al: Anomalies of the tracheobronchial tree in patients with esophageal atresia. *J Pediatr Surg* 1996;31:258-262.

Watersen BJ, Bonham Carter RE, Aberdeen E: Esophageal atresia: tracheoesophageal fistula. A study of survival in 218 infants. *Lancet* 1962;1:819-822.

Tracheal Stenosis

Dunham ME, Holinger LD, Backer CL, et al: Management of severe congenital tracheal stenosis. *Ann Otol Rhinol Laryngol* 1994;103:351-356.

Lam WW, Tam PK, Chan FL, et al: Esophageal atresia and tracheal stenosis: use of three-dimensional CT and virtual bronchoscopy in neonates, infants and children. *AJR Am J Roentgenol* 2000;174:1009-1012.

Tracheobronchomalacia

Altman KW, Wetmore RF, Marsh RR: Congenital airway abnormalities requiring tracheotomy: a profile of 56 patients and their diagnoses over a 9-year period. *Int J Pediatr Otorhinolaryngol* 1997;41:199-206.

Saltzberg AM: Congenital malformations of the lower respiratory tract. In: Kendig EL, Chernick V, eds. *Disorders of the Respiratory Tract in Children*. Philadelphia, WB Saunders Co, p 169, 1983.

Sotomayor JL, Godinez RI, Borden S, et al: Large airway collapse due to acquired tracheobronchomalacia in infancy. *Am J Dis Child* 1986;140:367-371.

Wiseman NE, Duncan PG, Cameron CB: Management of tracheobronchomalacia with continuous positive airway pressure. *J Pediatr Surg* 1985;20:489.

Trancheal Agenesis

van Veenendaal MB, Liem KD, Marres HA: Congenital absence of the trachea. *Eur J Pediatr* 2000;159:8-13.

Vascular Rings

Bakker DA, Berger RM, Witsenburg M, et al: Vascular rings: a rare cause of common respiratory symptoms. *Acta Paediatr* 1999;88:947-952.

Eklof O, et al: Arterial anomalies causing compression of the trachea and/or the esophagus. *Acta Paediatr Scand* 1971;60:81.

Hendren WH, Kim SH: Pediatric thoracic surgery. In: Scarpelli EM, Auld PAM, Goldman HS, eds. *Pulmonary Disease of the Fetus and Newborn and Child*. Philadelphia, Lea & Febiger, 1978, p 166.

Wychulis AR, Kincaid OW, Weidman WH, et al: Congenital vascular ring: surgical considerations and results of operation. *Mayo Clin Proc* 1971;46:182.

Chapter 9

Control of Breathing in Neonates

C ontrol of breathing can be viewed as a simple feedback loop. Respiratory drive originates in a central site (the initiator), and signals are transmitted via afferent pathways to the respiratory pump mechanism (the responder). The goal is rhythmic, rather than oscillatory, breathing. Information about the response of the respiratory pump is relayed back to the initiator, and subsequent signals are adjusted accordingly. This feedback loop is facilitated by certain modifiers that promote more precise adjustment of control of breathing. These modifiers include temperature, circulation time, and carbon dioxide sensitivity. If this closed loop is opened, rhythmic breathing cannot be maintained. If modifier information is faulty or incomplete, oscillatory breathing will result as the system makes constant readjustments while searching for the correct feedback state. Clinically, control-of-breathing disorders are characterized by various degrees of periodic breathing or frank apnea.

Central Control of Respiration

Stable control of breathing in babies is determined by three factors: central respiratory drive, maintenance of airway patency, and the proper functioning of the respiratory pump.

The respiratory center in the brainstem is the initiator of rhythmic signals to breathe. Fetal respiratory control is characterized by periodic breathing alternating with periods of apnea. Fetal breathing is accompanied by heart rate variability, an important sign of fetal well-being. It is not surprising that the fetus delivered prematurely continues to exhibit periodic breathing and apnea in the postnatal state. Gestational age is the most important factor determining rhythmic respiratory control in newborns. Central respiratory drive is periodic in immature infants but improves progressively with increasing maturation. In the immature infant, certain modifiers may act to further destabilize control of breathing.

Sleep State

Control of breathing is most disorganized and periodic during REM sleep. About 65% of sleep time is REM sleep in prematures, making them vulnerable to apnea, particularly of a diurnal nature.

Temperature

A stable thermal environment promotes rhythmic breathing while thermal fluctuations promote apnea. Up to 90% of apneic episodes in prematures occur during fluctuations in the thermal environment. About 65% occur during increases in air temperature, with the rest occurring when air temperature is decreasing.

Chemoreceptor Function

Although chemoreceptor function is present in the newborn, it is easily exhausted. Central nervous system (CNS) carbon dioxide responsiveness is blunted in immature infants. Hypoxia and hypercarbia act as central respiratory depressants, with this response persisting up to 52 weeks postconception. It is essential to maintain adequate baseline oxygenation in any infant with apnea. Drugs such as doxapram potentiate chemoreceptor function.

Circulatory Time

Although poorly understood in the neonate, circulatory time is a factor in determining CNS carbon dioxide sensitivity and adaptability to changes in P_{CO_2}.

Lung Volume

The maintenance of an ideal resting lung volume (or the functional residual capacity [FRC]) enhances rhythmic respiratory drive, while a low lung volume exacerbates periodic breathing and apnea. The maintenance of lung volume is one function of the respiratory pump.

Other Influences

Several centers have reported an increase in apnea frequency among very-low-birth-weight infants following immunizations.

Airway Patency and Airway Receptors

The upper and lower airway tree conducts the flow of respiratory gases between the environment and the alveolar-capillary interface. A complex set of neuromuscular functions and reflexes protects upper airway patency. These develop at different rates throughout gestation and may be temporarily depressed by illness or drugs. Like other components of control of breathing, maintenance of airway patency is primarily a function of gestational age but may be modified by additional factors. Disorders of upper airway function such as nasal obstruction or hypopharyngeal collapse produce obstructive apnea.

The Nose

Newborn infants are considered obligate nasal breathers and thus depend on nasal patency for adequate ventilation. About 30% of term infants, however, demonstrate mixed oronasal breathing during quiet and REM sleep. About 40% respond to airway occlusion with sustained oral breathing, although with reduced tidal volume. In the premature, however, compensatory mechanisms are poor, and nasal obstruction commonly precipitates apnea. Nasal obstruction is particularly common after nasotracheal intubation, nasal continuous positive airway pressure (CPAP), or prolonged use of nasogastric tubes.

Hypopharyngeal Function

Intact hypopharyngeal function is the most important factor in the maintenance of upper airway patency in infants. The hypopharynx is a collapsible tube subjected to negative pressure during inspiration and is normally kept open during inspiration by active contraction of a system of hypopharyngeal muscles. Failure of adequate integration of this complex function leads to pharyngeal collapse, the chief cause of obstructive apnea in infants. When hypopharyngeal muscle tone is poor, the upper airway collapses at pressures only slightly below atmospheric (-0.7 cm H_2O). Integration of pharyngeal muscle function is reduced during sleep, and a complete lack of resting tone may be observed during REM sleep. This increases the level of resting airway obstruction during sleep and exacerbates pharyngeal collapse during tidal breathing. Flexion of the neck further compromises airway patency. The primary effect of nasal CPAP in the management of apnea of prematurity is opposing pharyngeal collapse. Administration of xanthines may also enhance the function of the hypopharyngeal musculature.

Larynx and Trachea

The larynx and trachea are more rigid than the hypopharynx and are more resistant to collapse. Laryngeal function may be impaired by immaturity, edema, or vocal cord dysfunction. Upper and lower tracheal stenosis is recognized with increasing frequency in association with intubation and ventilator management, especially suction catheter-related injuries.

The Respiratory Pump

The respiratory pump mechanism consists of the lungs, the chest cage, and the diaphragm, along with the associated intercostal muscles and accessory muscles of respiration. The respiratory pump serves two important functions in control of breathing. One is to maintain an adequate resting lung volume that facilitates rhythmic respiratory drive. An ideal lung volume also allows each breath to be taken from an efficient point on the pressure-volume curve and serves as a reservoir for continued respiratory gas exchange between tidal breaths. The pump's second function is to facilitate adequate minute ventilation and maintain normal arterial oxygen and

carbon dioxide tensions, thus providing normal chemoreceptor feedback for rhythmic central respiratory drive. Function
of the respiratory pump is closely related to gestational age,
with immaturity of the mechanism being a major contributor
to apnea of prematurity.

Bony Thorax

Ribs are rigid structures that lift the chest cage and expand its volume when the intercostal muscles contract during inspiration. In the immature infant, ribs are thin and poorly
mineralized. These pliable structures are unable to resist the
retractive forces of the lung and chest wall and thus fail to
maintain an adequate resting lung volume, adequate tidal
volume, or effective distribution of ventilation.

The Intercostal Muscles

These muscles contract to expand the chest cage during
inspiration. In addition, they maintain resting tone at end
expiration to promote the continuous negative pleural pressure necessary to maintain functional residual capacity. This
mechanism is disorganized during REM sleep in premature
infants, resulting in loss of chest wall stability, loss of lung
volume, and exacerbation of apnea. These effects of immaturity can be opposed by the use of CPAP and xanthines.

The Diaphragm

The diaphragm, in conjunction with the rib cage and intercostal muscles, promotes uniform expansion of the internal thoracic volume. This promotes efficient tidal breathing
and distribution of ventilation. Function of the diaphragm
may be impaired by reduction in muscle mass or contractile
strength, by the supine posture, or by REM sleep in small
prematures. Strength of contraction and efficiency of resting
tone are enhanced by xanthines.

Apnea

Apnea of prematurity is the chief disorder of control of
breathing in the neonate. It occurs in nearly 25% of preterm
infants and in 75% of preterm infants weighing <1,000 g.

Table 1: Conditions That Can Destabilize Control of Breathing in the Neonate

- Hypoxemia
- Septicemia
- Antepartum magnesium sulfate
- Fetal asphyxia
- Congenital central nervous system anomalies
- Intracranial hemorrhage
- Prostaglandin E infusion
- Antepartum narcotics or general anesthesia
- Metabolic disease (eg, hypoglycemia, urea cycle disorder, organic aciduria, medium-chain acyl-CoA dehydrogenase deficiency)

Physiology

Apnea frequency increases with decreasing gestational age, particularly below 34 weeks. Apnea may be central or obstructive, but in premature infants it is usually mixed, with about 60% central and 40% obstructive episodes.

Apnea is defined as complete cessation of breathing for 20 seconds or longer and is frequently associated with periodic breathing. Periodic breathing involves episodes of progressive diminution of rate and depth of breathing, several seconds of absent breathing, and then subsequent return of respirations to baseline. Apnea and periodic breathing may or may not be accompanied by changes in heart rate or state of oxygenation.

Differential Diagnosis

Apnea of prematurity is the most common control-of-breathing disorder in the neonate, but other pathologic conditions must be considered when apnea occurs, especially in mature infants. If a previously stable preterm infant begins having frequent episodes of apnea, the conditions stated in Table 1 must be considered. Such infants should be promptly evaluated for stability of the thermal environment, adequacy of resting oxygenation, and status of hemoglobin concentration and caffeine or theophylline levels. If no obvious abnormality is found, infection should be strongly suspected. Apnea in a term infant is considered pathologic and always deserves investigation.

Management

Central respiratory drive and maintenance of upper airway patency are poorly integrated in infants less than 32 to 34 weeks' gestation. Thus, the incidence of apnea is high in such infants, and little improvement can be expected until further maturation occurs. Meanwhile, these infants are extremely vulnerable to the effects of the modifying conditions discussed earlier. Even at a postconceptional age of 34 to 36 weeks, the introduction of feeding may be accompanied by hypoxemia, cyanosis, and bradycardia. These are not episodes of apnea, and they occur during the waking state. They do, however, involve the same immature pharyngeal mechanisms that contribute to obstructive apnea and, like apnea, they improve with maturation.

Improved understanding of control of breathing in infants has led to the introduction of effective management tools. These are particularly effective in dealing with apnea of prematurity. Decisions to treat are based on frequency of episodes and whether they produce bradycardia or hypoxemia or require significant intervention.

General measures

All infants with apnea should be nursed in a stable thermal environment, which is best provided by a servocontrolled radiant warmer or incubator. It is critical to avoid flexion of the neck and airway closure. Adequate baseline oxygenation must be ensured in the infant with apnea during waking and

Table 2: Comparison of Methylxanthines

	Theophylline	Caffeine citrate
Mechanism	Increase respiratory rate and tidal volume	Increases respiratory rate and minute ventilation
Route	IV: theophylline PO: theophylline	IV: caffeine PO: caffeine
Loading dose	5 mg/kg	20 mg/kg
Starting maintenance dose	2 mg/kg/dose q 6-8 h	5 mg/kg/dose q.d.
Therapeutic range	Narrow: 7-13 mg/L	Wide: 8-20 mg/L
Approximate half-life	20 hours	100 hours
Time to steady state	5 days	14 days
Side effects	Tachycardia Irritability GI intolerance	Rare

sleep. This can be done by placing the infant on a $TcPo_2$ monitor or pulse oximeter with a strip recording for several hours and noting specific events. Low-flow supplemental oxygen may be needed in some infants with apnea, but oxygen monitoring is essential and hyperoxemia must be avoided. Nasal patency must be maintained.

Xanthines

These agents enhance rhythmic respiratory drive, improve carbon dioxide response, reduce REM sleep, enhance resting pharyngeal muscle tone, and strengthen force of contraction of the diaphragm. They exert effects on almost all components of the control-of-breathing loop. There is a linear dose-response relationship for theophylline, with decreasing frequency of apnea as serum level increases. More than 75% of episodes of apnea of prematurity can be abolished or significantly modified by xanthine therapy alone.

Theophylline

This methylxanthine increases respiratory rate and tidal volume, but its effect on respiratory rate is greater. It increases heart rate as well (see Table 2 for doses and side effects). Serum levels should be monitored once steady state is achieved. Therapeutic range is 7 to 13 mg/L with increasing control of apnea as levels increase. Because of a narrow therapeutic index, side effects or signs of toxicity may be seen at or above levels of 14 to 16 mg/L.

Caffeine citrate

Caffeine increases respiratory rate and minute ventilation with little effect on tidal volume or heart rate. It has the benefits of long half-life, wide therapeutic index, and reduced cardiovascular effects. Side effects commonly seen with theophylline (tachycardia, arousal, and gastrointestinal intolerance) are rare with caffeine.

Doxapram

Doxapram is an analeptic agent with potent respiratory and CNS stimulant properties. The drug also potentiates peripheral chemoreceptor activity. It is administered by continuous intravenous infusion at dosages of 0.5 to 1.5 mg/kg/h. At infusion rates greater than 1.5 mg/kg/h, the incidence of hypertension and CNS symptoms increases significantly. Because of potential toxicity, doxapram should be reserved for infants with refractory apnea of prematurity and significant hypoxemia who have failed other measures.

Nasal CPAP

Nasal CPAP reduces the incidence of obstructive apnea in prematures by opposing pharyngeal collapse. Central respiratory drive may also be enhanced by alterations in the Hering-Breuer deflation reflex. The technique also aids in maintaining an adequate resting lung volume. It is most effective when used with caffeine or theophylline. Delivery is optimal using short, silastic, double nasal prongs that minimize nasal trauma and have the lowest flow resistance. CPAP should be initiated with 5 to 6 cm H_2O pressure and system flow rates of 5 L/min. Pressures can be increased progressively up to 10 to 12 cm H_2O as needed to achieve adequate control of breathing. Changing of tubes and nasal suctioning should be minimized. Some immature infants requiring CPAP for control of apnea continue to need it until they reach a gestational age of 32 to 34 weeks, when pharyngeal muscle control usually matures.

Anemia

Anemia, particularly the progressive physiologic anemia of prematurity, may be associated with increased frequency or severity of apnea. Transfusion of packed red blood cells reduces the frequency of apnea in many prematures, although neither the incidence of apnea nor the response to transfusion is related to the hematocrit or the severity of anemia.

By James M. Adams, MD

Suggested Readings

Botham SJ, Isaacs D, Henderson-Smart DJ: Incidence of apnoea and bradycardia in preterm infants following DTPw and Hib immunization: a prospective study. *J Paediatr Child Health* 1997;33:418-421.

Czervinske M, Durbin CG, Gall TJ: Resistance to gas flow across 14 CPAP devices for newborns. *Respir Care* 1986;31:18.

Erenberg A, Leff R, Wynne B, et al: Results of the first double blind placebo controlled study of caffeine citrate for the treatment of apnea of prematurity. *Pediatr* 1998;102:756.

Martin RJ, Miller MJ, Waldemar CA: Pathogenesis of apnea in preterm infants. *J Pediatr* 1986;109:733.

Martin RJ, Nearman HS, Katona PG, et al: The effect of a low continuous positive airway pressure on the reflex control of respiration in the preterm infant. *J Pediatr* 1977;90:976.

Mathew OP: Maintenance of upper airway patency. *J Pediatr* 1985;106:863.

Miller MJ, Waldemar CA, Martin RJ: Continuous positive airway pressure selectively reduces obstructive apnea in preterm infants. *J Pediatr* 1985;106:91.

Muttitt SC, Tierney AJ, Finer NN: The dose response of theophylline in the treatment of apnea of prematurity. *J Pediatr* 1988;112:115.

Perlstein PH, Edwards NK, Sutherland JM: Apnea in premature infants and incubator-air-temperature changes. *N Engl J Med* 1970;282:461.

Wilson SL, Thach BT, Brouillette RT, et al: Influence of upper airway pressure and posture. *J Appl Physiol* 1980;48:500.

Chapter 10

Respiratory Therapy — General Considerations

Initial Stabilization

Inadequate transition from fetal to neonatal life is one of the most common causes of respiratory insufficiency in the newborn. Birth is a complicated process that requires the infant to make the transition from:

- a thermally stable environment to a relatively cold one;
- the placenta as the major organ of gas exchange to the lung;
- the parallel circulation of the fetal heart to the series circulation of the adult; and
- a continuous placental source of nutrition to an intermittent enteral one.

Thermal Transition

Remember that the newborn baby is wet and naked. Its attempts to generate heat use up oxygen and glucose, both of which may be in short supply. Place the baby on a radiant warmer, and dry the baby with warmed towels. Drying can also stimulate the mildly depressed infant. When drying the extremely delicate skin of the premature infant, gently dab the skin to prevent abrasions.

Respiratory Transition

The conducting pathway for air exchange must be clear, and the mechanics for moving air in and out of the lungs must be functioning.

Establish the airway

Secretions of fetal lung fluid, meconium, or amniotic fluid should be removed with brief (10 to 15 seconds) suctioning

> ## Table 1: Indications for Intubation (AHA/AAP Guidelines)
>
> - Prolonged positive pressure ventilation
> - Ineffective bag-and-mask ventilation
> - Requirement for chest compressions for circulatory support
> - Requirement for tracheal suctioning (see *Meconium Aspiration Syndrome* section, Chapter 4)
> - Congenital diaphragmatic hernia

of the nasopharynx and mouth. Prolonged or repetitive suctioning can occlude the airway and stimulate a vagal reflex. The stomach contents may be aspirated after effective ventilation is established. While suctioning will be sufficient for most infants, some will require endotracheal intubation to establish a stable airway (Table 1).

Establish ventilation

The following steps should be performed in the delivery room immediately after birth:

(1) Assess ventilation by observing chest movement and listening for air exchange.

(2) If inadequate, ventilate with either bag and mask or bag and endotracheal tube (ETT). Bag-and-mask ventilation is the mainstay of neonatal resuscitation and must be practiced. Obtaining an adequate seal without injuring the facial structures of the delicate premature takes practice and attention to detail.

(3) The bag should be compressed gently with just enough pressure to see the chest rise. As the resuscitation proceeds, the pressure required to inflate the chest should decrease as air sacs are recruited. If bag-

and-mask ventilation is carried out longer than 2 minutes, an orogastric tube should be placed.

(4) Breaths should be given at the rate of 40 to 60 per minute with 90% to 100% oxygen.

(5) Reassess adequacy of ventilation: Is the thorax moving symmetrically up and down with each breath? Is air entry heard symmetrically on each side of the chest? Is the baby pink, and/or is there an acceptable measurement of arterial oxygen tension (Pao_2) or Sao_2?

If these criteria are not met, you must:

(a) recheck the seal on the mask;

(b) adjust the position of the infant's head;

(c) check for secretions in the airway;

(d) suspect some mechanical impediment to ventilation, such as pneumothorax, diaphragmatic hernia, or chylothorax; or,

(e) if the infant required intubation, check ETT placement by direct visualization.

Most infants will establish stable ventilation in the delivery room. The single most common cause of failure is an inadequate airway. If in doubt, repeat steps a to e.

Circulatory Transition

In most infants, heart rate and blood pressure increase with adequate ventilation and oxygenation. Circulatory support usually takes the form of chest compressions, volume replacement, or medications.

Chest compressions

Chest compressions are indicated if, after 30 seconds of effective positive pressure ventilation with 100% oxygen, the heart rate is below 60. Chest compressions should always be given in conjunction with positive pressure ventilation. Once the heart rate is above 60, chest compressions should be discontinued. Compressions should depress the lower third of the sternum to a depth approximately one third the anteroposterior diameter of the chest. Chest compressions are coordinated with breaths in a ratio of 3:1 at a rate of 90 com-

Table 2: Causes of Persistent Circulatory Insufficiency

- Volume loss from bleeding
- Myocardial dysfunction accompanying asphyxia
- Redistribution of intravascular volume secondary to sepsis

pressions and 30 breaths per minute. This is often counted 'one and two and three and breathe.' Compressions can be performed with the balls of the thumbs with the hands circling the chest, or with the tips of the middle and index or ring finger. To prevent injury, care should be taken to press directly on the sternum and not to the sides. Compressions should be stopped every 30 seconds to determine the heart rate. If possible, the infant should be intubated.

Volume replacement

For infants with a clear history of blood loss or sepsis and signs of poor cardiac output, including pallor and weak pulses, volume replacement with 10 to 20 cc/kg of crystalloid/colloid (normal saline, Ringer's lactate, 5% albumin, or O-negative blood) is clearly justified. For the asphyxiated infant without a history of volume loss, circulatory insufficiency may be the result of poor myocardial contractility (Table 2). While administration of volume may improve cardiac output in these patients, it may also raise venous pressures and worsen pulmonary edema. Rapid volume infusions may cause surges in cerebral blood flow and increase the risk of intraventricular hemorrhage (IVH) in premature infants. For this population, correction of hypovolemia should proceed cautiously. Any infant needing circulatory support should have an umbilical venous catheter inserted. Premature infants are also particularly prone to circulatory insufficiency secondary to excessively aggressive use of high pressure or long inspiratory time ventilation (see *Lung and Heart Interaction* section, Chapter 2). For these infants, therapy is directed at decreasing ventilator pressures and at judicious volume replacement.

Medications

If the infant's heart rate remains below 60 despite adequate ventilation with 100% oxygen and chest compressions for at least 30 seconds, or if the infant is born without a heart rate, then medications should be given:

(1) Epinephrine: 0.1 to 0.3 mL/kg of a 1:10,000 solution is given into the ETT or umbilical venous catheter, but never through an umbilical artery catheter. The dose can be repeated every 5 minutes.

(2) Sodium bicarbonate: 2 mEq/kg of a 0.5 mEq/mL solution at a rate no faster than 1 mEq/kg/min is given to correct documented or assumed metabolic acidosis. If the metabolic acidosis persists, the dose may be repeated.

(3) Naloxone hydrochloride: 0.1 mg/kg of this narcotic antagonist is given to infants with respiratory depression and maternal narcotic administration within 4 hours of delivery. Observe the infant closely after administration because the narcotic may have a longer half-life than the antagonist.

Neither atropine nor calcium administration is indicated in the delivery room.

Nutrition Source

If the infant requires only minimal intervention to accomplish a successful transition and has a stable cardiorespiratory system, feeding either at the mother's breast or by bottle can be initiated as soon as feasible (see *Nutritional Support* section, Chapter 11). If the infant has any cardiovascular instability that might be worsened by feeding or might inhibit feeding, start an intravenous infusion of glucose. Begin with 4 to 6 mg/kg/min of glucose delivery, and adjust according to the initial glucose level. If the glucose is less than 40 mg/dL, give a bolus of 2.0 mL/kg of 10%

glucose intravenously over 5 minutes. Repeat the bolus and increase the maintenance glucose delivery if repeat serum glucose levels persist at less than 40 mg/dL.

Stabilization of Infants ≤28 Weeks' Gestation

Resuscitation and stabilization of extremely premature infants require special care. Some of the measures that may reduce the risk of intraventricular hemorrhage include:

(1) Maintaining a neutral thermal environment
(2) Providing adequate oxygenation and ventilation
(3) Administering prophylactic surfactant
(4) Preventing apnea
(5) Avoiding rapid volume expansion
(6) Minimizing stressful, noxious procedures
(7) Eliminating unnecessary, rough handling

By Alicia A. Moïse, MD, and Alfred L. Gest, MD

Oxygen Use and Monitoring

Oxygen is a primary tool in acute cardiopulmonary care and represents one of the few beneficial interventions in reducing death and morbidity in neonates. Like all such modalities, however, it has both risks and benefits.

Physiology

The principal goal of acute cardiopulmonary care is maintenance of adequate tissue oxygenation. Adequacy of oxygenation depends on a complex interrelationship of diffusion, transport, and circulatory factors as summarized in Table 3.

Tissue hypoxia occurs when circulatory oxygen delivery can no longer support minimal use. At this point, oxygen consumption falls below basal metabolic rate, anaerobic metabolism supervenes, and lactic acidemia appears. If the process continues, cell death will occur. (For more information, see *Oxygen Transport and Alveolar Ventilation* section, Chapter 2.)

Oxygen Administration

Oxygen is the most frequently used drug in the neonatal intensive care unit. Its use requires a physician's order, which

Table 3: Maintenance of Adequate Tissue Oxygenation				
Type of Hypoxia				
	Hypoxic	**Anemic**	**Hypokinetic**	**Histotoxic**
Pao$_2$	low	normal	normal	normal
Hgb	normal	low	normal	normal
Cao$_2$	low	low	normal	normal
Circulation	normal	normal	low	normal
Other				metabolic block or cell toxin

must state how it is to be administered and monitored. In emergency situations, oxygen may be administered in amounts sufficient to abolish cyanosis. The American Academy of Pediatrics (AAP)/American Heart Association (AHA) Neonatal Resuscitation Program recommends that 100% O$_2$ be given at 5 L/min flow, using a simple flowmeter and oxygen tubing that can be connected to a manual resuscitator bag, if needed. Oxygen is administered directly by holding the tubing 1/4 to 1/2 inch from the nose of the infant. As soon as this immediate goal has been achieved, monitoring can be initiated to more accurately establish the state of oxygenation and determine further needs.

The role of oxygen in the delivery room is particularly important. At birth, pulmonary vascular resistance is high, and its subsequent fall is critical to successful postnatal cardiopulmonary adaptation. The establishment of effective ventilation and normal alveolar Po$_2$ values at birth is a critical determinant of postnatal transition. Oxygen is a potent pulmonary vasodilator. If apnea or bradycardia occurs at delivery, bag-

and-mask ventilation should be initiated immediately. Even if spontaneous breathing is adequate, oxygen should be initiated promptly if cyanosis is present and continued until specific monitoring clarifies the underlying state of oxygenation.

Subsequent use of oxygen can be accomplished using a variety of devices, including a head hood, a nasal cannula, or a positive pressure device. In all circumstances, the inspired gas mixture should be heated and humidified. The oxygen hood is often used during the acute management of infants with respiratory distress. Its primary advantages are ease of use, precision of delivery, and availability of a wide range of oxygen concentrations. Spontaneously breathing infants with chronic oxygen needs may be managed with a low-flow nasal cannula using 100% oxygen at 1/8 to 2 L/min flow. Humidification of this system is also required. Use of a nasal cannula offers the advantage of promoting parental bonding and verbal and visual stimulation. However, because of the inability to control the oxygen concentration delivered, it provides unrestricted delivery of oxygen and is not suitable for infants at risk for retinopathy of prematurity. The nasal cannula should be reserved for delivery of low concentrations of oxygen to patients requiring oxygen therapy for prolonged periods of time after retinal vascularization is complete. Typically, these are infants with established bronchopulmonary dysplasia (BPD), especially those requiring oxygen administration at home (Table 4).

Oxygen Monitoring

When oxygen is administered, clinicians must periodically monitor inspired O_2 concentration and estimate arterial oxygen tension or content. Frequency and type of monitoring depend on the nature and severity of the disease process, birth weight, and gestational age. Monitoring is made more difficult by the fact that no clear relationship has been established between any specific laboratory value and adequacy of tissue oxygenation.

Arterial Oxygen Tension

The Pao_2 measured under steady-state conditions is now the gold standard for monitoring the status of central oxygen-

Table 4: Characteristics of Oxygen Delivery Methods

Characteristics	Hood	Cannula
Duration of use	acute*	chronic**
System flow	8-10 L/min	0.25-1.0 L/min
F_{IO_2} delivery range	0.21-1.0	0.21-0.4
Measured F_{IO_2}	accurate	not possible
Humidification	yes	yes
Heated gas flow	yes	no
Temp range—incubator	equal to incubator‡	
Temp range—warmer	36°-36.5° C	
Maintenance required	low	moderate
Easy visibility of patient	moderate	high
Enhances bonding	no	yes
Allows infant to be fed	no	yes
Adaptable for home use	no	yes

* Preferred for infants still at risk for retinopathy of prematurity.
** Use for infants requiring chronic oxygen therapy with complete retinal vascularization.
‡ Temperatures are chosen to reduce condensation in connector tubing.

ation. The Pa_{O_2} is a particularly important measurement in the management of parenchymal lung disease. Pa_{O_2}, and the inspired O_2 concentration necessary to achieve it, is the best clinical pulmonary function test available in the newborn because it directly reflects efficiency of gas exchange in the lung. A low Pa_{O_2} or high F_{IO_2} implies poor gas transfer, while more favorable values suggest improvement in lung function. Most sources consider 50 to 80 mm Hg to be the usual range for newborn Pao_2. Under conditions of the controlled nursery environment, however, a Pao_2 less than 50 mm Hg may be acceptable and compatible with normal tissue oxygenation. Circulatory status and hemoglobin concentration must be considered in such circumstances.

Although universally used, Pao_2 monitoring has recognized shortcomings. Pao_2 values are most valid when blood gas samples are obtained from indwelling catheters under quiet, resting conditions. When percutaneous puncture is necessary (ie, in older infants), agitation may occur, and values obtained may not reflect steady-state conditions. It is also necessary to appreciate that arterial Po_2 values vary considerably throughout the day in sick neonates. Intermittent sampling produces only a limited view of a single point in time.

Transcutaneous oxygen monitor

Transcutaneous oxygen ($TcPo_2$) monitors are useful for judging trends in oxygenation during management of acute lung disease. These monitors measure skin surface Po_2 (not Pao_2), which, under proper conditions, is closely correlated with arterial Po_2. The $TcPo_2$ sensor combines a miniature blood gas electrode with a servo-controlled heater. The sensor is applied to the skin in a way that excludes any effect of environmental air on values measured. The technique depends on heating the skin at the sensor site to 43.5° to 44.0°C. This increases the tissue Po_2 as oxygen diffuses to the skin surface. With these operating temperatures and proper calibration, skin surface Po_2 at the electrode site correlates closely with central arterial Po_2.

In certain clinical circumstances, however, correlation is poor and $TcPo_2$ may underestimate Pao_2. Such conditions include circulatory insufficiency, inadequate electrode temperature, improper calibration and lack of user expertise, patient age greater than 10 weeks (skin thickness factor), and use of vasodilator agents. Maturation and thickening of skin with increasing postnatal age limit the use of this technique largely to neonates. All of these artifacts of measurement result in underestimation of arterial Po_2.

Under usual circumstances, $TcPo_2$ should be in the 40 to 80 mm Hg range. There is a time lag between measured $TcPo_2$ and Pao_2 values. As a result, oxygen concentration should not be continuously raised and lowered in attempts to 'chase' fluctuating $TcPo_2$ values. The Fio_2 and management plan selected should be designed to minimize fluctuations of $TcPo_2$ values as much as possible without constant manipulation of Fio_2.

Pulse oximeter

Pulse oximetry is useful for monitoring trends in oxygenation. This technique is less complex and does not require calibration or the level of user sophistication that $TcPo_2$ monitors do. The technique measures peripheral hemoglobin-O_2 saturation (Spo_2), which, in most instances, is well correlated with central saturation (Sao_2). Movement artifacts may, at times, severely limit the applicability of this technique. Artifacts of saturation measurement may also occur in the presence of high-intensity light, >50% fetal hemoglobin, and some radiant warmers. Pulse oximetry does not measure the Pao_2 and, thus, is relatively insensitive in detecting hyperoxemia. This is particularly important in the small premature infant. In acute lung disease, the range of desirable hemoglobin saturation as measured by the pulse oximeter is 85% to 95%. Under such circumstances, arterial oxygen content will be acceptable and hyperoxemia will rarely occur. For older infants, see *Bronchopulmonary Dysplasia* section, Chapter 5.

Capillary blood sampling

Capillary blood gas determinations have been used in the clinical setting to estimate adequacy of oxygenation, but this technique tends to underestimate Pao_2. These measurements require extensive warming of extremities (43° to 44°C), free-flowing puncture, and strictly anaerobic collection. Such conditions are difficult to reproduce in the clinical setting. For this reason, capillary sampling is not recommended as a tool for oxygen monitoring.

Summary

Oxygen administration is best carried out using a combination of monitoring techniques. Such an approach minimizes the shortcomings of each and allows a clinician the most balanced view of overall status of tissue oxygenation while optimizing patient safety.

By Joseph A. Garcia-Prats, MD, and James M. Adams, MD

Management of the Airway

All forms of positive pressure respiratory support require unrestricted access to the infant's airway. This access can be gained using a face mask, endotracheal tube, or nasal prongs.

Bag-and-Mask Ventilation
Indications

Ventilatory support delivered by a face mask is now reserved for emergency situations, such as the delivery room management of apneic infants. The source of positive pressure support is either an anesthesia bag or a self-inflating bag.

Technique

Mastery of bag-and-mask positive pressure ventilation equips the physician for emergency management of infants with compromised cardiopulmonary function. Its indications are for apnea and for respiratory failure. The required equipment includes a soft face mask of the appropriate size (term and preterm) and a source of positive pressure support (bag). Proper placement of the mask over the infant's face to cover the nose and mouth (not the eyes) takes practice and close attention. The ability to troubleshoot equipment failure in an emergency and familiarity with each component of the self-inflating bag (Table 5) are important. For more information, see *Initial Stabilization* section, this chapter.

Table 5: Components of the Self-Inflating Bag

Component	Function
Air inlet	Draws in air during release of bag
	With no reservoir, maximum F_{IO_2} is 0.4
Oxygen inlet	Connect green O_2 tubing and set flow at 8-10 L/min
	Connect O_2 source to blender for specified F_{IO_2}
Patient outlet	Connects to the mask or endotracheal tube
	May add pressure manometer via special adapter
Valve assembly	Controls the pressure pop-off of the bag
	Valve usually set to pop off at 30-35 cm H_2O
Oxygen reservoir	Connected at the air inlet to deliver F_{IO_2} of 1.0
	Always connect during emergency situations

Endotracheal Intubation
Indications

Placement of an ETT is indicated for prolonged positive pressure ventilation for infants with respiratory failure. In addition, intubation is required in the delivery room when bag-and-mask ventilation is ineffective, if tracheal suctioning is required, or if diaphragmatic hernia is suspected (see *Initial Stabilization* section, this chapter).

Table 6: Endotracheal Intubation

Infant Weight (g)	Tube Size Inner Diameter (mm)	Distance Lip to Tip (cm)
500-999	2.5	<7
1,000-1,999	3.0	7-8
2,000-2,999	3.5	8-9
3,000-3,999	3.5-4.0	9-10

Technique

Equipment. Preparation for the procedure requires a proper-sized ETT (Table 6), a laryngoscope and blade (usually Miller 0 or 1), suction equipment, precut tape, scissors, a bag and mask, and an oxygen source.

Tube placement. Many supervised intubations are required to gain proficiency. Each attempt at tube placement should never last more than 20 seconds. Stand at the head of the infant with the laryngoscope in your left hand, and stabilize the infant's head with your right hand. Slide the laryngoscope blade over the tongue until the tip of the blade rests in the vallecula. Lift the blade slightly to move the epiglottis out of the way and insert the tube with your right hand.

Watch the tube go through the cords to the black lines of the cord guide. The tip will be 1 to 2 cm below the cords.

Continue to hold the tube firmly at the lips and remove the laryngoscope. Note where the centimeter marks on the tube line up with the gum of the infant. Optimal position is 6 cm plus the baby's weight in kg following the 7-8-9 rule (ie, 8 cm for a 2-kg baby) (Table 6). A low tube that preferentially ventilates only one lung produces the risk of unilateral lung rupture and may be more dangerous than a high tube. Position the bevel of the tube anteriorly for optimal air flow.

Figure 1: Proper method for endotracheal tube placement. See text for explanation.

Auscultate over both sides of the chest and over the stomach to ensure that breath sounds are heard symmetrically over the chest. Watch for symmetric expansion of the chest with inspiration, and confirm tube position with a chest radiograph. The tip of the tube should lie halfway between the clavicles and the carina.

Tape the tube with two pieces of elastic tape, which should be wound around the tube only once. Stoma adhesive can be used to protect the skin of the face from the tape. To hold the baby and tube while another person tapes, cup the baby's head in one palm, hold the tube with the thumb and forefinger of the same hand, and then gently press the tube against the roof of the mouth with the forefinger of the other hand (Figure 1).

Precautions

Tube position. Be cautious about tube placement. A tube that is too low will slide in and out of one mainstem bronchus with changes in head position. This will result in relative overinflation of one lung and may precipitate air leaks. Mainstem bronchus intubation can also lead to a maldistribution of administered surfactant, resulting in unilateral hyaline membrane disease (HMD) and unilateral lung overdistention. A tube that is too high may become easily displaced with head movements or with suctioning.

Tube size. The size of the ETT should be appropriate for the size of the infant (Table 6) and should allow for an audible air leak. A tube that fits too snugly significantly increases the risk of tracheal stenosis. On the other hand, the resistance to airflow in the tube increases with the fourth or fifth power of the radius, so that small changes in tube diameter may increase resistance to gas flow substantially. These size limitations mean that it would be difficult to deliver the high flows necessary to ventilate a 4.0-kg infant through a 2.5-mm ETT.

Type of tube. Orotracheal intubation is recommended because of concerns about nasal deformities after long-term nasotracheal intubation and because the tip of the tube remains more stable with changes in head position.

Complications. Prolonged orotracheal intubation may cause palatal grooving and may interfere with dentition. Subglottic stenosis occurs in as many as 10% of survivors of prolonged intubation. The risk of subglottic stenosis is related to the duration of intubation, the number of reintubations, and the size of the ETT relative to the size of the infant.

Tracheobronchial Suctioning
Indications

The requirements for tracheal suctioning vary with the type of lung disease. Infants with HMD and transient tachypnea of the newborn (TTN) have few secretions during the acute stage of their disease. Therefore, the need for suctioning is minimal, especially since suctioning is associated with significant physiologic derangements, including hypoxia, hypercarbia, and hypertension, and may increase the risk of intraventricular hemorrhage. In this group of infants, indications for suctioning include visible secretions in the ETT, coarse breath sounds, and loss of chest wall movement while receiving mechanical venti-

Table 7: Considerations When Suctioning Infants

Physician's order	Indicate frequency of suctioning and special needs.
Suction catheter	# 6 French for 2.5 or 3.0 tubes, # 8 French for 3.5 or 4.0 tubes.
Resuscitation bag	Connect to O_2 source and to blender. Use if ventilator rate is <20/min, if infant is on CPAP, or if infant is not tolerating procedure.
Wall suction	Set at continuous and at 80 mm Hg.
Sterile saline	Instill 3-6 drops in tube to loosen secretions. Use either bag or ventilator for 30 seconds to distribute.

lation. In infants with meconium aspiration or bacterial pneumonia, or in older infants with chronic lung disease, secretions can be a problem and routine suctioning is required.

Technique

Suctioning should be performed using sterile technique and using the largest catheter that fits easily down the ETT (Table 7). Suctioning through a port on the ETT adapter may prevent some of the physiologic derangements associated with suctioning. A few drops of saline instilled into the airway may help loosen tenacious secretions. Because the suction catheter can damage airway epithelium, the catheter should *not* be inserted beyond the tip of the ETT. The distance to the tip of the ETT should be recorded and posted in a convenient location at the bedside so that caregivers will know how far to insert the suction catheter. If hand-bagging accompanies suctioning, a pressure manometer must be attached to the bag to prevent delivery of excessive positive pressure.

Table 8: Technique for Placing and Securing Nasal Prongs for CPAP

- In small premature infants, nasal prongs may remain in place best when placed upside down in the nose.

- Tape prongs in a secure manner (Elastoplast® tape works well). Do not secure prongs with occlusive bands that encircle the head.

- Position the infant's head to the side to minimize traction on the nose from ventilator tubing.

- Because prongs may be needed for a prolonged period, avoid trauma to the nose and posterior pharynx.

- Change nasal prongs only when an increased work of breathing is noticed, when sudden episodes of apnea appear, or when there are other clinical signs of nasal obstruction.

- Suction nasopharynx as needed to maintain airway patency, usually every 6 to 8 hours.

Nasal Prongs
Indications

Nasal prongs are used to deliver continuous positive airway pressure (CPAP). Nasal CPAP is used:

- to maintain lung volume in preterm infants with chest wall instability;
- to support the upper airway of preterm infants to prevent obstructive apnea; and
- to prevent small airway closure in preterm and term infants with chronic lung disease.

Technique

A variety of nasal prongs are available for administration of nasal CPAP. Prongs must have a low resistance to gas flow and should be easy to stabilize. Flow through the system should be 4 to 5 L/min, and the gas should be warmed and humidified. Excessive flow rates can cause drying or irritation to the nose or posterior pharynx. Placement and maintenance of nasal prongs can be aided by the technique in Table 8.

Complications

Complications from use of nasal prongs are rare. Occasionally, nasal deformities may result if the prongs are too large or applied too tightly. Frequent nasal suctioning may result in mucosal injury and nasal obstruction.

By Joseph A. Garcia-Prats, MD, and James M. Adams, MD

Surfactant Administration

Indications

Intratracheal administration of exogenous surfactant has been shown to reduce the severity of respiratory distress and mortality in infants. Surfactant therapy is now considered routine for treating and preventing HMD in infants.

Surfactant may be given as a preventive or prophylactic treatment or as a rescue intervention after HMD is established. Available evidence based on cost analysis and clinical outcomes such as death and pneumothorax suggests that surfactant should be given routinely as a prophylactic strategy to infants <30 weeks' gestation or to infants <1,250 g with evidence of surfactant deficiency. When used as prophylactic treatment, surfactant should be given as soon after birth as possible, preferably within 15 minutes of delivery. When given as a rescue treatment, a reasonable guideline is to administer surfactant when the infant reaches an arterial to alveolar oxygen (a/A) ratio of 0.22 or less. Typically, this is an infant who requires greater than 35% oxygen to maintain a Pao_2 of 50 to 80 mm Hg.

Surfactant deficiency or inactivation may be important in some forms of respiratory distress in full-term newborns. Surfactant has been used in infants with meconium aspiration and diaphragmatic hernia with encouraging results, but the studies have been uncontrolled, and the number of patients involved is too small at this time to make a recommendation.

Dose and Interval
Survanta®
Prophylaxis. The dose for Survanta® is 4 mL/kg (100 mg phospholipids/kg), and up to three additional doses may be given at least 6 hours apart, if needed clinically. Additional doses are given if the infant remains intubated and requires at least 30% inspired oxygen to maintain adequate oxygenation.

Rescue. The first dose is given as soon as possible after the diagnosis of HMD, preferably before 8 hours of age. Subsequent doses are administered as described for prophylaxis.

Exosurf®
Prophylaxis. The dose for Exosurf® is 5 mL/kg (67.5 mg/kg colfosceril palmitate), and second and third doses may be given 12 and 24 hours later to those infants with continued oxygen or ventilatory needs.

Rescue. Two doses of 5 mL/kg are given 12 hours apart. The first dose is given as soon as possible after the diagnosis of HMD.

Infasurf®
Prophylaxis. The dose for Infasurf® is 3 mL/kg (approximately 100 mg phospholipid/kg). Two additional doses 12 hours apart may be given if the infant is still intubated and requires an inspired oxygen concentration of at least 30% to maintain adequate oxygenation.

Rescue. Up to three 3-mL doses 12 hours apart can be administered for treatment of HMD. The initial dose should be given as soon as possible after the diagnosis is made.

Curosurf®
Rescue. Curosurf® is recommended for infants with respiratory distress syndrome and an oxygen requirement >0.6 when less than 15 hours of age. The initial dose is 2.5 mL/kg (approximately 200 mg phospholipid/kg) followed by 1.25 mL/kg every 12 hours for a total of up to 3 doses.

Techniques of Administration
Although the four surfactants most commonly given in the United States are administered somewhat differently,

the underlying principle is that they should be administered as rapidly as possible without producing undue respiratory compromise in order to achieve maximum distribution in the lung.

The approved method of giving Survanta® involves placing a 5-French catheter into the ETT until it protrudes slightly at the end of the ETT. Alternatively, the catheter can be placed through a neonatal suction adapter so that mechanical ventilation is not interrupted. The surfactant is then delivered in 4 different aliquots, while the patient is positioned differently for the delivery of each aliquot. The positions are as follows: (1) head and body inclined slightly down, head turned to the right; (2) head and body inclined slightly down, head turned to the left; (3) head and body inclined slightly up, head turned to the right; and (4) head and body inclined slightly up, head turned to the left. The infant should be ventilated for 30 seconds after each aliquot.

Infasurf® is administered in a manner similar to Survanta® except that it is given in 2 aliquots instead of 4. With each aliquot, the infant is positioned with either the left or the right side dependent, and 20 to 30 breaths are given during the instillation. There should be a brief pause between the aliquots to assess cardiorespiratory status.

Curosurf® is also administered in 2 aliquots, with the infant positioned either left or right side dependent for each aliquot. It is recommended that the ventilator rate be initially changed to between 40 and 60 breaths per minute with a 0.5-second inspiratory time. The surfactant is then given via a 5-French end-hole catheter cut to a length of 8 cm. The infant is then manually ventilated between 40 and 60 times per minute in 100% oxygen for 1 minute. After restabilization, the other side is made dependent and the remaining aliquot given.

For Exosurf®, the infant's ETT is fitted with a special ETT adapter with a side port that is supplied with the surfactant. Therefore, the surfactant is administered without interrupting mechanical ventilation.

Exosurf® is administered in 2 half doses (2.5 mL/kg) while the infant is in midline. The instillation should be timed with inhalation and given over 1 to 2 minutes. After the first half dose is given, the baby's head and torso are turned 45° to the right for 30 seconds. Mechanical ventilation should not be interrupted. The infant is returned to the midline and the second half dose is given in an identical manner, except that after the dose is given, the infant is turned 45° to the left.

Precautions
Before dosing
Ensure adequate positioning of the ETT by auscultation, visualization of chest expansion, and noting the centimeter marks on the ETT at the gum (Table 2). It is not necessary to confirm with a chest x-ray because this may unnecessarily delay surfactant administration. Any suctioning of the ETT should be performed before instillation.

During dosing
Monitor chest expansion. Decreased movement may represent obstruction of the airway by the surfactant. The dose may be slowed temporarily until movement returns or the peak inspiratory pressure (PIP) increases to overcome the obstruction.

Monitor for decrease in oxygenation as determined by noninvasive oxygen monitors or visible cyanosis. Determine if chest expansion is diminished; if so, proceed as above or, if movement is good, increase FIO_2.

Agitation may result from either of the above or the handling required for instillation. Sedation with a narcotic such as morphine may be beneficial before subsequent dosing.

After dosing
Pay close attention to changes in chest expansion, noninvasive oxygen monitors, and arterial blood gases for the first 30 minutes to 1 hour. Rapid changes in compliance may require frequent changes in PIP, FIO_2, positive end-expiratory pressure (PEEP), and rate; otherwise, overdistention

of the lung may occur, leading to possible pneumothoraces or pulmonary interstitial emphysema.

Do not suction the patient for 2 hours after surfactant administration unless absolutely necessary.

Complications

Transient bradycardia and oxygen desaturation complicate about 10% of doses. Reflux of surfactant into the ETT, pallor, vasoconstriction, hypotension, ETT blockage, hypertension, hypocarbia, hypercarbia, and apnea occur with less than 1% of doses. Special attention needs to be given to chest rise and oxygenation during surfactant administration. The peak inflation pressure and inspired oxygen concentration may need to be temporarily increased to permit optimal delivery of surfactant and to prevent respiratory compromise. Similarly, after surfactant delivery, these two parameters may need to be rapidly decreased to prevent overdistention, lung injury, and hyperoxia. Because of these adverse effects and the complexity and inconvenience of the approved methods of dosing, some clinicians have altered the method of surfactant delivery. It has been shown that administration of two fractional doses of Survanta® through a catheter inserted through the suction valve is as effective and safe as the current regimen that requires removal of the infant from the ventilator. Administration of Exosurf® by continuous infusion results in less loss of chest wall movement than does bolus administration. However, compelling data from experiments in animals suggest that continuous infusion may not be as effective. Therefore, it is our policy to administer the surfactants according to the instructions on the package insert until additional efficacy data are available.

By Alicia A. Moïse, MD, and Alfred L. Gest, MD

Positive Pressure Ventilatory Support

Positive pressure ventilatory support is used in preterm and term infants to improve oxygenation and ventilation, to support

> **Table 9: Types of Positive Pressure Ventilatory Support**
>
> - Continuous positive airway pressure (CPAP)
> - Intermittent positive pressure ventilation (IPPV)
> - Synchronized intermittent mandatory ventilation (SIMV)
> - High-frequency ventilation (HFV)
>   - High-frequency jet ventilation (HFJV)
>   - High-frequency oscillatory ventilation (HFOV)

lung volume, and to prevent and treat apnea. The various types of positive pressure ventilatory support are listed in Table 9.

Continuous Positive Airway Pressure

CPAP is a technique for maintaining end-expiratory airway pressure greater than atmospheric pressure (ie, CPAP is PEEP for the spontaneously breathing infant).

Physiology

In infants receiving CPAP, proximal airway pressure is usually maintained 4 to 12 cm H_2O above atmospheric pressure. CPAP has these physiologic effects:

Support of resting lung volume. In infants with loss of resting lung volume because of chest wall instability (see *Chronic Pulmonary Insufficiency of Prematurity* section, Chapter 5) or diaphragm dysfunction (eg, paralysis, eventration), CPAP increases resting lung volume and improves oxygenation and ventilation.

Maintenance of upper airway patency. In preterm infants with poorly supported upper airways, nasal CPAP increases pressure in the posterior pharynx, prevents airway closure during inspiration, and helps prevent obstructive apnea. Similarly, in infants with chronic lung disease and damage to large central airways (trachea and mainstem bronchi),

CPAP helps maintain airway patency and reduce airway resistance, particularly during expiration.

Improved distribution of ventilation. In infants with parenchymal lung disease, the lung can be divided into a well-ventilated compartment and an open but poorly ventilated compartment. Pao_2 is determined by the alveolar oxygen tension in the poorly ventilated compartment, by the size of this compartment relative to the well-ventilated compartment, and by the distribution of blood flow between the well-ventilated compartment, the poorly ventilated compartment, and the shunt (see $\dot{V}a/\dot{Q}$ *Relationships* section, Chapter 2, and *Hyaline Membrane Disease* section, Chapter 4). The only way to improve arterial oxygenation in infants with parenchymal lung disease is to improve oxygenation in the poorly ventilated compartment of the lung. Much of the ventilatory impairment in the poorly ventilated compartment is the result of increased resistance to gas flow in airways supplying these lung units. Application of CPAP dilates these airways, lowers resistance to gas flow, and improves ventilation. As a result, Pao_2 increases and hypoxia is relieved.

Technique

CPAP can be applied via nasal prongs or an ETT. Treatment of hypoxia in infants with severe parenchymal lung disease such as HMD often requires relatively high levels of end-expiratory pressure, 6 to 10 cm H_2O. In this group of infants, end-expiratory pressure is initially set at 5 cm H_2O with increases in increments of 1 to 2 cm to a maximum of 10 cm. While increasing end-expiratory pressure will virtually always increase Pao_2, it also overdistends the lung and may impair ventilation. If $Paco_2$ increases significantly with increased end-expiratory pressures, the infant is probably receiving too much CPAP.

The use of CPAP to prevent obstructive apnea usually requires lower levels of end-expiratory pressure, 4 to 8 cm H_2O. When CPAP is delivered by nasal prongs, there is often a flow of gas from the CPAP circuit into the nose and nasopharynx and out through the mouth. Therefore, the end-expiratory pressure in the nasopharynx and central airways is always lower than the pressure measured at the proximal airway. The magnitude of this pressure difference will be determined to a large extent by the resistance to gas flow through the nasal prongs. With very small prongs (those used for 500- to 750-g infants) this resistance may be very high and the proximal airway pressure may have to be set high, 8 to 12 cm H_2O, to maintain even relatively modest levels of end-expiratory pressure in the airways. With CPAP delivered via an ETT, there is no flow at end expiration, and end-expiratory pressures in the central airways are similar to those measured at the proximal airway.

Precautions

The mechanical complications related to endotracheal intubation and the use of nasal prongs are described in the *Management of the Airway* section, this chapter. Other complications related to CPAP are rare, and almost all are the result of alveolar overdistention. Levels of end-expiratory pressure must be tailored to the severity of the parenchymal lung disease. If the end-expiratory pressure is too high, the more normal alveoli will be overdistended. Alveolar overdistention increases the risk of air leak and may impair right ventricular filling and blood flow through the lung (see *Lung and Heart Interaction* section, Chapter 2). An increase in $Paco_2$ with increases in end-expiratory pressure is often a warning of alveolar overdistention.

By Thomas N. Hansen, MD

Intermittent Positive Pressure Ventilation

The use of intermittent positive pressure ventilation (IPPV) has markedly improved survival for infants with respiratory failure. However, optimal use of IPPV requires the physician to have a firm understanding of how the ventilator interacts with the lung to improve oxygenation and ventilation.

Physiology

Infant ventilator. Most infant ventilators provide intermittent mandatory ventilation (IMV). In Figure 2, airway

Figure 2: Time-cycled pressure-limited infant ventilator with airway pressure displayed graphically. See text for description. (Adapted from Hansen TN, Corbet AJ. In: Taeusch HW, et al, eds. *Schaffer and Avery's Diseases of the Newborn*. 6th ed. Philadelphia, WB Saunders, 1991.)

pressure (Paw) is displayed graphically over time. The infant's lungs are displayed as dashed lines increasing in volume over time. Gas flows into the ventilator circuit continuously, allowing the infant to take spontaneous breaths between ventilator breaths. PEEP is generated by a flow resistor on the exhalation limb of the circuit. A positive pressure breath is generated by closing the exhalation valve for a preset period, the inspiratory time (Ti), and allowing pressure to build within the circuit. The rate at which this pressure builds is determined by the rate of gas flow into the circuit (system flow). If system flow is high, the inspiratory wave form resembles a square wave (Figure 2). The magnitude of the increase in circuit pressure is measured at the proximal airway. The maximum pressure delivered, PIP, is limited by venting excess pressure to the atmosphere. During a positive

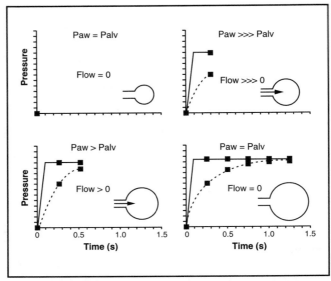

Figure 3: Determinants of gas flow into the lung. See text for description. Airway pressure Paw (solid line), alveolar pressure Palv (dashed line).

pressure breath, airway pressure exceeds alveolar pressure (Palv), gas flows into the infant's lungs, and the lung volume increases. The respiratory rate or the number of breaths per minute is determined by both Ti and the expiratory time (Te):

$$\text{respiratory rate} = 60/(Ti + Te).$$

Mean airway pressure (MAP) is the average airway pressure throughout the respiratory cycle and can be increased by increasing PIP, Ti, or PEEP. If the pressure waveform resembles a square wave, MAP can be calculated:

$$MAP = (PIP - PEEP) \times (Ti/[Ti + Te]) + PEEP$$

Figure 4: Lung volume above FRC as a function of time during a positive pressure breath. See text for description.

Determinants of gas flow into the lung

Alveolar pressure. Immediately before a positive pressure breath, Paw equals Palv, and there is no gas flow into the lung (Figure 3).

At the beginning of the positive pressure breath, airway pressure increases rapidly to the PIP. At this point, Paw is much greater than Palv, the driving pressure for gas flow (Paw - Palv) is large, and gas flows rapidly into the lungs. As gas flows into the lungs, the volume of gas in the lungs increases. Since Palv and lung volume are directly related (Palv = volume/compliance), as volume increases, so does Palv. Therefore, over time, Palv will become closer to Paw and the driving pressure for gas flow will decrease. Eventually, Palv will equal Paw and gas flow will cease. The point at which Palv equals Paw marks the official end of inspiration.

Lung volume. In the *Lung Mechanics* section of Chapter 2, positive pressure inflation of the lung was used as an example of a special solution to the equation of motion. While this solution does not strictly apply to the shorter in-

Table 10: Volume Above FRC as a Function of Time for the Lung in Figure 4

Ti (sec)	Time constants	Volume % Vmax	Volume (mL)
0.1	1	63%	15.8
0.2	2	86%	21.6
0.3	3	95%	23.7
0.4	4	98%	24.5
0.5	5	99%	24.8

spiratory times used with conventional mechanical ventilation, Paw is still constant over much of inspiration. Therefore, the volume of gas in the lung above functional residual capacity (FRC) over time is given by $V(t) = Vmax (1 - e^{-t/R \times C})$ (Figure 4).

In Figure 4, the lung is inflated with a PIP of 25 cm H_2O. Obviously, at time zero, the volume of gas in the lung above FRC is zero. If inspiratory time is prolonged sufficiently (>5 time constants), then Palv = Paw, gas flow into the lung will cease, and inspiration will end. The volume of gas in the lung above FRC at this time, Vmax, is the product of PIP and the respiratory system compliance. At time points between these two extremes, the volume of gas in the lung will be determined by Vmax (Paw and compliance) and the respiratory time constant (compliance and resistance). See Table 10 for examples.

Increases or decreases in resistance will affect the rate of inflation but will not alter the ultimate lung volume. Changes in compliance, however, will affect the ultimate lung volume and the rate of inflation to that volume.

Figure 5: The illustration on the left depicts a two-compartment lung. A is a well-ventilated compartment with a normal airway resistance and compliance, while compartment B is an open but severely underventilated compartment with a reduced compliance and an increased airway resistance. In B, lung compliance is reduced so that during positive pressure inflation, the ultimate lung volume (VmaxB) is less than in the well-ventilated compartment (VmaxA). More importantly, the increase in airway resistance outweighs the decrease in compliance, so the inspiratory time constant is prolonged and compartment B inflates more slowly.

Determinants of oxygenation

Cause of hypoxemia. As stated earlier (see $\dot{V}_A/\dot{Q}$ *Relationships* section, Chapter 2, and *Hyaline Membrane Disease* section, Chapter 4), in infants with parenchymal lung disease, the Pao_2 is determined by the oxygen tension in open but poorly ventilated lung units. In the case of pure $\dot{V}_A/\dot{Q}$ mismatch, continued perfusion of open but poorly ventilated lung units with very low alveolar oxygen tensions results in arterial hypoxemia. In infants with HMD, a reduction in alveolar oxygen tension in open but poorly ventilated lung units results in local vasoconstriction, redirection of blood flow through right-to-left shunt pathways, and arterial hypoxemia secondary to right-to-left shunt. In both instances, the only way to improve Pao_2 is to improve alveolar oxygen tension in open but poorly ventilated lung units. The only way mechanical ventilation can

Table 11: Efficiency of Ventilator Variables on Pao$_2$

Variable	n	Corr. Coef.	$\Delta Po_2/\Delta MAP$	P
PEEP	34	0.55	6.08	<0.001
PIP	40	0.51	5.07	<0.001
I/E	26	0.41	1.90	<0.05

MAP was increased by increasing either PEEP, PIP, or Ti, expressed as inspiratory to expiratory time ratio (I/E) in this study. For any given change in MAP, PEEP produced the greatest increase in arterial oxygen tension, PaO$_2$, followed by increases in PIP and finally by increases in Ti (Stewart, 1981).

increase the alveolar oxygen tension in open but poorly ventilated lung units is by improving their ventilation.

In infants with parenchymal lung disease, ventilation to open, poorly ventilated lung units is reduced because of an increased airway resistance and decreased lung compliance (Figure 5).

Effects of mechanical ventilation on oxygenation. Increasing MAP by increasing Ti, PIP, or PEEP increases arterial Po$_2$ in infants with parenchymal lung disease (Table 11). This implies that increasing any of the components of MAP improves ventilation of open but severely underventilated lung units. However, as seen in Table 11, increases in PEEP are more efficient in increasing Pao$_2$, followed by increases in PIP and finally increases in Ti. The reasons for these differences in efficiency can be understood by exploring the effects of changes in PIP, Ti, and PEEP on oxygenation (Figures 6 and 7).

Increasing MAP by increasing Ti, or, to a lesser extent, PIP, will result in overdistention of normal lung units (Figure 6). As discussed in the *Lung and Heart Interaction* section of Chapter 2, alveolar overdistention will compress intra-alveolar vessels and divert blood flow through the right-to-

Figure 6: Effects of increases in Ti and PIP on volume delivered to well-ventilated (WV) and poorly ventilated (PV) lung units. Increasing Ti from 0.2 second to 0.5 second allows more time for gas to flow into PV lung units, increasing alveolar Po_2, hence arterial Po_2. However, because of their shorter time constant, WV lung units become even more distended. Increasing PIP (dashed curves) increases the maximum volume of inflation in PV lung units, hence the volume delivered at any given Ti. The increase in delivered volume increases alveolar Po_2, hence arterial Po_2. Again, this effect is magnified in the normally com-

pliant WV lung units, resulting in alveolar overdistention, although to a lesser degree than that produced by increasing Ti. (Adapted from Hansen TN, Corbet AJ. In: Taeusch HW, et al, eds. *Schaffer and Avery's Diseases of the Newborn*. 6th ed. Philadelphia, WB Saunders, 1991.)

left shunt. This increase in right-to-left shunt blunts the increase in oxygenation resulting from improved alveolar Po_2 in poorly ventilated lung units and blunts the overall increase in arterial Po_2. Since PEEP results in less alveolar overdistention, there is less redirection of blood flow away from well-ventilated lung units, and any given increase in MAP results in a greater increase in arterial Po_2.

Alveolar overdistention also increases the risk of alveolar rupture and air block (see *Air Block* section, Chapter 5). Based on the discussion above, one would predict that the incidence

Figure 7: Effects of increased PEEP on ventilation. Increasing MAP by increasing PEEP splints small airways open, decreases airway resistance, decreases the time constant, and allows more gas to enter poorly ventilated lung units for any given PIP or Ti. Since airways supplying well-ventilated lung units are

already maximally dilated, PEEP will have little effect on ventilation to this lung compartment.

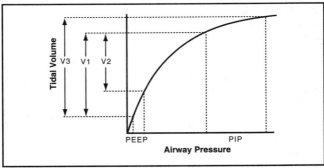

Figure 8: During positive pressure ventilation, the airway pressure cycles between PEEP and PIP. The cyclical changes in airway pressure result in cyclical changes in lung volume, the tidal volume. A plot of the pressure volume curve for the lung relates changes in pressure to changes in volume. As shown on this curve, any increase in PEEP at a constant PIP will reduce tidal volume, while any increase in PIP at a constant PEEP will increase tidal volume. However, since the pressure-volume curve tends to flatten at higher lung volumes, the ability to raise tidal volume by increasing PIP is limited. (Adapted from Hansen TN, Corbet AJ. In: Taeusch HW, et al, eds. *Schaffer and Avery's Diseases of the Newborn.* 6th ed. Philadelphia, WB Saunders, 1991.)

Table 12: Methods of Altering Pa$_{CO_2}$

	PEEP	PIP	RR
to ⇓ Pa$_{CO_2}$	⇓	⇑	⇑
to ⇑ Pa$_{CO_2}$	⇑	⇓	⇓

of air block would be reduced by relying on PEEP to improve oxygenation rather than increasing Ti (or to a lesser extent, increasing PIP). In fact, several studies have now shown that methods of mechanical ventilation that use short Ti have a markedly reduced incidence of pneumothorax.

Determinants of ventilation. The Pa$_{CO_2}$ is determined by the rate of CO_2 production divided by the alveolar ventilation. Alveolar ventilation is equal to respiratory rate times the difference between tidal volume and dead-space volume. If dead-space volume and CO_2 production are relatively constant, Pa$_{CO_2}$ is inversely proportional to both the respiratory rate and the tidal volume. For the most part, tidal volume is proportional to the difference between PIP and PEEP (Figure 8).

The effects of mechanical ventilation on the Pa$_{CO_2}$ are summarized in Table 12. If Ti is less than 3 time constants, increasing Ti will increase tidal volume but at the expense of overdistention of more normal lung units. It is possible to lower the Pa$_{CO_2}$ by increasing the respirator rate rather than by altering ventilator pressures. However, as the respirator rate increases, the absolute time allotted for expiration decreases (see *Lung Mechanics* section, Chapter 2). If expiratory time decreases to less than 3 time constants for expiration, gas trapping and alveolar overdistention may occur.

Techniques

Indications for mechanical ventilation. Many infants <30 completed weeks' gestation ultimately require mechanical ventilation. Because of this, and because of data sug-

Table 13: Initial Ventilator Settings	
Rate	60 breaths/min
System flow	8-10 L/min
FIO_2	⇑10%
Ti	0.2 sec
PIP	25 cm H_2O
PEEP	5 cm H_2O

gesting that early intubation in this population reduces mortality, many clinicians routinely intubate all such infants (see *Initial Stabilization* section, this chapter). Larger infants are ventilated for apnea or for being unable to maintain a Pao_2 greater than 50 torr on a continuous distending pressure of 10 to 12 cm H_2O and 100% oxygen. We do not normally ventilate spontaneously breathing older infants just to control $Paco_2$.

Ventilator settings

Goals of mechanical ventilation. The overall goals of mechanical ventilation are to maintain adequate tissue oxygenation, maintain an intact circulation, and allow recovery without causing additional lung injury.

More specifically, we attempt to maintain the arterial Po_2 between 50 and 80 torr, although we will accept an arterial Po_2 between 40 and 50 torr if there is evidence of adequate oxygen delivery to the tissues. Recent evidence suggests that attempts to rigidly control the $Paco_2$ increase the risk of lung injury. We do not routinely try to lower the $Paco_2$ below 40 torr, and we often tolerate values of $Paco_2$ between 50 and 80 torr.

Initial ventilator settings. Typically, FIO_2 is set 10% greater than the FIO_2 the patient was receiving before institution of mechanical ventilation (Table 13). Ventilator gas

Table 14: Subsequent Ventilator Settings

Pao_2	$Paco_2$	PEEP	PIP
low	low	⇑	
low	high		⇑
high	high	⇓	
high	low		⇓

should be warmed to 34° to 36° C and humidified to greater than 90% to prevent excessive water loss from the respiratory tract and to prevent lung injury from exposure to cold, dry air. This requires a heated nebulizer with heated ventilator circuits to prevent condensation in the ventilator tubing.

Subsequent ventilator settings. Hypoxia should be treated initially by increasing Fio_2. If this is not successful, then MAP must be increased. MAP should be increased by increasing PEEP, especially if the $Paco_2$ is not elevated (realizing that increasing PEEP will reduce the tidal volume). Increased PIP will increase both MAP and tidal volume and may be useful in those situations that require additional control of $Paco_2$. If at all possible, MAP should not be increased by increasing Ti because of the risk of alveolar overdistention and air leak. To allow sufficient time for exhalation, respirator rate usually is not increased to greater than 80 to 100 breaths/min.

Weaning is accomplished as shown in Table 14. For infants less than 30 weeks' gestation, when PIP is less than 25 cm H_2O and Fio_2 is less than 0.30, the respirator rate is slowly decreased to 15 to 20 breaths/min, and the infant is weaned directly to nasal CPAP. In this group of infants, respirator rates of less than 15 breaths/min, or endotracheal CPAP, are unlikely to succeed because of the high resistance of the 2.5-mm ETT. For the infant who cannot wean from the ventilator because of apnea or chronic lung disease, we use a respirator rate of 20 to 30 breaths/min and prolong the Ti to allow better distribution of ventilation through damaged airways (see *Bronchopulmonary Dysplasia* section, Chapter 5).

Infants >30 weeks' gestation can be weaned to endotracheal CPAP when PIP is <25 cm H_2O and FiO_2 is <0.40 and then to an oxygen hood when they require <5 cm H_2O of end-expiratory pressure.

Ancillary support. Endotracheal intubation and maintenance of the ETT are examined in detail in the section on *Management of the Airway*, this chapter.

Neuromuscular blockers may shorten the course of HMD and reduce periods of nonoptimal oxygenation and raised intracranial pressure associated with mechanical ventilation. In addition, there is some evidence that paralysis may reduce the incidence of intracranial hemorrhage in small preterm infants with HMD and fluctuating blood pressures (see *Lung and Heart Interaction* section, Chapter 2). However, neuromuscular blockade decreases dynamic lung compliance, increases airway resistance, and removes any contribution of the infant's own respiratory effort from tidal breathing, thereby often requiring that PIP be increased. In addition, neuromuscular blockade results in significant fluid retention and makes management of fluid balance more difficult. We typically sedate ventilated infants with morphine or fentanyl and reserve neuromuscular blockade for infants requiring high ventilator pressures (>30 cm H_2O).

Complications of therapy

The most serious complications of mechanical ventilation are related to prolonged endotracheal intubation, air leaks, and BPD and are all examined in Chapter 5.

Necrotizing tracheobronchitis is a necrotic inflammatory process involving the trachea and mainstem bronchi in neonates requiring mechanical ventilation. It is thought to result from drying of the tracheal mucosa secondary to inadequate humidification in the presence of high rates of gas flow and high concentrations of oxygen. Sloughing of the tracheal epithelium with occlusion of the distal trachea causes symptoms of airway obstruction, including hyperexpansion on chest radiograph and poor chest movement. Treatment may require emergency bronchoscopy.

Atelectasis occasionally occurs after extubation from mechanical ventilation and in some instances may reflect injury to the bronchi from suction catheters. In small preterm infants, postextubation atelectasis may be prevented by weaning to nasal CPAP.

By Thomas N. Hansen, MD

Synchronized Intermittent Mandatory Ventilation

Frequent asynchrony of spontaneous and conventional IMV breaths in sick neonates may result in ventilation breaths out of phase with the infant's own respiratory efforts. Asynchrony of spontaneous and conventional IMV breaths in sick neonates has been associated with impaired gas exchange, gas trapping, increased ventilatory support, increased barotrauma, increased use of sedation or paralysis, and increased variability of cerebral blood flow velocity. Previous attempts to synchronize IMV breaths with spontaneous respirations failed because triggering devices were insensitive. In recent years, newer, more sensitive devices have been developed to detect respirations. These devices detect inspiration by measuring: (1) airflow through the ETT using a hot-wire anemometer, (2) airflow through the ETT using a variable-orifice pneumotachometer, (3) changes in chest wall impedance using a cardiorespiratory monitor, or (4) diaphragm movements using a balloon-like pressure capsule taped to the abdomen.

Synchronized intermittent mandatory ventilation (SIMV) systems approved by the Food and Drug Administration (FDA) for use in newborns have a visual display that indicates spontaneous breaths and whether mechanical breaths are triggered or controlled. Most of the available systems have SIMV and assist-control (A/C) modes. In the SIMV mode, spontaneous breaths trigger the ventilator to maintain the preset rate; during apnea, controlled breaths are delivered at the preset rate. In the A/C mode, every spontaneous breath triggers a mechanical breath, and controlled breaths are delivered at the preset rate during apnea. Clinicians must be aware of potential problems that can increase asynchrony in all systems, including autocycling (inappropriate triggering of the ventilator due to artifact) and sensors missing spontaneous breaths. The time delay from the onset of a spontaneous breath to the rise in airway pressure following the triggered mechanical breath is known as the response time and typically ranges between 20 to 100 ms. In general, ventilators that have short response times are more sensitive to a patient's respiratory efforts, but they are also more prone to sense artifacts and autocycle.

Autocycling occurs when pressure or flow changes not related to respiratory movements trigger the ventilator. This can happen when there is an air leak around the ETT or in the respiratory circuit or when the to-and-fro movement of the condensation in the respiratory tubing creates pressure or flow changes. Thoracic distortion and movement artifacts are also sources of autocycling. Cardiac impulses can create interference in the signal detection. These difficulties are especially notable in extremely small premature infants, who may inefficiently and inconsistently trigger the ventilator and are at most risk for hyperventilation and barotrauma caused by autocycling. Appropriate weaning strategies depending on the patient's clinical condition, respiratory effort, and response to the weaning of ventilator support create additional challenges. Weaning of peak inspiratory pressures can follow conventional IMV strategies, but weaning of rate might cause the infant to increase spontaneous respiratory effort. Other ventilatory modalities, such as pressure support, may need to be added to ensure that the infant's work of breathing is not unduly increased by greater spontaneous effort.

There is a physiologic rationale for improvement in the outcome of mechanical ventilation when patient and ventilator breaths are synchronized. A recent meta-analysis comparing patient-triggered ventilation and conventional ventilation demonstrated a shorter duration of ventilation in the patient-triggered ventilation group (weighted mean difference -45.2 hours, 95% CI -78.3 to -12.1). Some investigators have also observed decreased (1) mean airway pressure, (2) F_{IO_2}, (3) fluctuation of cerebral blood flow velocity, (4) work of breathing, and (5) number of unit doses of sedatives and analgesics; however, long-term benefits such as less chronic lung disease, less intraventricular hemorrhage, and less air leak syndrome are yet to be proven.

In conclusion, many systems that attempt to synchronize the delivery of controlled breaths with spontaneous breaths are available. Although these systems appear to be beneficial in some patients, their indications and long-term benefits are not yet well defined. Clinicians who use these systems must become familiar with their individual designs, strategies, and potential problems.

By Caraciolo J. Fernandes, MD, George T. Mandy, MD, and Leonard E. Weisman, MD

High-Frequency Jet Ventilation

The jet ventilator has been used to treat the major complication of mechanical ventilation, pulmonary interstitial emphysema (PIE), while minimizing the effect of intrathoracic pressure variations on cardiovascular function.

Physiology

For conventional ventilators, alveolar ventilation is equal to respirator rate times tidal volume minus dead-space volume. High-frequency jet ventilation (HFJV) achieves normal to subnormal Pa_{CO_2} using tidal volumes far less than dead-space volume pulsed at very high respirator rates (60 to 600 cycles per second). The ventilator delivers a high-pressure 'puff' of gas through a small-bore cannula positioned in the airway at the proximal end of the ETT. These puffs of gas entrain additional gas as they jet down the center of the airway lumen. While the actual volume of gas delivered is unknown, it is clear that alveolar ventilation occurs with volumes considerably less than conventional, minimizing alveolar overdistention and air leak. Oxygenation remains proportional to MAP. Since HFJV dramatically reduces $Paco_2$ using lower MAP than conventional ventilators, it is a less effective oxygenator. In other words, use of HFJV at the low lung volumes needed to treat air block magnifies the jet's poor ability to recruit alveoli. For this reason, background conventional ventilation is often required to avoid atelectasis. The only FDA-approved indication for HFJV is for treatment of PIE, but some centers use it for infants with meconium aspiration syndrome and severe respiratory failure. Recent studies have demonstrated a poorer outcome (defined as either grade 4 IVH, cystic periventricular leukomalacia, or death) associated with HFJV use in preterm infants compared with infants managed with conventional ventilators.

Complications

The potential complications of HFJV include the need for reintubation with a special, larger ETT with two ports, one for delivering the jet of gas and the other for monitoring airway pressure; difficulty in maintaining normal FRC; and necrotizing tracheitis (may have been minimized by newer systems of improved humidification).

By Joseph A. Garcia-Prats, MD, and Thomas N. Hansen, MD

High-Frequency Oscillatory Ventilation

High-frequency oscillatory ventilation (HFOV) was initially proposed as an alternative to conventional ventilation in an attempt to accomplish adequate oxygenation and ventilation at low tidal volumes. Although it was intended to reduce barotrauma and the development of chronic lung disease, it has been used more recently as rescue therapy where conventional ventilation has failed.

Physiology

Types of ventilators. High-frequency oscillators (HFOs) use a piston diaphragm to oscillate a bias flow of gas and generate an active movement of gas in and out of the lung. They use very small tidal volumes (usually less than dead space) and rely on a bias flow of gas to flush CO_2 out of the system and maintain a supply of fresh gas at the proximal end of the ETT. Operator-controlled parameters include MAP, frequency, and piston amplitude. Frequency is commonly set at 10 to 15 Hz, and Ti is set at 33%, providing an I:E ratio of 1:2. Alterations in MAP primarily influence oxygenation, while changes in piston amplitude primarily affect ventilation.

Some high-frequency flow interrupter (HFFI) ventilators perform physiologically equivalent to HFOs. HFFI ventilators use pneumatic valves, controlled mechanically or by a microprocessor, to generate pressure oscillations in the patient circuit. These oscillations occur around normal IMV breaths. Although exhalation is predominantly passive, a Venturi system in the exhalation valve generates a negative pressure swing during expiration to enhance lung emptying. In the high-frequency ventilation mode, the operator controls amplitude and frequency. Pressure amplitude varies around the IMV pressure that determines the MAP.

Mechanisms of gas exchange. HFOV, like conventional ventilation, increases Pao_2 by increasing ventilation to open, poorly ventilated lung units. The increase in Pao_2 depends on an increase in MAP. Whether HFOV can produce increases in oxygen comparable to those obtained with conventional ventilators at the same MAP remains to be determined. HFOV, like HFJV, is highly effective at removing CO_2 even at tidal volumes much less than dead space volume. The rate of CO_2 removal is tidal volume dependent, and tidal volume is also frequency dependent, so that CO_2 removal is proportional to the respiratory frequency times the tidal volume squared. The mechanism by which HFOV accomplishes CO_2

removal has not been determined, but there are several possible explanations:

- bulk convection of gas may occur in alveoli located near central airways;
- HFOV may facilitate molecular diffusion of gas within the terminal lung units;
- gas exchange may occur between lung units with uneven time constants (pendelluft);
- currents of gas flow may be set up with forward flow of fresh gas down the center of the airway and a net backward flow of alveolar/airway gas up the airway; and
- enhanced dispersion of both turbulent and laminar streams of gas flow (Taylor dispersion) may occur at high frequencies.

Indications

HMD. HFOV of experimental animals with HMD results in less lung injury than conventional ventilation. However, six randomized controlled trials comparing HFOV to conventional ventilation have been unable to demonstrate consistent differences in mortality, incidence of air leak, or incidence of BPD. In three of these trials, the incidence of severe IVH was greater in those infants receiving HFOV. Hence, inconsistent pulmonary benefits and concerns over increased neurologic complications continue to dampen enthusiasm for HFOV as a primary mode of ventilation for preterm infants with HMD.

PIE. Although some clinical data suggest that HFOV may be beneficial in treating preterm infants with PIE and respiratory failure, no randomized controlled trials have been performed to substantiate these clinical observations. In contrast, in a large randomized trial, the use of HFJV has been shown to be superior to conventional mechanical ventilation in the treatment of infants with PIE. Like HFJV, HFOV uses very small tidal volumes and should minimize alveolar distention.

Term infants with respiratory failure. Data supporting the use of HFOV in term infants with respiratory failure are limited. However, several retrospective studies and one prospective randomized trial have observed that HFOV improves gas exchange and reduces the need for extracorporeal membrane oxygenation (ECMO) in infants with severe respiratory failure. Infants with homogeneous lung diseases (respiratory distress syndrome, pneumonia) seem to respond to HFOV more often than those with a more heterogenous lung disease (eg, meconium aspiration syndrome).

Recent data also suggest that HFOV can augment the response to inhaled nitric oxide when an effective lung recruitment strategy is applied. In one large prospective randomized trial, the response rate for HFOV plus nitric oxide was significantly higher than that for either therapy alone, particularly in infants with respiratory distress syndrome or meconium aspiration syndrome.

In summary, the use of HFOV for infants with HMD is still controversial. At present, HFOV should probably be reserved for treatment of preterm infants with PIE and for term infants who are approaching ECMO criteria.

Techniques

Although each ventilator has individual design and performance characteristics, the management principles are similar.

Frequency settings. The optimal frequency results in minimal pressure swings and adequate gas exchange. In preterm infants, most investigators choose a frequency range between 10 and 15 Hz.

Tidal volume. Tidal volume is determined by observing chest wall movement and measuring blood gas tensions.

MAP. Oxygenation is determined by MAP. Typically, clinicians start with a MAP equal to or greater than that used on the conventional ventilator. MAP is increased incrementally until adequate oxygenation is achieved and the lungs appear adequately inflated on chest radiograph. HFOV is ineffective at recruiting atelectatic alveoli. Therefore, sighs must be given when the patient is initially placed on HFOV and after disconnection for suctioning. The sigh should be administered at a PIP similar to that used on the conventional ventilator.

Complications

Possible complications of HFOV include gas trapping, impairment of cardiovascular function, and an unexplained increased risk of IVH. Gas trapping is a major concern. At high frequencies, expiration may be shorter to the point that Te is less than 3 time constants, and gas trapping may occur. This may be a particular problem with ventilators that use a fixed Ti/Te. The interaction between the heart and lungs during HFOV is largely mediated by MAP and compliance of the respiratory system. Cardiac function may be impaired during HFOV as the MAP is elevated. The association between HFOV and IVH is primarily influenced by the HIFI trial. Meta-analysis of more recent studies, particularly those that used a high lung volume approach, suggests that HFOV is not associated with an increased risk of IVH. However, until this issue is resolved, HFOV should be used cautiously in infants <31 weeks' gestation in the first 3 days after birth.

By Donough J. O'Donovan, MD, Leonard E. Weisman, MD, and Thomas N. Hansen, MD

Nonventilatory Management of Respiratory Failure

Inhaled Nitric Oxide

Inhaled nitric oxide (iNO) can improve oxygenation in near-term babies who have failed conventional therapies for respiratory failure due to persistent pulmonary hypertension of the newborn (PPHN) and its associated diseases. The use of iNO in these infants also reduces the need for ECMO.

Physiology

Nitric oxide (NO) has been identified as an endogenous vasodilator. It is synthesized via NO synthase by the oxidation of the guanido nitrogen of L-arginine. NO then activates guanylate cyclase, leading to the production of cyclic guanosine monophosphate and subsequent vascular relaxation.

The physical properties of NO make it an excellent agent for the treatment of PPHN. It exists as a gas at room temperature and freely diffuses through cells. At very low concentrations (1 to 80 ppm), iNO has been shown in animal studies to relax pulmonary blood vessels, thereby reducing resistance, increasing pulmonary blood flow, and improving oxygenation. iNO has no effects on the systemic circulation. Once in the bloodstream, iNO binds tightly to hemoglobin, oxidizing the iron to form methemoglobin.

Indications

Randomized controlled trials support the use of iNO in term and near-term infants who are hypoxic, are on mechanical ventilation, and have an oxygen index (OI) >25. For these infants, iNO improves oxygenation in 50% and reduces the need for ECMO. No reduction of mortality has been seen with the use of iNO. Earlier use of iNO at a lower OI and, therefore, lesser illness severity is under investigation.

One clinical trial examined the use of iNO in infants with congenital diaphragmatic hernia. iNO was not beneficial in these infants.

The use of iNO in premature infants is controversial. Although there is improvement in oxygenation, improvement in long-term outcome has not been demonstrated.

Technique

iNO is administered to term and near-term infants with respiratory failure on mechanical ventilation. When iNO is blended into the infant's breathing circuit, great care must be taken to monitor its concentration and effects. Studies support the use of iNO in doses of 10 to 80 ppm. A dose-response trial demonstrated no difference in response between 5 and 80 ppm of iNO. Therefore, iNO should be administered at the lowest effective dose. Typically, iNO is started at 10 to 20 ppm and actively weaned when there is an effective response. Levels of NO, nitrogen dioxide (NO_2), and oxygen in the breathing circuit should be continuously monitored.

Precautions

The side effects of iNO are related to the dose and total exposure. Methemoglobin levels must be monitored, and methemoglobinemia can occur with high doses of iNO (≥80 ppm). If methemoglobin levels exceed 5%, iNO should be weaned or discontinued, and treatment with methylene blue (1 to 2 mg/kg) or ascorbic acid (100 mg/dose) should be considered. NO reacts with oxygen to form NO_2, exposure to which can cause pulmonary edema and bronchiolitis obliterans. NO_2 levels in the ventilator circuit should be monitored and kept below 5 ppm.

By Mary E. Wearden, MD, and Michael R. Gomez, MD

Extracorporeal Membrane Oxygenation

Severe respiratory or cardiovascular failure in an infant that does not respond to usual aggressive medical therapy has high mortality and high morbidity rates for the survivors. ECMO techniques can support an infant's ventilation and circulation, thereby allowing healing of the condition responsible for the illness.

Indications

Great care must be taken to select the appropriate candidates for ECMO therapy. In general, ECMO is most likely to be successful in infants with:

- gestational age ≥34 weeks; infants <34 weeks who are placed on ECMO and heparinized have a prohibitive risk of intracerebral hemorrhage;
- weight ≥2.0 kg; smaller infants require smaller cannulas, limiting ECMO flow;
- no preexisting bleeding disorders; systemic anticoagulation is necessary for ECMO and will be difficult to control with preexisting bleeding;
- reversible underlying disease; older infants with chronic lung diseases or conditions not likely to resolve in less than 2 weeks are less likely to benefit from ECMO; and
- normal hearts; infants should have a cardiac ultrasound examination before being placed on ECMO. The presence of congenital heart disease is no longer a contrain-

dication to ECMO. ECMO can be used to stabilize infants with anomalous venous drainage before surgery and can be used to support infants with pulmonary hypertension postoperatively.

ECMO is typically used to treat respiratory failure from meconium aspiration syndrome, respiratory distress syndrome, pneumonia and sepsis, PPHN, and selected forms of congenital heart disease, both preoperatively and postoperatively. The benefits of ECMO to infants with congenital diaphragmatic hernia remain controversial.

ECMO criteria are designed to select those infants with a high risk of death or severe adverse outcome. Although there is some variation among centers, criteria usually include some measure of inadequate oxygenation despite maximal support. Since ventilatory expertise and outcomes vary among institutions, each program may have to develop its own ECMO criteria. In general, these include criteria that identify infants with an 80% mortality.

Technique

ECMO is not a cure for cardiorespiratory failure. It simply supports ventilation or circulation until the organs recover. There are two general techniques for ECMO: venoarterial and venovenous. Both techniques use the same basic ECMO system, consisting of a roller pump, membrane oxygenator, and heat exchanger connected in series and primed with heparinized blood.

For venoarterial ECMO, a catheter is inserted in the right internal jugular vein with its tip in the right atrium, and another catheter is inserted in the right common carotid artery with its tip in the arch of the aorta. The infant is anticoagulated with a bolus of heparin and is connected to the circuit. Poorly oxygenated blood is drained from the right atrium; pumped through the ECMO system, where oxygen is added and carbon dioxide is removed; and then returned to the aorta via the right internal carotid artery, thus bypassing the entire pulmonary circulation. After the infant is connected to the circuit, the flow is slowly increased to about 150 mL/kg/min, after which the mechanical ventilator can be reduced to decrease the exposure to oxygen toxicity, barotrauma, and volutrauma. Typical settings may be 30% oxygen and low respiratory rate and PIP so that the lung can begin to recover. The Pao_2 is maintained between 50 to 70 mm Hg by adjusting the ECMO flow. The infant receives a continuous infusion of heparin to maintain a clotting time 2 to 3 times normal. Platelets are transfused to maintain the platelet count above 100,000/mm³. After 4 to 5 days of ECMO, when there is evidence that the underlying condition is improving, the infant is weaned by gradually reducing the circuit flow while the ventilator settings are increased as needed. After a brief trial off, the infant can be decannulated. In addition to supporting oxygenation and providing for CO_2 removal, venoarterial ECMO offers considerable circulatory support.

Venovenous ECMO is also performed by draining blood from the right atrium, but the oxygenated blood is then returned to the venous system either by a second cannula site or a double-lumen cannula in the right atrium. This technique is not true bypass. Although it can support oxygenation and accomplishes CO_2 removal, it typically does not support circulation. Also, because of some venous recirculation, it is less efficient at oxygen delivery than venoarterial ECMO. The advantage of venovenous ECMO is that the carotid artery is spared.

Outcome

From 1981 through 1995, more than 13,974 infants received ECMO therapy, with a 73% overall survival in a group with a high predicted mortality. The best survival rate, approaching 90%, is in infants with medical conditions (meconium aspiration, pulmonary hypertension); the poorest survival rate (58%) is in infants with the surgical condition of diaphragmatic hernia. A recent randomized controlled trial conducted in the United Kingdom demonstrated a reduced risk of death or severe disability when ECMO was available to infants with severe lung diseases.

Complications

The most serious complications of ECMO are related to the central nervous system, with intracranial bleeding or cerebral infarcts occurring in 17% of infants. Other, less frequent complications include sepsis, hemorrhage at surgical or gastrointestinal sites, and complications related to the ECMO circuit, especially clots. Because infants who require ECMO have severe underlying cardiopulmonary disturbances, the effects on neurologic outcome are difficult to determine. Follow-up has not identified any unique complications among ECMO survivors, but only follow-up into adulthood will determine the ultimate effects of neck vessel ligation.

By Alicia A. Moïse, MD, and Michael R. Gomez, MD

Suggested Readings

Initial Stabilization

Bloom RS, Cropley C, and the AHA/AAP Neonatal Resuscitation Steering Committee, eds. *Textbook of Neonatal Resuscitation.* American Heart Association and American Academy of Pediatrics, 1995.

Disorders of the neonate. Part II: In: Winters RW, ed. *The Body Fluids in Pediatrics.* Boston, Little, Brown Co, 1973, pp 185-348.

Goddard-Finegold J: Experimental models of intraventricular hemorrhage. In: Pape KE, Wigglesworth JS, eds. *Perinatal Brain Lesions.* Boston, Blackwell Scientific Publications, 1989, pp 115-133.

Oxygen Use and Monitoring

Adams JM, Murfin K, Mort J, et al: Detection of hyperoxemia in neonates by a new pulse oximeter. *Neonatal Intensive Care* 1994;42-45.

Brunstler I, Enders A, Versmold HT: Skin surface Pco_2 monitoring in newborn infants in shock: effect of hypotension and electrode temperature. *J Pediatr* 1982;100:454.

Bucher HU, Fanconi S, Baeckert P, et al: Hyperoxemia in newborn infants: detection by pulse oximetry. *Pediatrics* 1989;84:226-230.

Clark JS, Votteri B, Ariagno RL, et al: Noninvasive assessment of blood gases. *Am Rev Respir Dis* 1992;145:220-232.

Cochran WD: Umbilical artery catheterization. In: Report of the 69th Ross Conference on Pediatric Research, *Iatrogenic Problems in Neonatal Intensive Care.* Columbus, Ross Laboratories, 1976.

Editorial: Blood gas monitors: justifiable enthusiasm with a note of caution. *Am J Respir Crit Care Med* 1994;149:850-851.

Hansen TN, Tooley WH: Skin surface carbon dioxide tension in sick infants. *Pediatrics* 1979;64:942.

Huch R, Huch A, Albani M, et al: Transcutaneous Po_2 monitoring in routine management of infants and children with cardiorespiratory problems. *Pediatrics* 1976;57:681.

Jackson JC, Truog WE, Watchko JF, et al: Efficacy of thromboresistant umbilical artery catheters in reducing aortic thrombosis and related complications. *J Pediatr* 1987;110:102.

Jennis MS, Peabody JL: Pulse oximetry: an alternative method for the assessment of oxygenation in newborn infants. *Pediatrics* 1987;79:524.

Landers S, Hansen TN: Skin surface oxygen monitoring. *Perinatol Neonatol* 1984;8:39.

Moïse A, Landers S, Fraley K: Colonization and infection of umbilical catheters in newborn infants. *Pediatr Res* 1986;20:400A. Abstract.

Neal WA, Reynolds JW, Jarvis CW, et al: Umbilical artery catheterization: demonstration of arterial thrombosis by aortography. *Pediatrics* 1972; 50:6.

Poets CF, Southall DP: Noninvasive monitoring of oxygenation in infants and children: practical considerations and areas of concern. *Pediatrics* 1994;93:737-744.

Poets CF, Wilken M, Seidenberg J, et al: Reliability of a pulse oximeter in the detection of hyperoxemia. *J Pediatr* 1993;122:87-90.

Pologe JA: Pulse oximetry: technical aspects of machine design. *Int Anesthesiol Clin* 1987;25:137.

Ramanathan R, Durand M, Larrazabal C: Pulse oximetry in very low birth weight infants with acute and chronic lung disease. *Pediatrics* 1987;79:612.

Rodriguez LR, Kotin N, Lowenthal D, et al: A study of pediatric house staff's knowledge of pulse oximetry. *Pediatrics* 1994;93:810-813.

Symanski MR, Fox HA: Umbilical vessel catheterization: indications, management, and evaluation of the technique. *J Pediatr* 1972;80:820.

Wukitsch MW: Pulse oximetry: historical review and Ohmeda functional analysis. *Int J Clin Monit Comput* 1987;4:161.

Management of the Airway

Bizzle TL, Kotas TV: Positive pressure hand ventilation: potential errors in estimating inflation pressures. *Pediatrics* 1983;72:122.

Cotton RT, Seid AB:. Management of the extubation problem in the premature child: anterior cricoid split as an alternative to tracheotomy. *Ann Otol Rhinol Laryngol* 1980;89:508.

Donn SM, Blane CE: Endotracheal tube movement in the preterm neonate: oral versus nasal intubation. *Ann Otol Rhinol Laryngol* 1985; 84:18.

Duke PM, Coulson JD, Santos JI, et al: Cleft palate associated with prolonged orotracheal intubation in infancy. *J Pediatr* 1976;89:990.

Fan LL, Flynn JW, Pathak DR: Risk factors predicting laryngeal injury in intubated neonates. *Crit Care Med* 1983;11:431.

Fanconi S, Duc G: Intratracheal suctioning in sick preterm infants: prevention of intracranial hypertension and cerebral hypoperfusion by muscle paralysis. *Pediatrics* 1987;79:538-543.

Greisen G, Frederiksen PS, Hertel J, et al: Catecholamine response to chest physiotherapy and endotracheal suctioning in preterm infants. *Acta Paediatr Scand* 1985;74:525.

Jung AL, Thomas GK: Stricture of the nasal vestibule: a complication of nasotracheal intubation in newborn infants. *J Pediatr* 1974;85:412.

McMillan DD, Rademaker AW, Buchan KA, et al: Benefits of orotracheal and nasotracheal intubation in neonates requiring ventilatory assistance. *Pediatrics* 1986;77:39.

Miller KE, Edwards DK, Hilton S, et al: Acquired lobar emphysema in premature infants with bronchopulmonary dysplasia: an iatrogenic disease? *Pediatr Radiol* 1981;138:589.

Moylan FMB, Seldin EB, Shannon DC, et al: Defective primary dentition in survivors of neonatal mechanical ventilation. *J Pediatr* 1980; 96:106.

Perlman J, Thach B: Respiratory origin of fluctuations in arterial blood pressure in premature infants with respiratory distress syndrome. *Pediatrics* 1988;81:399-403.

Sherman JM, Lowitt S, Stephenson C, et al: Factors influencing acquired subglottic stenosis in infants. *J Pediatr* 1986;109:322.

Simbruner G, Coradello H, Fodor M, et al: Effect of tracheal suction on oxygenation, circulation, and lung mechanics in newborn infants. *Arch Dis Child* 1981;56:326.

Tarnow-Mordi W: Is routine endotracheal suction justified? *Arch Dis Child* 1991;66:374-375.

Wimberley PD, Lou HC, Pedersen H, et al: Hypertensive peaks in the pathogenesis of intraventricular hemorrhage in the newborn. Abolition by phenobarbitone sedation. *Acta Paediatr Scand* 1982;71:537-542.

Wung JT, Driscoll JM, Epstein RA, et al: A new device for CPAP by nasal route. *Crit Care Med* 1975;3:76.

Surfactant Administration

Bloom BT, Delmore P, Kattwinkel J: Surfactant prophylaxis increases costs at > 30 weeks. *Pediatr Res* 1994;35:1286A.

Bloom BT, Kattwinkel J, Hall RT, et al: Comparison of Infasurf (calf lung surfactant extract) to Survanta (beractant) in the treatment and prevention of respiratory distress syndrome. *Pediatrics* 1997;100:31-38.

Clark RH, Auten RL, Peabody J: A comparison of the outcomes of neonates treated with two different natural surfactants. *J Pediatr* 2001;139:828-831.

Curosurf package insert. Napa, California: Dey, February 2000.

Exosurf package insert. Research Triangle Park, North Carolina: Glaxo Wellcome Inc, January 1998.

Hudak ML, Martin DJ, Egan EA, et al: A multicenter randomized masked comparison trial of synthetic surfactant versus calf lung surfactant extract in the prevention of neonatal respiratory distress syndrome. *Pediatrics* 1997;100:39-50.

Infasurf package insert. Amherst, New York: Forest Pharmaceuticals, Inc, July 1998.

Lendig JW, Notter RH, Cox C, et al: A comparison of surfactant as immediate prophylaxis and as rescue therapy in newborns of less than 30 weeks' gestation. *N Engl J Med* 1991;324:865-871.

Segerer H, Van Gelder W, Angenent FWM, et al: Pulmonary distribution and efficacy of exogenous surfactant in lung-lavaged rabbits are influenced by the instillation technique. *Pediatr Res* 1993;34:490-494.

Sitler CG, Turnage CS, McFadden BE, et al: Pump administration of exogenous surfactant: effects on oxygenation, heart rate, and chest wall movement of premature infants. *J Perinatol* 1993;13:197.

Soll RF, McQueen MC: *Respiratory Distress Syndrome in Effective Care of the Newborn Infant.* Oxford University Press, 1992, pp 325-355.

Speer CP, Robertson B, Curstedt T, et al: Randomized European multicenter trial of surfactant replacement therapy for severe neonatal respiratory distress syndrome: single versus multiple doses of Curosurf. *Pediatrics* 1992;89:13-20.

Surfactant replacement therapy for severe neonatal respiratory distress syndrome: an international randomized clinical trial. Collaborative European Multicenter Study Group. *Pediatrics* 1988 Nov;82:683-91.

Survanta® package insert. Columbus, Ohio: Ross Products Division of Abbott Laboratories, October 1999.

Ueda T, Ikegami M, Rider ED, et al: Distribution of surfactant and ventilation in surfactant-treated preterm lambs. *J Appl Physiol* 1994;76:45-55.

Zola EM, Gunkel JH, Chan RK, et al: Comparison of three dosing procedures for administration of bovine surfactant to neonates with respiratory distress syndrome. *J Pediatr* 1993;122:453-459.

Positive Pressure Ventilatory Support

Bhutani VK, Abbasi S, Sivieri EM: Continuous skeletal muscle paralysis: effect on neonatal pulmonary mechanics. *Pediatrics* 1988;81:419.

Bland RD, Kim MH, Light MJ, et al: High frequency mechanical ventilation in severe hyaline membrane disease. An alternative treatment? *Crit Care Med* 1980;8:275-280.

Boros SJ, Matalon SV, Ewald R, et al: The effect of independent variations in inspiratory-expiratory ratio and end expiratory pressure during mechanical ventilation in hyaline membrane disease: the significance of mean airway pressure. *J Pediatr* 1977;91:794.

Chan V, Greenough A: Inspiratory and expiratory times for infants ventilator-dependent beyond the first week. *Acta Paediatr* 1994;83:1022.

Chatburn RL: Physiologic and methodologic issues regarding humidity therapy. *J Pediatr* 1989;114:416-420.

Crone RK, Favorito J: The effects of pancuronium bromide on infants with hyaline membrane disease. *J Pediatr* 1980;97:991.

Drew JH: Immediate intubation at birth of the very-low-birth-weight infant. *Am J Dis Child* 1982;136:207-210.

Edberg KE, Sandberg K, Silberberg A, et al: Lung volume, gas mixing, and mechanics of breathing in mechanically ventilated very low birth weight infants with idiopathic respiratory distress syndrome. *Pediatr Res* 1991; 30:496-500.

Enhorning G, Holm BA: Disruption of pulmonary surfactant's ability to maintain openness of a narrow tube. *J Appl Physiol* 1993;74:2922-2927.

Feihl F, Perret C: Permissive hypercapnia. How permissive should we be? *Am J Respir Crit Care Med* 1994;150:1722-1737.

Finer NN, Tomney PM: Controlled evaluation of muscle relaxation in the ventilated neonate. *Pediatrics* 1981;67:641.

Hansen TN, Corbet AJ, Kenny JD, et al: Effects of oxygen and constant positive pressure breathing on aADCO$_2$ in hyaline membrane disease. *Pediatr Res* 1979;13:1167.

Hansen TN, Corbet AJ: Principles of respiratory monitoring and therapy. In: Ballard R, Taeusch W, eds. *Schaffer's Diseases of the Newborn.* WB Saunders, 1991, pp 488-498.

Hanssler L, Tennhoff W, Roll C: Membrane humidification—a new method for humidification of respiratory gases in ventilator treatment of neonates. *Arch Dis Child* 1992;67:1182-1184.

Heicher DA, Kasting DS, Harrod JR: Prospective clinical comparison of two methods for mechanical ventilation of neonates: rapid rate and short inspiratory time versus slow rate and long inspiratory time. *J Pediatr* 1981; 98:957.

Henry GW, Stevens DC, Schreiner RL: Respiratory paralysis to improve oxygenation and mortality in large newborn infants with respiratory distress. *J Pediatr Surg* 1979;14:761.

Herman S, Reynolds EO: Methods for improving oxygenation in infants mechanically ventilated for severe hyaline membrane disease. *Arch Dis Child* 1973;48:612-617.

John E, Ermocilla R, Golden J, et al: Effects of gas temperature and particulate water on rabbit lungs during ventilation. *Pediatr Res* 1980;14:1186-1191.

Kano S, Lanteri CJ, Pemberton PJ, et al: Fast versus slow ventilation for neonates. *Am Rev Respir Dis* 1993;148:578-584.

Landers S, Hansen TN, Corbet AJ, et al: Optimal constant positive airway pressure assessed by aADCO$_2$ in hyaline membrane disease. *Pediatr Res* 1986;20:884-889.

Lesouef PN, England SJ, Bryan AC: Total resistance of the respiratory system in preterm infants with and without an endotracheal tube. *J Pediatr* 1984;104:108.

Levene MI, Quinn M: Use of sedatives and muscle relaxants in newborn babies receiving mechanical ventilation. *Arch Dis Child* 1992;67:870-873.

Liu M, Wang L, Li E, et al: Pulmonary surfactant will secure free airflow through a narrow tube. *J Appl Physiol* 1991;71:742-748.

Pietsch JB, Nagaraj HS, Groff DB: Necrotizing tracheobronchitis: a new indication for emergency bronchoscopy in the neonate. *J Pediatr Surg* 1985; 20:391.

Pollitzer MJ, Reynolds EO, Shaw DG: Pancuronium during mechanical ventilation speeds recovery of lungs of infants with hyaline membrane disease. *Lancet* 1981;1:346-348.

Primhak RA: Factors associated with pulmonary air leak in premature infants receiving mechanical ventilation. *J Pediatr* 1983;102:764.

Richardson P, Pace WR, Valdes E, et al: Time dependence of lung mechanics in preterm lambs. *Pediatr Res* 1992;31:276-279.

Sandberg K, Edberg KE, Benton W, et al: Surfactant improves gas mixing and alveolar ventilation in preterm lambs. *Pediatr Res* 1991;30:181-189.

Schreiner MS, Downes JJ, Kettrick RG, et al: Chronic respiratory failure in infants with prolonged ventilator dependency. *JAMA* 1987;258:3398.

Simbruner G: Inadvertent positive end-expiratory pressure in mechanically ventilated newborn infants: detection and effect on lung mechanics and gas exchange. *J Pediatr* 1986;108:589.

Spitzer AR, Fox WW: Postextubation atelectasis—the role of oral versus nasal endotracheal tubes. *J Pediatr* 1982;100:806.

Stewart AR, Finer NN, Peters KL: Effects of alterations of inspiratory and expiratory pressures and inspiratory/expiratory ratios on mean airway pressure, blood gases, and intracranial pressure. *Pediatrics* 1981;67:474.

Tarnow-Mordi WO, Griffiths ERP, Wilkinson AR: Low inspired gas temperature and respiratory complications in very low birth weight infants. *J Pediatr* 1989;114:438-442.

UK Collaborative Collective Trial Group: UK collaborative randomized trial of neonatal ECMO. *Lancet* 1996;348:75-82.

Vilstrup C, Gommers D, Bos JA, et al: Natural surfactant instilled in premature lambs increases lung volume and improves ventilation homogeneity within five minutes. *Pediatr Res* 1992;32:595-599.

Vilstrup CT, Bjorklund LJ, Larsson A, et al: Functional residual capacity and ventilation homogeneity in mechanically ventilated small neonates. *J Appl Physiol* 1992;73:276-283.

Wung JT, Driscoll JM, Epstein RA, et al: A new device for CPAP by nasal route. *Crit Care Med* 1975;3:76.

Wung JT: Respiratory management for low birth weight infants. *Neonatal Intensive Care* 1994;January/February:32-33.

Synchronized Intermittent Mandatory Ventilation

Baumer JH: International randomised controlled trial of patient triggered ventilation in neonatal respiratory distress syndrome. *Arch Dis Child Fetal Neonatal Ed* 2000;82:F5-F10.

Beresford MW, Shaw NJ, Manning D: Randomised controlled trial of patient triggered and conventional fast rate ventilation in neonatal respiratory distress syndrome. *Arch Dis Child Fetal Neonatal Ed* 2000;82:F14-F18.

Bernstein G, Mannino FL, Heldt GP, et al: Randomized multicenter trial comparing synchronized and conventional intermittent mandatory ventilation in neonates. *J Pediatr* 1996;128:453-463.

Bernstein G, Cleary JP, Heldt GP, et al: Response time and reliability of three neonatal patient-triggered ventilators. *Am Rev Respir Dis* 1993;148:358-364.

Bernstein G, Heldt GP, Mannino FL: Increased and more consistent tidal volumes during synchronized intermittent mandatory ventilation in newborn infants. *Am J Respir Crit Care Med* 1994;150:1444-1448.

Cleary JP, Bernstein G, Mannino FL, et al: Improved oxygenation during synchronized intermittent mandatory ventilation in neonates with respiratory distress syndrome: a randomized, crossover study. *J Pediatr* 1995; 126:407-411.

Dimitriou G, Greenough A, Laubscher B, et al: Comparison of airway pressure-triggered and airflow-triggered ventilation in very immature infants. *Acta Paediatr* 1998;87:1256-1260.

Donn SM, Nicks JJ, Becker MA: Flow-synchronized ventilation of preterm infants with respiratory distress syndrome. *J Perinatol* 1994;14:90-94.

Donn SM, Sinha SK: Controversies in patient-triggered ventilation. *Clin Perinatol* 1998;25:49-61.

Greenough A, Milner AD, Dimitriou G: Synchronized mechanical ventilation for respiratory support in newborn infants. *Cochrane Database Syst Rev* 2000;(2):CD000456.

Hird MF, Greenough A: Randomized trial of patient triggered ventilation versus high frequency positive pressure ventilation in acute respiratory distress. *J Perinat Med* 1991;19:379-384.

Hummler H, Gerhardt T, Gonzalez A, et al: Influence of different methods of synchronized mechanical ventilation on ventilation, gas exchange, patient effort, and blood pressure fluctuations in premature neonates. *Pediatr Pulmonol* 1996;22:305-313.

Jarreau PH, Moriette G, Mussat P, et al: Patient-triggered ventilation decreases the work of breathing in neonates. *Am J Respir Crit Care Med* 1996; 153:1176-1181.

Laubscher B, Greenough A, Kavadia V: Comparison of body surface and airway triggered ventilation in extremely premature infants. *Acta Paediatr* 1997;86:102-104.

Rennie JM, South M, Morely CJ: Cerebral blood flow velocity variability in infants receiving assisted ventilation. *Arch Dis Child* 1987;62:1247.

Schulze A, Gerhardt T, Musante G, et al: Proportional assist ventilation in low birth weight infants with acute respiratory disease: a comparison to assist/control and conventional mechanical ventilation. *J Pediatr* 1999;135:339-344.

Visveshwara N, Freeman B, Peck M, et al: Patient-triggered synchronized assisted ventilation of newborns: report of a preliminary study and three years' experience. *J Perinatol* 1991;11:347-354.

High-Frequency Jet Ventilation

Boros SJ, Mammel MD, Coleman JM: Neonatal high-frequency jet ventilation: four years' experience. *Pediatrics* 1985;75:657.

Carlo WA, Beoglos A, Chatburn RL, et al: High-frequency jet ventilation in neonatal pulmonary hypertension. *Am J Dis Child* 1989;143:233.

Carlo WA, Chatburn RL, Martin RJ, et al: Decrease in airway pressure during high-frequency jet ventilation in infants with respiratory distress syndrome. *J Pediatr* 1984;04:101.

Froese AB, Bryan AC: State of the art: high-frequency ventilation. *Am Rev Respir Dis* 1987;135:1363-1374.

Keszler M, Donn SM, Bucciarelli RL, et al: Multicenter controlled trial comparing high-frequency jet ventilation and conventional mechanical ventilation in newborn infants with pulmonary interstitial emphysema. *J Pediatr* 1991;119:85-93.

Mammel MC, Gordon MJ, Connett JE, et al: Comparison of high-frequency jet ventilation and conventional mechanical ventilation in a meconium aspiration model. *J Pediatr* 1983;103:630.

Slutsky AS: Nonconventional methods of ventilation. *Am Rev Respir Dis* 1988;138:175.

Trindade W, Goldberg RN, Bancalari E, et al: Conventional vs high-frequency jet ventilation in a piglet model of meconium aspiration: comparison of pulmonary and hemodynamic effects. *Pediatrics* 1985;107:115.

Wiswell, TE, Graziani LJ, Kornhauser MS, et al: High-frequency jet ventilation in the early management of respiratory distress syndrome is associated with a greater risk for adverse outcomes. *Pediatrics* 1996;98:1035-1043.

High-Frequency Oscillatory Ventilation

Bancalari A, Gerhardt T, Bancalari E, et al: Gas trapping with high-frequency ventilation: jet versus oscillatory ventilation. *J Pediatr* 1987;110:617-622.

Bryan AC, Froese AB: Reflections on the HiFi trial. *Pediatrics* 1991;87:565-567.

Carter JM, Gerstmann DR, Clark RH, et al: High-frequency oscillatory ventilation and extracorporeal membrane oxygenation for the treatment of acute neonatal respiratory failure. *Pediatrics* 1990;85:159-164.

Clark RH, Dykes FD, Bachman TE, et al: Intraventricular hemorrhage and high-frequency ventilation: a meta-analysis of prospective clinical trials. *Pediatrics* 1996;98:1058-1061.

Clark RH, Gerstmann DR, Null DM, et al: Prospective randomized comparison of high frequency oscillatory and conventional ventilation in respiratory distress syndrome. *Pediatrics* 1992;89:5-12.

Clark RH, Gerstmann DR, Null DM: Pulmonary interstitial emphysema treated by high frequency oscillatory ventilation. *Crit Care Med* 1986;14:926-930.

Clark RH, Yoder BA, Sell MS: Prospective, randomized comparison of high-frequency oscillation and conventional ventilation in candidates for extracorporeal membrane oxygenation. *J Pediatr* 1994;24:447-454.

Cools F, Offringa M: Meta-analysis of elective high-frequency ventilation in preterm infants with respiratory distress syndrome. *Arch Dis Child Fetal Neonatal Ed* 1999;80:F15-F20.

deLemos R, Yoder B, McCurnin D, et al: The use of high-frequency oscillatory ventilation (HFOV) and extracorporeal membrane oxygenation (ECMO) in the management of the term/near term infant with respiratory failure. *Early Hum Dev* 1992;29:299-303.

Frantz ID, Wethammer J, Stark AR: High-frequency ventilation in premature infants with lung disease: adequate gas exchange at low tracheal pressure. *Pediatrics* 1983;71:483-488.

Frantz ID: High-frequency ventilation. In: *Neonatal Respiratory Diseases.* Associates in Medical Marketing Co., Newtown, PA, 1995;5:1.

Froese AB, Butler PO, Fletcher WA, et al: High-frequency oscillatory ventilation in premature infants with respiratory failure: a preliminary report. *Anesth Analg* 1987;66:814-824.

Gerstmann DR, DeLemos RA, Coalson JJ, et al: Influence of ventilatory technique on pulmonary baro-injury in baboons with hyaline membrane disease. *Pediatr Pulmonol* 1988;5:82-91.

Gerstmann DR, Minton SD, Stoddard RA, et al: The Provo multicenter early-HFOV trial: improved pulmonary and clinical outcomes in respiratory distress syndrome. *Pediatrics* 1996;98:1044-1057.

Hamilton PP, Onayemi A, Smyth JA, et al: Comparison of conventional and high frequency ventilation: oxygenation and lung pathology. *J Appl Physiol* 1983;55:131-138.

HiFi Study Group: High-frequency oscillatory ventilation compared with conventional mechanical ventilation in the treatment of respiratory failure in preterm infants. *N Engl J Med* 1989;320:88-93.

HiFO Study Group. Randomized study of high-frequency oscillatory ventilation in infants with severe respiratory distress syndrome. *J Pediatr* 1993; 122:609-619.

Keszler M, Donn SM, Bucciarelli RL, et al: Multicenter controlled trial comparing high-frequency jet ventilation and conventional mechanical ventilation in newborn infants with pulmonary interstitial emphysema. *J Pediatr* 1991;119:85-93.

Kinsella JP, Truog WE, Walsh WF, et al: Randomized, multicenter trial of inhaled nitric oxide and high-frequency oscillatory ventilation in severe, persistent pulmonary hypertension of the newborn. *J Pediatr* 1997;131: 55-62.

Marchak BE, Thompson WK, Duffty P, et al: Treatment of RDS by high-frequency oscillatory ventilation: a preliminary report. *J Pediatr* 1981; 99: 287-292.

Ogawa Y, Miyasaka K, Kawano T, et al: A multicenter randomized trial of high-frequency oscillatory ventilation as compared with conventional mechanical ventilation in preterm infants with respiratory failure. *Early Hum Dev* 1993;32:1-10.

Plavka R, Kopecky P, Sebron V, et al: A prospective randomized comparison of conventional mechanical ventilation and very early high frequency oscillatory ventilation in extremely premature newborns with respiratory distress syndrome. *Intensive Care Med* 1999;25:68-75.

Rettwitz-Volk W, Veldman A, Roth B, et al: A prospective, randomized, multicenter trial of high-frequency oscillatory ventilation compared with conventional ventilation in preterm infants with respiratory distress syndrome receiving surfactant. *J Pediatr* 1998;132:249-254.

Simma B, Fritz M, Fink C, et al: Conventional ventilation versus high-frequency oscillation: hemodynamic effects in newborn babies. *Crit Care Med* 2000;28:227-231.

Slutsky AS: Nonconventional methods of ventilation. *Am Rev Respir Dis* 1988;138:175.

Extracorporeal Membrane Oxygenation

Bartlett RH, Roloff DW, Cornell RG, et al: Extracorporeal circulation in neonatal respiratory failure: a prospective randomized study. *J Pediatr* 1985; 76:479.

Campbell LR, Bunyapen C, Holmes GL, et al: Right common carotid artery ligation in extracorporeal membrane oxygenation. *J Pediatr* 1988;113:110.

Cilley RE, Zwischenberger JB, Andrews AF, et al: Intracranial hemorrhage during extracorporeal membrane oxygenation in neonates. *J Pediatr* 1986;78:699.

Cornish JD, Heiss KF, Clark RH, et al: Efficacy of venovenous extracorporeal membrane oxygenation for neonates with respiratory and circulatory compromise. *J Pediatr* 1993;122:105-109.

Hirschl RB, Schumacher RE, Snedecor SN, et al: The efficacy of extracorporeal life support in premature and low birth weight newborns. *J Pediatr Surg* 1993;28:1336-1341.

Hocker JR, Simpson PM, Rabalais GP, et al: Extracorporeal membrane oxygenation and early-onset group B streptococcal sepsis. *Pediatrics* 1992;89:1-4.

Hofkosh D, Thompson AE, Nozza RJ, et al: Ten years of extracorporeal membrane oxygenation: neurodevelopmental outcome. *Pediatrics* 1991; 87:549-555.

Kanto WP: A decade of experience with neonatal extracorporeal membrane oxygenation. *J Pediatr* 1994;124:335-347.

Ogawa Y, Miyasaka K, Kawano T, et al: A multicenter randomized trial of high-frequency oscillatory ventilation as compared with conventional mechanical ventilation in preterm infants with respiratory failure. *Early Hum Dev* 1993;32:1-10.

O'Rourke PP, Crone RK, Vacanti JP, et al: Extracorporeal membrane oxygenation and conventional medical therapy in neonates with persistent pulmonary hypertension of the newborn: a prospective randomized study. *Pediatrics* 1989;84:957-963.

O'Rourke PP, Lillehei CW, Crone RK, et al: The effect of extracorporeal membrane oxygenation on the survival of neonates with high-risk congenital diaphragmatic hernia: 45 cases from a single institution. *J Pediatr Surg* 1991;36:147-152.

Ortega M, Ramos AD, Platzker AC, et al: Early prediction of ultimate outcome in newborn infants with severe respiratory failure. *J Pediatr* 1988; 113:744-747.

Wildin SR, Landry SH, Zwischenberger JB: Prospective, controlled study of developmental outcome in survivors of extracorporeal membrane oxygenation: the first 24 months. *Pediatrics* 1994;93:404-408.

Nitric Oxide

Donn SM: Alternatives to ECMO. *Arch Dis Child* 1994;70:F81-F83.

Edwards AD: The pharmacology of inhaled nitric oxide. *Arch Dis Child* 1995;72:F127-F130.

Finer NN, Etches PC, Kamstra B, et al: Inhaled nitric oxide in infants referred for extracorporeal membrane oxygenation: dose response. *J Pediatr* 1993;124:302-307.

Karamanoukian HL, Glick PL, Wilcox DT, et al: Pathophysiology of congenital diaphragmatic hernia. VIII. Inhaled nitric oxide requires exogenous surfactant therapy in the lamb model of congenital diaphragmatic hernia. *J Pediatr Surg* 1995;30:1-4.

Kinsella JP, Ivy DD, Abman SH: Inhaled nitric oxide improves gas exchange and lowers pulmonary vascular resistance in severe experimental hyaline membrane disease. *Pediatr Res* 1994;36:402-408.

Kinsella JP, McQueston JA, Rosenberg AA, et al: Hemodynamic effects of exogenous nitric oxide in ovine transitional pulmonary circulation. *Am J Physiol* 1992;263:H875-H880.

Kinsella JP, McQueston JA, Rosenberg AA, et al: Hemodynamic effects of exogenous nitric oxide in ovine transitional pulmonary circulation. *Am J Physiol* 1992;875-880.

Kinsella JP, Neish SR, Shaffer E, et al: Low-dose inhalational nitric oxide in persistent pulmonary hypertension of the newborn. *Lancet* 1992; 340:819-820.

Kinsella JP, Truog WE, Walsh WF, et al: Randomized, multicenter trial of inhaled nitric oxide and high-frequency oscillatory ventilation in severe, persistent pulmonary hypertension of the newborn. *J Pediatr* 1997;131:55-62.

Roberts JD Jr, Fineman JR, Morin FC III, et al: Inhaled nitric oxide and persistent pulmonary hypertension of the newborn. The Inhaled Nitric Oxide Study Group. *N Engl J Med* 1997;336:605-610.

Roberts JD, Polaner DM, Lang P, et al: Inhaled nitric oxide in persistent pulmonary hypertension of the newborn. *Lancet* 1992;340:818-819.

Shah N, Jacob T, Exler R, et al: Inhaled nitric oxide in congenital diaphragmatic hernia. *J Pediatr Surg* 1994;29:1010-1015.

Walker MW, Kinter MT, Roberts RJ, et al: Nitric oxide-induced cytotoxicity: involvement of cellular resistance to oxidative stress and the role of glutathione in protection. *Pediatr Res* 1995;37:41-49.

Zayek M, Cleveland D, Morin FC: Treatment of persistent pulmonary hypertension in the newborn lamb by inhaled nitric oxide. *J Pediatr* 1993; 122:743-750.

Chapter 11

Nutritional and Gastrointestinal Support for the Infant With Respiratory Distress

Nutritional Support

Nutrition is integral to the management of the infant with respiratory distress. Malnutrition affects respiratory function by impairment of cellular reactions, protective antioxidant mechanisms, immune defenses, and lung development. In addition, excessive carbohydrate administration may increase the workload of the lung. Consequently, it may be difficult to wean an infant with compromised lung function from ventilatory support if attention is not paid to nutritional well-being.

To achieve rates of nutrient accretion (Table 1) similar to those of the fetus, optimal acute and chronic nutrition for high-risk neonates must be maintained. In providing this nutritional support, the clinician must consider the neonate's limited body stores, increased energy expenditure, and potential nutrient-therapy interactions. The goal of nutritional support is to enable a body-weight gain of approximately 15 g/kg/d or, for neonates older than 35 weeks' gestation, ≥20 g/d.

This section focuses on the guidelines for the acute and chronic nutritional management of high-risk neonates, most of whom require respiratory support. This population includes the very-low-birth-weight (VLBW) infant (<1,500 g) and the larger, more mature infant with bronchopulmonary dysplasia (BPD).

Parenteral Nutrition

Immaturity or severe illness usually requires that total parenteral nutrition (TPN) be used as the initial mode of nutrition for the high-risk neonate. This support provides intravenous (IV) glucose, synthetic amino acids, electrolytes, minerals, vitamins, and lipids.

If begun within the first 3 days after birth, glucose plus amino acids has been shown to reverse negative nitrogen balance, increase protein synthesis rate, and elevate the serum concentrations of essential amino acids better than solutions containing only glucose. The amino acid solutions containing the greatest percentage of essential amino acids are currently Trophamine® and Aminosyn-PF®. These mixtures also appear to improve the solubility of calcium and phosphorus.

Inadequate intakes of calcium and phosphorus can lead to undermineralized bone, rickets, and fractures. Consequently, parenteral solutions must maintain good solubility and delivery of these minerals. Careful attention to factors influencing the solubility of calcium and phosphorus (eg, pH, temperature, calcium and phosphorus concentration, amino acid source and concentration) is a priority.

It is controversial whether the amino acid cysteine (supplemented as hydrochloride, 30 to 40 mg/g amino acids) is essential for high-risk neonates; nonetheless, addition of this amino acid lowers the pH, favoring the solubility of calcium and phosphorus. Occasionally, this results in a mild metabolic acidosis, which is treated with sodium or potassium acetate (1 to 3 mEq/dL); the use of sodium bicarbonate must be avoided in TPN solutions. To optimize solubility while the solution is mixed, phosphorus should be added before calcium.

Inadequate provision of essential fatty acids may affect growth, produce essential fatty acid deficiency, and hinder the production of pulmonary surfactants. Contemporary lipid infusions contain 10% or 20% lipid (1.1 kcal/mL and

Table 1: Comparison of Suggested Parenteral and Enteral Fluid, Energy, and Nutrient Intakes for Low-Birth-Weight Infants

Component (units)	Parenteral Intake (unit/kg/d)	Enteral Intake (unit/kg/d)
Water (mL)	150	150
Energy (kcal)	80-100	120-130
Protein (g)	3.0-3.5	3.5
Fat (g)	1-4	5-7
Carbohydrate (g)	16	12-14
Vitamin A (IU)	500	700-2,000
Vitamin D (IU)	160	400 IU/d
Vitamin E (IU)	2.8	5-25 IU/d
Vitamin K (μg)	80	7-9*
Thiamin (vitamin B_1) (μg)	350	20-40 μg/d
Riboflavin (vitamin B_2) (μg)	150	60 μg/d
Pyridoxine (vitamin B_6) (μg)	180	35-60 μg/d
Vitamin B_{12} (μg)	0.3	0.1-0.5 μg/d
Niacin (mg)	6.8	0.8 mg/d
Folic acid (μg)	56	50 μg/d
Sodium (mEq)	2-4	2-8
Potassium (mEq)	2-3	2-3
Chloride (mEq)	2-3	2-3
Calcium (mg)	80-120	200-220
Phosphorus (mg)	60-90	100-110

Component (units)	Parenteral Intake (unit/kg/d)	Enteral Intake (unit/kg/d)
Magnesium (mg)	9-10	7-10
Zinc (μg)	350-450	1,000-2,000
Copper (μg)	65	65-300
Chromium (μg)	0.4	0.1-0.4
Manganese (μg)	10	7.5
Selenium (μg)	2	1-2

*Vitamin K, 0.5 to 1.0 mg at birth.

The following conversion factors are used:

Ca	40 mg = 1 mmol = 2 mEq
P	31 mg = 1 mmol
Mg	24 mg = 1 mmol = 2 mEq
Na	23 mg = 1 mmol = 1 mEq
K	39 mg = 1 mmol = 1 mEq
Cl	35 mg = 1 mmol = 1 mEq
Vitamin A	1 μg retinol = 3.33 IU vitamin A = 6 μg β-carotene = 1.83 μg retinyl palmitate = 1 retinol equivalent
Vitamin E	1 mg α-tocopherol = 1 IU vitamin E
Vitamin D	1 μg vitamin D (cholecalciferol) = 40 IU vitamin D (cholecalciferol)
Niacin	1 mg niacin = 1 niacin equivalent = 60 mg tryptophan

Schanler RJ: The low-birth-weight infant. In Walker WA, Watkins JB: *Nutrition in Pediatrics.* 2nd ed. Malden, MA, Blackwell Science, Inc, 1996. p. 393.

Table 2: Energy Distribution From Total Parental Nutrition*

Component	kcal/dL	mL/kg per day	kcal/kg per day	% kcal
Glucose (12.5%)	42.5	130	55.3	52%
Amino acids (2.4%)	9.6	—	11.4	11%
Lipids (20.0%)	—	20	40.0	37%
Totals	**52.1**	**150**	**106.7**	**100%**

*Maintain similar balance of nonprotein calories

2.0 kcal/mL, respectively) in blends of soy and safflower oils, predominantly as the essential fatty acids linoleic and linolenic acids. A 20% lipid emulsion infused throughout a 24-hour period produces lower serum triglycerides than a 10% emulsion, despite similar lipid intakes.

Twenty percent intralipid emulsion is usually initiated no later than the fifth day after birth at 5 mL/kg/d (1 g/kg/d) and advanced by increments of 5 to 10 mL/kg/d (1 to 2 g/kg/d), with a goal of 20 mL/kg/d (4 g/kg/d). Triglyceride concentrations should be monitored carefully in infants with severe respiratory disease. Infants on extracorporeal membrane oxygenation (ECMO) may require a separate IV for lipids, since lipids may cause cracked hubs when infused through the ECMO circuit.

Peripheral TPN solutions of 12.5% glucose and 2.2% amino acids infused at 130 mL/kg/d, when coadministered with IV lipid at 4 g/kg/d (20 mL/kg/d), provide a balanced distribution of calories and optimal weight gain (Tables 2 and 3). The quantity of protein, however, may be increased (up to 4 g/kg/d) during times of increased losses or increased nitrogen demands, such as those following necrotizing enterocolitis (NEC) or gastrointestinal surgery.

The distribution of lipid calories is important and should parallel that in enteral nutrition—approximately 45% to 50% glucose, 40% to 50% lipid, and 10% to 15% protein. There are 3.4 kcal/g in glucose, 9 kcal/g in lipid, and 4 kcal/g in amino acid. High-glucose-containing TPN solutions (glucose providing more than 50% of calories or >12 mg/kg/min) may increase carbon dioxide production and raise the P_{CO_2}.

Nursery guidelines for TPN should specify biochemical monitoring to avoid toxicity or deficiencies (Table 4). These should include protein and calorie status (albumin and blood urea nitrogen [BUN]) and renal (BUN, creatinine, and electrolytes), bone (calcium, magnesium, phosphorus, and alkaline phosphatase), and liver function tests (fractionated bilirubins, alanine transaminase [ALT], and gamma glutaryl transferase [GGT]).

Enteral Nutrition

Enteral nutrition should be initiated as soon as clinical stability allows. The TPN-associated risks of cholestatic jaundice, undermineralized bone, and infection are lessened with enteral feeding. Small volumes of 'trophic' milk feedings (10 to 20 mL/kg/d) can safely be initiated in most infants once physiologic stability in the infant is achieved—as early as the first few days after birth—even in conjunction with mechanical ventilation or indwelling umbilical catheters. For the high-risk neonate, enteral nutrition has been shown to stimulate gastrointestinal trophic hormones, motor activity, and intestinal development and to improve feeding tolerance, growth, and biochemical markers of nutritional status. As the infant matures and feeding tolerance improves, the volume is advanced in increments of 10 to 20 mL/kg/d to achieve full enteral feeding of 150 mL/kg/d. As milk volume increases, the TPN fluids are diminished accordingly.

Table 3: Neonatal Parenteral Nutrition*

	per 100 mL	per 130 mL/kg/d
Glucose (g)	12.5	16.25
Amino acids (g)	2.4	3.1
NaCl (mEq)	2.6	3.4
Ca gluconate (mEq)	3.0	3.9
Ca gluconate (mg Ca)	60	78
$MgSO_4$ (mEq)	0.5	0.65
$MgSO_4$ (mg)	6.0	7.8
K_2PO_4 (mmol P)	1.5	1.95
K_2PO_4 (mg P)	46	60
K_2PO_4 (mEq K)	2.2	2.9
KCl (mEq)	0.2	0.26
Total K (mEq)	(2.4)	(3.1)
Cysteine HCl	30 mg/g amino acids	30 mg/g amino acids

Vitamins will be added daily as 40% of a vial of M.V.I.® Pediatric (per kg) for infants <2.5 kg, and 1 vial for infants >2.5 kg.
Heparin is added to a concentration of 1 U/mL.
20% Intralipid (50% linoleic acid), 2.0 kcal/mL.

* Note: This is one example of a neonatal parenteral nutrition solution in a hospital that uses standard solutions. Other institutions may use different standard solutions or individual solutions for each infant.

Methods of enteral feeding

Milk is administered via orogastric, nasogastric, or transpyloric feeding tubes until the infant is sufficiently mature to coordinate sucking, swallowing, and breathing. There are advantages and disadvantages to each tube-feeding

Contents of 1 Vial (5 mL) of M.V.I.® Pediatric

Vitamin A	2,300 IU (690 µg)	Biotin	20 µg
Vitamin D	400 IU (10 µg)	Thiamin (B_1)	1.2 mg
Vitamin E	7 IU (7 mg)	Riboflavin (B_2)	1.4 mg
Vitamin K	200 µg	Niacin	17 mg
Vitamin C	80 mg	Pyridoxine (B_6)	1.0 mg
Pantothenic acid	5 mg	Folic acid	140 µg
		Vitamin B_{12}	1.0 µg

Information provided by Astra Pharmaceutical Products, Westborough, MA.

Daily Trace Element Requirements

Trace elements	Infant <2.5 kg (µg/kg/d)	Infant >2.5 kg (µg/kg/d)
Zinc	400	250; 100 if >3 mos
Copper	40	10
Chromium	0.4	0.1
Manganese	10	2.5
Selenium	2	1.5

Greene HL, Hambidge KM, Schanler R, et al: Guidelines for the use of vitamins, trace elements, calcium, magnesium, and phosphorus in infants and children receiving total parenteral nutrition: report of the Subcommittee on Pediatric Parenteral Nutrient Requirements from the Committee on Clinical Practice Issues of the American Society for Clinical Nutrition. *Am J Clin Nutr* 1988;48:1324-1342.

method. When compared with the transpyloric method, gastric feedings result in increased fat absorption (through stimulation of gastric lipase), increased potassium absorption, decreased risk of bacterial overgrowth and intestinal perforation, and decreased need for radiographic verification of tube

Table 4: Labs–Infants on TPN Exclusively

	Initially	Short-term	Long-term
Urine glucose	q void	q.d.	q.d.
Triglyceride	4 hours after each change in infusion rate, then (depending if jaundice, SGA*, sepsis, or severe cardiopulmonary disease):		
	q.o.d.	twice weekly	q wk
Lytes, glucose	q.d.	twice weekly	q wk
BUN, creatinine	q.d.	twice weekly	q wk then q o wk
Calcium	∅	q wk	q o wk
Mg, PO$_4$, and Alk Phos	∅	q wk	q o wk
Albumin (and prealbumin)	∅	q wk	q o wk
Bilirubin U/C, ALT, GGT	∅	q o wk	q o wk

*SGA = small for gestational age

position. Transpyloric feedings are used in infants who have failed the orogastric method, usually because of dysmotility and poor gastric emptying. This method may decrease the risk of milk aspiration.

Milk may be infused either continuously or intermittently (every 2 to 4 hours). The continuous infusion method has been assumed to be associated with lower energy expenditure, improved pulmonary function, and greater nutrient absorption. However, more recent studies found better feeding tolerance and weight gain with no adverse effect on pulmonary function in VLBW infants fed by the intermittent bolus method. Also, gastrointestinal hormonal stimulation and glucose tolerance have been shown to be more physiologic when the intermittent feeding method is used. Thus, for VLBW infants at this institution, feedings are now initiated with the intermittent bolus method. As the infant achieves physiologic stability, nonnutritive feeding and skin-to-skin contact between the parent and infant are introduced to prepare the infant to learn to feed orally. Oral feeding generally is introduced after attainment of complete tube feeding but more often is not completely achieved until 35 weeks. Infants older than 35 weeks and greater than 2,000 g body weight can usually achieve all oral feedings.

Human milk

Human milk is the most frequent choice of feeding in most nurseries. Data are emerging to suggest that human milk improves nutrient absorption, stimulates gastrointestinal function, and benefits host defense. The protein composition is whey dominant (70% whey, 30% casein) (Tables 5 and 6). The whey-protein fraction tends to be more soluble and more easily digested compared with casein, and it contains the host-defense proteins: lactoferrin, secretory IgA, and lysozyme. Milk produced during the initial 2 to 4 weeks of lactation, or preterm milk, usually has a greater protein content than term milk, but this declines during lactation. Therefore, optimal intakes of protein may be a concern after the first 2 weeks of feeding.

Fat absorption from human milk generally is excellent because of the presence of human milk lipase and the unique packaging of fatty acids in the fat globule (the particular arrangement of fatty acids on the glycerol backbone improves their availability for enzymatic cleavage). The presence of cholesterol is important for membrane stability. Very-long-chain polyunsaturated fatty acids (eg, docosahexaenoic acid [DHA], arachidonic acid), which are present in human milk,

Table 5: Nutritional Components of Human Milk, Fortified Human Milk, and Commercial Formula

	Human Milk	Fortified Human Milk	Premie Formulas*	Term Formulas*		
Energy (kcal/oz)	~20	~24	24	20	24	27
(kcal/dL)	~67	~81	81	67	81	91
Protein (g/dL)	1.0	2.0	2.4	1.4	1.7	1.9
Protein calories (%)	6%	10%	12%	8%	8%	8%
Fat (g/dL)	3.5	3.9	4.0	3.5	4.31	4.8
MCT (%)	2	11	40-50	2	2	2
Fat calories (%)	52%	45%	44%	48%	48%	48%
Carbohydrate (g/dL)	7.0	8.8	8.9	7.3	8.9	9.9
Lactose (%)	100	80	40-50	100	100	100
CHO calories (%)	42%	45%	44%	43%	43%	43%
Calcium (mg/dL)	26	143	131	52	63	71
Phosphorus (mg/dL)	14	81	67	35	43	48
Sodium (mEq/dL)	0.9	1.5	1.3	0.8	1.0	1.1
Potassium (mEq/dL)	1.3	2.9	2.1	1.9	2.3	2.5
Chloride (mEq/dL)	1.6	2.6	2.0	1.2	1.4	1.6
Zinc (mg/dL)	0.3	1.3	1.2	0.5	0.8	0.9
Iron (mg/dL) (fortified)	0.03	0.35	1.4	1.2	1.5	1.6

but not bovine milk, are membrane constituents with a predilection for retinal membranes. Red blood cell concentrations of DHA, for example, remain elevated in infants fed human milk, but decline rapidly with formula feeding. In VLBW infants, an association has been seen between increased dietary DHA and visual evoked responses.

The concentration of fat in human milk rises during a single milk expression. The higher-fat-containing hind milk

Enriched Formulas*				Fortified Human Milk + Enriched	Premie 24 + Enriched*
22	24	27	30	30	30
74	81	91	100	100	100
2.0	2.2	2.5	2.7	2.9	2.8
11%	11%	11%	11%	11%	11%
4.0	4.3	4.9	5.6	5.3	5.3
20-25	20-25	20-25	20-25	40-50	40-50
48%	48%	48%	48%	47%	48%
7.8	8.7	9.6	10.4	10.5	10.8
40-50	40-50	40-50	40-50	40-50	40-50
42%	42%	42%	42%	42%	41%
83	97	102	106	165	161
48	53	58	63	93	87
1.1	1.2	1.4	1.4	1.9	1.7
2.0-2.7†	2.2-2.9†	2.5-3.3†	2.7-3.7†	3.6-3.8†	2.7-3.4†
1.6	1.8	2.0	2.2	3.1	2.4
0.9	1.0	1.1	1.2	1.6	1.5
1.3	1.5	1.6	1.8	0.83	1.8

(continued on next page)

often is used in high-risk infants to provide a greater energy intake and to promote weight gain. Mothers can be taught to fractionate their milk collection and bring only the hind milk to the nursery. (Mothers discard the first 2 to 3 minutes of milk that is expressed from each breast. The subsequently expressed milk is hind milk.)

Mineral absorption from human milk is high, but the quantity of calcium, phosphorus, and sodium is inadequate to meet

Table 5: Nutritional Components of Human Milk, Fortified Human Milk, and Commercial Formula
(continued)

	Human Milk	Fortified Human Milk	Premie Formulas*	Term Formulas*		
Vitamin D (IU/dL)	2	122	218	42	49	55
Vitamin A (IU/dL)	390	1,010	1,008	206	244	273
Renal solute (mOsm/dL)	7.0	14.3	15.1	9.8	11.5	12.8
Osmolality (mOsm/kg H_2O)	260	350	310	270	360	415

Fortified Human Milk = Similac® Human Milk Fortifier (HMF)
Premie Formulas = Similac® Special Care (Ross), Enfamil® Premature (Mead Johnson)
Term Formulas = Enfamil® (Mead Johnson), Similac® (Ross)
Enriched Formulas = NeoSure® (Ross), EnfaCare™ (Mead Johnson)
Fortified Human Milk + Enriched = Human Milk + 4 packets Similac® HMF per 100 mL, plus NeoSure® (Ross) or EnfaCare™ (Mead Johnson) [4 g/dL]

the greater needs of the VLBW infant, the infant who has chronically received TPN, or the infant who requires restricted fluid intake. For this reason, a multicomponent fortifier containing energy, protein, calcium, phosphorus, sodium, and multivitamins should be added to the milk (Tables 5 and 6). It is not uncommon for infants to require 160 to 200 mL/kg/d of fortified human milk. Human milk fortification continues until the infant reaches 2,000 g body weight and 35 weeks' postmenstrual age or until the infant achieves successful full oral feeding.

Optimizing nutrition with human milk fortifiers is important because human milk may have profound benefits

Enriched Formulas*				Fortified Human Milk + Enriched	Premie 24 + Enriched*
56	65	69	71	138	183
336	360	414	465	450	1,090
13.2	14.2	16.0	17.8	24.7	22.1
255	280	320	350	500	559

Premie 24 + Enriched = Similac® Special Care (Ross) or Enfamil®
Premature (Mead Johnson) + NeoSure® (Ross) or EnfaCare™
(Mead Johnson) [4 g/dL]
*   Numbers given are averages of the products listed.
†   Range of potassium (Ross > Mead Johnson)

for the high-risk infant's gastrointestinal function and host defense. A variety of proteins, peptides, hormones, and specific growth factors are responsible for better feeding tolerance and gastric emptying than those of formula-fed infants. In a recent study, VLBW infants fed fortified human milk had a lower incidence of late-onset sepsis and NEC and were discharged from the hospital earlier than infants fed preterm formula.

Commercial formulas

Several state-of-the-art enteral formulas are designed specifically for the high-risk neonate to avoid nutrient deficits and to compensate for the effects of immature intestinal function

Table 6: Nutrient Intakes From Milks for Premature Infants

	FEBM	Premie Formula 24	Enriched Formula 22
Volume (mL/kg/d)	150	150	150
Energy (kcal/kg/d)	120	120	110
Protein (g/kg/d)	3.0	3.5	3.0
% calories	10%	11%	11%
Fat (g/kg/d)	5.9	6.3	6.0
% calories	45%	47%	48%
Carbohydrate (g/kg/d)	13.2	13.2	12
% calories	45%	42%	41%
Calcium (mg/kg/d)	215	207	126
Phosphorus (mg/kg/d)	122	111	72
Sodium (mEq/kg/d)	2.25	1.8	1.7
Potassium (mEq/kg/d)	4.44	3.2-4.1*	3.0-4.1*
Chloride (mEq/kg/d)	3.9	2.9	2.6
Zinc (mg/kg/d)	2.0	1.8	1.4
Iron (mg/kg/d)–fortified	0.5	2.1	2.0
Vitamin D (IU/kg/d)	183	255	84
Vitamin A (IU/kg/d)	1,515	1,512	506

FEBM (fortified expressed breast milk)—Similac® Human Milk Fortifier/Enfamil® Human Milk Fortifier; 4 packets per 100 mL human milk.

(Tables 5 and 6). The quantity and quality of the nutrients are increased to match the high rate of fetal nutrient accretion. All products contain protein exceeding 3 g/kg/d. Most formulas have a whey:casein ratio of 60:40. Approximately 50% of the long-chain fats are replaced by medium-chain fatty acids. The

FEBM + Enriched 30	Premie 24 + Enriched 30	Enriched Formula 30
120	120	120
120	120	120
3.5	3.4	3.2
12%	11%	11%
6.3	6.4	6.6
47%	48%	48%
12.6	13.0	12.7
41%	41%	41%
199	193	136
112	104	78
2.4	2.1	1.7
4.3-4.6*	3.2-4.1*	3.2-4.4*
3.7	2.8	2.6
1.92	1.74	1.6
1.0	2.2	2.2
166	220	91
1,313	1,313	550

Premie Formula—Enfamil® Premature Formula/Similac® Special Care
Enriched Formula—NeoSure® (Ross)/EnfaCare™ (Mead Johnson)
*Range of potassium (Ross > Mead Johnson)

lactose content is reduced to approximately 50% by the addition of glucose polymers to lessen the osmolality and to accommodate the premature infant's immature lactase activity. All preterm formulas contain abundant calcium and phosphorus and an appropriate osmolality and renal solute load.

Table 7: Selected Enteral Dietary Supplements

Additive	Caloric content	Source
Glucose	3.4 kcal/g	dextrose
Polycose® powder (R)	3.8 kcal/g	glucose polymers
Polycose® liquid (R)	2.0 kcal/mL	glucose polymers
Corn oil	8.4 kcal/mL	LCT (34% EFA)
MCT oil (MJ)	7.7 kcal/mL	MCT (0% EFA)
Casec (MJ)	0.88 g protein/g	calcium caseinate
ProMod® (R)	0.76 g protein/g	whey protein concentrate

MCT = medium-chain triglycerides
LCT = long-chain triglycerides
EFA = essential fatty acids
R = Ross
MJ = Mead Johnson

Recognizing the nutritional quantity and quality differences among formulas for preterm infants and formulas for full-term infants is important. The latter contain significantly lower quantities of protein, calcium, phosphorus, vitamins, and trace elements. Soy-based formulas are not recommended for low-birth-weight infants because of poor protein quality and diminished mineral absorption. The hydrolysate-based formulas also have low levels of many minerals and generally are derived solely from casein.

Casein contains more aromatic and sulfur-containing amino acids, which are more difficult for the low-birth-weight infant to metabolize.

To achieve adequate weight gain, 150 to 160 mL/kg/d of milk is generally needed. The preterm formulas are initially administered in small volumes of 10 to 20 mL/kg/d; subsequently, the volume is increased by stepwise increments of 10 to 20 mL/kg/d.

Micronutrient Supplementation

Occasionally, supplementation with macronutrients (calories and protein; Table 7), or micronutrients (vitamins, minerals, and trace elements) may be necessary to provide an adequate intake and weight gain.

Infants on 150 to 160 mL/kg/d fortified human milk, Similac® Special Care with Iron (SSC), or Enfamil® Premature Formula with Iron (EPF) generally receive adequate amounts of calories, protein, vitamins, and trace elements (infants fed fortified human milk may require 180 to 200 mL/kg/d).

Iron can be provided using Fer-In-Sol® at 2 mg/kg/d elemental iron for infants on fortified human milk by 1 month of age.

Postdischarge Nutrition

Nutrition should always be discussed during discharge planning. Certain key questions need to be answered so that an appropriate nutrition plan can be devised. Some studies have shown that the use of enriched formulas fed to 12 months' corrected age is associated with improved growth.

More often, especially in infants with BPD, adequate intake is not achieved and biochemical markers of nutritional status reveal deficits. These infants cannot be discharged on a routine diet. If the infant is fed only formula, the enriched formulas (NeoSure® or EnfaCare™) can provide multinutrient needs. These formulas can be concentrated to 24- to 30-kcal/oz formulations to meet the need for fluid restriction. The

Table 8: Nutritional Assessment of the High-Risk Neonate

Growth		
Body weight gain	Plot on growth grid	daily
Rate of weight gain	15 g/kg/d or ≥20 g/d	weekly
Length	1 cm/wk	weekly
Head circumference	1 cm/wk	weekly
Biochemical		
Protein status	Albumin	q o wk
	BUN	q o wk
	Prealbumin	as needed
Mineral status	Ca, P, Alk Phos	q o wk
Anemia	Hemoglobin	weekly
	Reticulocyte count	weekly
Cholestasis	Fract. bilirubin ALT, GGT	>1 month on TPN
Poor growth with good intake	Zinc, Vitamin A	as needed

breast-feeding infant needs further attention. Unrestricted breast-feeding plus two to three feedings of the enriched formula, prepared as 24- to 30-kcal/oz formulations, may suffice. In all cases, follow-up visits for nutritional status are recommended at 1 week and 1 month after discharge. Rates of growth should exceed 20 g/d for weight and 0.7 cm/week for length and head circumference. Biochemical monitoring to assess mineral and protein status is indicated at these follow-up visits.

Table 9: Concentrating Infant Formula to 27 kcal/oz

	Standard 27	20 kcal + Oil	20 kcal + Polycose
Energy	90 kcal/dL	90 kcal/dL	90 kcal/dL
Fat	4.8 g/dL	6.6 g/dL	3.6 g/dL
	48% total cal	65% total cal	36% total cal
Carbo-hydrate	9.5 g/dL	6.7 g/dL	14.9 g/dL
	42% total cal	30% total cal	66% total cal
Protein	2.5 g/dL	1.4 g/dL	1.4 g/dL
	11% total cal	6% total cal	6% total cal

Note that the percentage of calories from protein is increased by concentrating a standard formula to 27 kcal/oz compared with adding calories as fat or carbohydrate. Adding only fat or carbohydrate results in an imbalance in calorie distribution.

Nutritional Assessment

Laboratory values and growth goals should be established and then routinely monitored when caring for high-risk neonates. Laboratory values used to monitor enteral nutrition include albumin, calcium, phosphorus, and alkaline phosphatase (initially every week, then every other week if feeding and clinical status have been stable) (Table 8). Monitoring prealbumin or BUN is helpful if assessment of acute changes in nutritional or clinical status is needed.

Finally, the high-risk infant should achieve an average weight gain of 15 g/kg/d during a week (or ≥20 g/d for the mature, >35 weeks' gestation infant), a head circumference gain of 1.0 cm per week, and serial increases in body or knee-to-heel length.

Chronic Nutritional Management

Chronic nutritional management is especially important in infants with BPD, who are often fluid restricted and receiving diuretics. Furthermore, the infant with BPD has increased energy expenditure and nutrient needs. With volume limitations of 100 to 130 mL/kg/d and increased metabolic demands, growth is often poor.

Calorie and protein supplements are available for addition to the infant's milk (Table 7). Caution is advised with this practice. Nutrient ratios (Table 9) can easily be altered inappropriately. Routine supplementation with glucose polymers, for example, can increase the carbohydrate load and can potentially increase the infant's respiratory quotient or cause lactic acidosis. Protein and other minerals important for linear skeletal growth can become diluted. For these reasons, multinutrient supplements should be used. These supplements may come in powder form, such as enriched formula powder (NeoSure® or EnfaCare™). The enriched formulas can be either added to fortified human milk or preterm formula or concentrated to provide 20- to 30-kcal/oz formulations. In infants with severe BPD who are over 6 months of age, selected formulas (30 kcal/oz) may be considered (see *Bronchopulmonary Dysplasia* section, Chapter 5). Solid foods using iron-enriched cereal and vitamin A-rich foods should also begin with 1 to 2 tsp/d to encourage development of oral motor skills.

Besides the usual parameters (Table 8), nutritional assessment should include the evaluation of fluid and electrolyte balance. Renal ultrasound imaging to rule out nephrocalcinosis and wrist radiographs to evaluate the possibility of rickets may also be warranted in some infants. Finally, growth goals should include chronologic and corrected age comparisons to national growth charts.

By Christina J. Valentine, MD, RD, Richard J. Schanler, MD, and Steven A. Abrams, MD

Gastrointestinal Support of Feeding Problems
Feeding Intolerance

The most common problem encountered when feeding VLBW infants is feeding intolerance. Markers commonly

Table 10: Commonly Used GI Medications

	Drug	Dose
Antacids and H₂ blockers	Aluminum hydroxide	0.5 to 1.0 mL/dose PO q 1 to 2 hours
	Aluminum hydroxide with magnesium hydroxide	0.5 to 1.0 mL/dose PO q 1 to 2 hours
	Ranitidine hydrochloride	1.5-2.0 mg/kg/dose q 6-12 hours PO 1.5 mg/kg dose q 6 hours IV
	Famotidine hydrochloride	0.5 mg/kg/dose q 8-12 hours PO/IV
Prokinetic agents	Metoclopramide hydrochloride	0.1 to 0.3 mg/kg/dose to max 0.5 mg/kg/dose q 6 to 8 hours PO,IV ac
	Bethanechol chloride	0.1 to 0.2 mg/kg/dose PO q 6 to 8 hours ac
Anticholestasis agents	Ursodiol (UDCA)	7.5 to 22.5 mg/kg/dose q 12 hours (stable in solution for 5 days after preparation)

used to evaluate this problem include the quantity of gastric residuals, incidence of emesis, and pattern of stooling. Signs of intolerance are residuals that are green, bloody, or greater than one half of the previous 3 hours' intake. *Any* occurrence of emesis is a concern, and the infant should be assessed.

A minimum initial evaluation should include an examination of the abdomen, the feeding tube placement, the baby's position, and a review of the child's medications. Stools that become frequent or loose, contain glucose, or have a low pH (<5.5) signal a need for evaluation for sepsis or intolerance of milk or medications.

If the initial evaluation is unremarkable, consideration should be given to decreasing the volume of feeds, changing the strength or type of milk, or changing the mode of feeding to a milk drip or a slow infusion over 60 to 120 minutes. Babies who have glucose-positive or acidic stools and who are shown to be sepsis-free should be investigated for the presence of malabsorption.

Gastroesophageal Reflux

Because of esophageal, antral, or duodenal dysfunction, many infants with chronic lung disease develop gastroesophageal reflux (GER). Although lower esophageal sphincter tone is decreased in preterm infants compared with term infants, GER in preterm infants appears to be related to transient increases in intra-abdominal pressure or abnormal duodenal activity. In addition, many congenital and acquired structural abnormalities of the gastrointestinal tract can present with vomiting. Thus, the initial evaluation of the infant with GER should include a barium swallow with visualization of the upper gastrointestinal tract. Because this radiographic study is performed under stressful artificial circumstances, it is not an adequate method to evaluate lower esophageal sphincter tone. If there are no anomalies and clinical evidence of reflux is present, a trial of histamine H_2-receptor antagonists or prokinetic agents is warranted (Table 10).

Intestinal Dysmotility

Delayed intestinal transit of nutrients is demonstrated by the presence of increased abdominal girth and poor stool output with or without the presence of gastric residuals. Better intestinal motor activity may be achieved by feeding full-strength, rather than dilute, formulas. Cereal or fiber may also enhance antral and intestinal motor activity, and prokinetic agents may improve transit (Table 10).

Ineffective Sucking

Although the sucking mechanism is present at 32 to 34 weeks' gestation, many infants who have chronic lung disease have difficulty sucking. Effective propulsion of oral nutrients requires that an infant exert both a coordinated effort and adequate strength of effort. To allow adequate opportunity for development of sucking skills, infants should be periodically offered 'pacifier practice,' or experience with nonnutritive sucking. At 32 to 34 weeks' gestation, oral feedings can be initiated. Infants who have difficulty establishing sucking skills may benefit from occupational therapy and speech pathology consultation and the establishment of a consistent feeding regimen.

Short Gut

Chronic inflammation, bacterial overgrowth, and malabsorption may occur in bowel-recovering NEC or surgical resection. The presence of acidic, glucose-positive stools and increased frequency or volume of stools may indicate that any or all of these problems exist. Smaller volume of milk drip feedings is frequently helpful. The clinician should consider zinc supplements and carefully follow protein nutrition laboratory values while maximizing protein delivery. Generally, it is more desirable in premature infants to continue using human milk or premature formulas; however, in some cases, predigested formulas are needed but may be a nutritional compromise. If intolerance persists when predigested formulas are fed, subspecialty consultation may be helpful.

Cholestasis

Cholestasis may occur in infants who have received chronic TPN. Introduction of small enteral feedings and decreased use of TPN may be helpful in reversing or reducing progression of cholestasis. Parenteral copper and manganese should be omitted or limited when cholestatis develops. Pharmacologic agents (Table 10) may also enhance hepatic clearance of bilirubin and reduce cholestasis.

By Diane Anderson, PhD, RD, CSP, FADA, and Carol L. Berseth, MD

Suggested Readings

Anderson DM, Kliegman RM: The relationship of neonatal alimentation practices to the occurrence of endemic necrotizing enterocolitis. *Am J Perinatol* 1991;8:62-67.

Anderson GC: Current knowledge about skin-to-skin (Kangaroo) care for preterm infants. *J Perinatol* 1991;11:216-226.

Berseth CL: Assessment in intestinal motility as a guide in the feeding management of the newborn. *Clin Perinatol* 1999;26:1007-1015.

Berseth CL, Nordyke CK: Manometry can predict feeding readiness in preterm infants. *Gastroenterology* 1992;103:1523-1528.

Biondillo (Hurst) N: *Breast-Feeding Your Hospitalized Baby.* Houston, Texas Children's Hospital, 1988.

Blondheim O, Abbasi S, Fox WW, et al: Effect of enteral gavage feeding rate on pulmonary functions of very low birth weight infants. *J Pediatr* 1993;122:751-754.

Brown RL, Wessel J, Warner BW: Nutrition considerations in the neonatal extracorporeal life support patient. *Nutr Clin Pract* 1994;9:22-27.

Carver JD, Wu PY, Hall RT, et al: Growth of preterm infants fed nutrient-enriched or term formula after hospital discharge. *Pediatrics* 2001;107:683-689.

DeVille K, Baker JH, Al-Tawil Y, et al: Motor responses and gastric emptying in preterm infants fed formula with varying concentrations and rates of infusion. *Am J Clin Nutr* 1989;68:103-108.

Edelman NH, Rucker RB, Peavy HH: Nutrition and the respiratory system. *Am Rev Respir Dis 1986*;134:347-352.

Friedman Z, Rosenberg A: Abnormal lung surfactant related to essential fatty acid deficiency in a neonate. *Pediatrics* 1979;63:855-859.

Gibson AT, Pearse RG, Wales JK: Knemometry and the assessment of growth in premature babies. *Arch Dis Child* 1993;69:498-504.

Grant J, Denne SC: Effect of intermittent versus continuous enteral feeding on energy expenditure in premature infants. *J Pediatr* 1991;118:928-932.

Hamill PV, Drizd TA, Johnson CL: Physical growth: National Center for Health Statistics percentiles. *Am J Clin Nutr* 1979;32:607-629.

Haumont D, Deckelbaum RJ, Richelle M, et al: Plasma lipid and plasma lipoprotein concentrations in low birth weight infants given parenteral nutrition with twenty or ten percent lipid emulsion. *J Pediatr* 1989;115:787.

Heird WC, Kashyap S, Gomez MR: Parenteral alimentation of the neonate. *Semin Perinatol* 1991;15:493-502.

Heldt GP: The effect of gavage feeding on the mechanics of the lung, chest wall, and diaphragm of preterm infants. *Pediatr Res* 1988;24:55-58.

Koenig WJ, Amarnath RP, Hench V, et al: Manometrics for preterm and term infants: a new tool for old questions. *Pediatrics* 1995;95:203-206.

Kurzner SI, Garg M, Bautista DB: Growth failure in infants with bronchopulmonary dysplasia: nutrition and elevated resting metabolic expenditure. *Pediatr* 1988;81:379-384.

Lucas A, Bishop NJ, King FJ, et al: Randomised trial of nutrition for preterm infants after discharge. *Arch Dis Child* 1992;67:324-327.

Macdonald PD, Skeoch CH, Carse H, et al: Randomized trial of continuous nasogastric, bolus nasogastric, and transpyloric feeding in infants of birth weight under 1400 g. *Arch Dis Child* 1992;67:429-431.

Meetze WH, Valentine C, McGuigan JE, et al: Gastrointestinal priming prior to full enteral nutrition in very low birth weight infants. *J Pediatr Gastroenterol Nutr* 1992;15:163-170.

Morales E, Craig LD, MacLean WC Jr: Dietary management of malnourished children with a new enteral feeding. *J Am Diet Assoc* 1991;91:1233.

Moskowitz SR, Pereira G, Spitzer A, et al: Prealbumin as a biochemical marker of nutritional adequacy in premature infants. *J Pediatr* 1983;102:749-753.

Neu J, Valentine C, Meetze W: Scientifically-based strategies for nutrition of the high-risk low birth weight infant. *Eur J Pediatr* 1990;150:2-13.

Orenstein SR: Controversies in pediatric gastroesophageal reflux. *J Pediatr Gastroenterol Nutr* 1992;14:338.

Rivera A Jr, Bell EF, Bier DM: Effect of intravenous amino acids on protein metabolism of preterm infants during the first three days of life. *Pediatr Res* 1993;33:106–111.

Schanler RJ: Suitability of human milk for the low-birthweight infant. *Clin Perinatol* 1995;22:207-222.

Schanler RJ, Shulman RJ, Lau C: Feeding strategies for premature infants: beneficial outcomes of feeding fortified human milk versus preterm formula. *Pediatrics* 1999;103:1150-1157.

Schanler RJ, Shulman RJ, Lau C, et al: Feeding strategies for premature infants: randomized trial of gastrointestinal priming and tube-feeding method. *Pediatrics* 1999;103:434-439.

Sondheimer JM: Gastroesophageal reflux: update on pathogenesis and diagnosis. *Pediatr Clin North Am* 1988;35:103.

Sosenko IRS, Frank L: Nutritional influences on lung development and protection against chronic lung disease. *Semin Perinatol* 1991;15:462-468.

Valentine CJ, Hurst NM, Schanler RJ: Hindmilk improves weight gain in low birth weight infants fed human milk. *J Pediatr Gastroenterol Nutr* 1994;18:474-477.

Vanderhoff JA: Short bowel syndrome. *Clin Perinatol* 1996;23:377-386.

Yunis KA, Oh W: Effects of intravenous glucose loading on oxygen consumption, carbon dioxide production, and resting energy expenditure in infants with bronchopulmonary dysplasia. *J Pediatr* 1989;115:127-132.

Ziegler EE: Trophic feeds. Nutrition of the very low birthweight infant. In: Ziegler EE, Lucas A, Moro GE: *Nestle Nutrition Workshop Series, Paediatric Programme.* Vol. 43, Nestec Ltd. Philadelphia, PA, Vevey/Lippincott Williams & Wilkins, 1999. pp. 233-244.

Chapter 12

Ethical Considerations

Parent-Physician Communication

Effective communication serves as a major cornerstone of support for parents during an infant's hospitalization. Initial parent-physician encounters are often limited to quick, informal discussions. But as soon as the infant is relatively stable, the physician should meet formally with the parents to achieve these goals: (1) to educate the parents in a general manner about their child's illness, (2) to identify the personal needs of the family and of others who may provide emotional support, (3) to clarify expectations for future communication and decision-making, (4) to identify key neonatal intensive care unit (NICU) personnel to the family, and (5) to demonstrate empathy and compassion. These formal meetings should occur in a calm environment away from the bedside to permit the parents and the physician to focus on the discussion; this is especially important for the initial encounter, which sets an important tone for the parent-physician interaction for the duration of the infant's hospitalization.

The acuity of the infant's care often determines the style of ongoing communication adopted by parents and the physician. Although communication can be provided informally by others caring for the infant, the physician should maintain consistent rapport with the family to ensure that accurate information is conveyed and to establish a sense of constancy and trust. Furthermore, the neonatologist must communicate with the infant's obstetrician and primary care pediatrician, because they often provide support to the family while the infant is acutely ill.

Table 1: Suggested Readings for Parents of Premature Infants

- Harrison H, Kositsky A: *The Premature Baby Book: A Parents' Guide to Coping and Caring in the First Years.* New York, St Martin's Press, 1983.

- Manginello FP, DiGeronimo TF: *Your Premature Baby. Everything You Need to Know About the Childbirth, Treatment, and Parenting of Premature Infants.* New York, John Wiley & Sons Inc, 1991.

- Shelov SP, Hannemann RE: *Caring for Your Baby and Young Child.* New York, Bantam Books, 1983.

- Dewyze J: *The Baby Came Early: A Moving Account of the Premature Birth of Her Child.* Ben-Simon Publications, 1986.

- Lafferty LE: *Born Early: A Premature Baby's Story for Children.* Songbird Publications, 1994.

- Murphy-Melas E, Tate D: *Watching Bradley Grow: A Story About Premature Birth.* Longstreet Press, 1996.

- Gotsch G: *Breastfeeding Your Premature Baby.* La Leche League International, 1990.

The physician should recognize that the family can develop any number of coping styles. Some may remain aloof, others may become confrontational, and still others may become overly dependent on caregivers. Although these adaptive styles may make communication difficult for the physician, consistent, ongoing interaction with the family should remain a priority in the daily care of the infant.

Extended family and friends can provide important support to the family. Family support should be buttressed by pastoral support, peer-support groups, social workers, and the infant's primary care providers. Personal family physicians can often provide additional background information and translate technical concepts. A library of consumer-oriented information is often available (Table 1).

Prenatal Counseling and Delivery Room Care

Many high-risk deliveries are identified prenatally, and neonatologists may be asked to provide consultation or parental education or to assist in decision making. When delivery is imminent, the physician's role is to prepare the family for the events that are anticipated at birth. Families may also wish to provide the neonatologist with specific directives about the extent of delivery room care for their infant. However, the physician should not make a commitment to the family to resuscitate or to withhold resuscitation until the infant can be evaluated.

Withholding Care

Do-Not-Resuscitate Orders

The process of informed consent requires that decision making be done in consultation with the family. These conversations should be routinely documented in the medical record. When the physician and parents agree that resuscitation should not be provided to an infant if cardiac arrest occurs, a note must be written in the chart attesting to the virtual futility of the infant's survival. Orders not to resuscitate the infant must be written in the chart by the attending physician and communicated to the staff. It should be emphasized to families that a do-not-resuscitate (DNR) order pertains only to this single aspect of care and that attention to other needs will continue to be provided.

Occasionally, parents and physicians disagree about treatment plans. Typically, these conflicts arise when families object to the continued provision or escalation of care. It is important that physicians thoroughly discuss their decision-making process with families and offer consultation for second opinions. Most pediatric hospitals offer consultation services to assist families and physicians in resolving these conflicts. While committee decisions are not legally binding, formal case review can give family members an opportunity to vent their frustrations and can permit the establishment of consensus. Sometimes, conflicts arise when families demand that ongoing or escalating care be provided despite physician recommendations to the contrary. These are special circumstances in which the physician has determined that continued care is futile and painful. Because it is difficult to determine what constitutes a futile situation in a way that can be universally applied, some hospitals now maintain guidelines and procedures to identify when ongoing care is futile or inappropriate. While these guidelines are sanctioned by law in some states, their legality has not been tested.

Withdrawing Life Support

Ideally, an atmosphere should be created that recognizes the dignity of the patient, minimizes the suffering of the infant, and provides emotional support for the family. The dying infant should be relieved of pain, and unnecessary support should be discontinued. Parents should be able to choose whether they prefer to be with the child in a private, hospice-like environment or to remain within the mainstream of the NICU. In addition, parents should participate in decisions concerning withdrawal of support (eg, ventilator). Regardless of the manner chosen for the infant to die, the process should be unhurried and orderly.

When an infant dies, several administrative details must be completed. Generally, families must be asked to consider organ donation and autopsy and to designate funeral arrangements. The physician must write a death note in the chart, designate the time of death, and complete the death certificate.

Questions and issues concerning the infant's care may continue after death. Therefore, posthumous contact is essential and can be provided by nurses, neonatologists, or family physicians by telephone or formal interview. If the grieving process appears to be dysfunctional, referral for counseling may be offered.

By Carol L. Berseth, MD, and Timothy R. Cooper, MD

Suggested Readings

American Academy of Pediatrics Committee on Bioethics. Ethics and the care of critically ill infants and children. *Pediatrics* 1996;98:149-152.

Berseth CL: Ethical dilemmas in the neonatal intensive care unit. *Mayo Clin Proc* 1987;62:67-72.

Brent DA: A death in the family: the pediatrician's role. *Pediatrics* 1983;72:645-651.

Evans AL, Brody BA: The do-not-resuscitate order in teaching hospitals. *JAMA* 1985;253:2236-2239.

Fost N, Crawford RE: Hospital ethics committees. Administrative aspects. *JAMA* 1985;253:2687-2692.

Halevy A, Brody BA: Brain death: reconciling definitions, criteria, and tests. *Ann Intern Med* 1993;119:519-525.

Halevy A, Brody BA: A multi-institution collaborative policy on medical futility. *JAMA* 1996;276:571-574.

Schneidarman LJ, Jecker NS, Johnsen AR: Medical futility: its meaning and ethical implications. *Ann Intern Med* 1990;112:949-954.

Chapter 13

Discharge Planning

Discharge Criteria

Every discharge must be considered individually, and active problems should be resolved or managed through outpatient care. Nevertheless, guidelines for discharge may be helpful. The following are minimum criteria for discharge:

1. Parents show evidence of consistent involvement and readiness for posthospital care, including any medication administration, cardiopulmonary resuscitation (CPR) training, and instruction in the use of home respiratory equipment as necessary for the infant's care.
2. Infant is medically stable and without any evidence of acute illness.
3. Infant has no evidence of apnea or bradycardia for 5 to 8 days before discharge if infant is to be discharged without a home apnea or bradycardia monitor.
4. Infant demonstrates the ability to take adequate feedings by mouth or tolerate enteral nutrition and has a sustained pattern of weight gain.
5. Infant has documentation of normal body temperature in an open crib with normal ambient temperature (24 to 25°C).
6. Social worker conducts predischarge social assessment of the home environment through interview with parents.
7. An appropriate primary care provider is identified for frequent outpatient follow-up after discharge to confirm sufficient weight gain.

Special Considerations

The following considerations should be taken into account when discharging preterm infants, regardless of whether they are healthy or medically fragile:

1. Supplemental oxygen over baseline requirements may be necessary with oral feedings. Baseline oxygen requirements at rest and with oral feeds may need to be determined with a multichannel monitoring study before discharge.

2. Since 1991, the American Academy of Pediatrics has recommended that preterm infants be monitored in car seats before hospital discharge. Recent studies have shown that about 18% of preterm infants may have evidence of oxygen desaturation, bradycardia, and/or apnea when in a car seat. If these problems are found, the infant may need repositioning in the seat with supports or need a different car seat, or travel with the infant may need to be limited.

3. Air travel for the first 6 months after discharge may be hazardous for high-risk preterm infants. These infants may need supplemental oxygen during air travel.

4. Routine immunizations are to be done before discharge based on the infant's chronologic age. They may include influenza, pneumococcus, and respiratory syncytial virus (RSV) immunoprophylaxis if warranted by the infant's medical history.

5. Specialty follow-up appointments with ophthalmologists, pulmonologists, and developmental pediatricians can be arranged before discharge and may enhance continuity of care. This follow-up will vary depending on each infant's needs.

6. Arrangements for home respiratory therapy or frequent nursing home visits, if necessary, should be made before discharge. This will help ensure the infant's smooth transition to the home environment.

Table 1: Considerations for Home Apnea Monitoring

- Persistent, symptomatic apnea at >36 weeks' postmenstrual age
- History of severe apparent life-threatening event and abnormal polysomnography
- Technology-dependent infant (eg, home mechanical ventilation)
- Home oxygen administration
- Central hypoventilation syndromes

Home Apnea Monitoring

The 1987 National Institutes of Health Consensus Conference on Infantile Apnea and Home Monitoring statement does not recommend routine monitoring or screening of normal term or preterm infants.

The normal median baseline oxygen saturation is 97.9% during sleep; however, normal infants also have apneic pauses and episodes of desaturation (<90% saturation) lasting more than 5 seconds. The median lowest saturation has been shown to be 83%, with the 10th and 90th percentiles equaling 78% and 87%, respectively. These episodes of desaturation are associated with periodic breathing and with apnea, and they seem to be normal physiologic occurrences.

In the past, home monitoring was considered in infants with persistent apnea or an apparent life-threatening event (ALTE) and in selected infants with a history of apnea of prematurity (Table 1). As many as 8% to 10% of infants discharged from the neonatal intensive care unit are sent home on an apnea monitor. However, as neither apnea of prematurity nor apnea during feedings predicts sudden infant death syndrome (SIDS), home monitoring of infants with these conditions is not warranted. Further, home monitoring has not been shown to improve infant mortality or morbidity. While apnea of prematurity usually resolves by 36 weeks' postmenstrual age (see *Control of Breathing in Neonates,* Chapter 9), some premature infants who are otherwise ready for discharge continue to have idiopathic apnea at this age. The relationship of apnea of prematurity and infantile apnea is not clear, but, again, there does not seem to be any relationship between apnea of infancy and SIDS. Infants discharged on home oxygen (see *Bronchopulmonary Dysplasia* section, Chapter 5) may benefit from home monitoring. Theoretically, the monitor will provide a warning should the nasal cannula become dislodged and the infant subsequently develop apnea or bradycardia. Infants with ALTE may also benefit from being monitored, but only those shown to have an abnormal polysomnography. More than two episodes of ALTE requiring 'resuscitation' by the caregiver should prompt consideration of Munchausen by proxy.

If home monitoring is performed, a recording monitor is preferred because it not only documents events, but also allows interpretation of alarm situations. Data from such devices have demonstrated that most alarm situations are not significant; thus, these monitors provide reassurance to physicians and parents. Home monitoring, even when used for specific, targeted groups, does not guarantee survival.

By Odell Wilson, MD

Car Seats

Before hospital discharge, a period of observation of the premature infant in a standard car safety seat is recommended. Infants with documented desaturation, apnea, or bradycardia in a semiupright position should travel in a supine or prone position in an alternative safety device. Alternative child restraint devices are available for these infants. Specific information on currently available restraint systems can be obtained from the American Academy of Pediatrics brochure

"Family Shopping Guide to Car Seats." Car safety seats with three-point harness systems and convertible car safety seats with five-point harness systems provide optimum comfort, fit, and positioning for the premature or small infant. A small infant should not be placed in a car safety seat with a shield, abdominal pad, or arm rest that could come into direct contact with the infant's face and neck during an impact. Premature infants should be transported in infant-only seats, not seats designed for babies who weigh >20 pounds.

By Michael E. Speer, MD

Respiratory Syncytial Virus Prophylaxis

RSV is the most important cause of bronchiolitis and pneumonia in infants and young children. In preterm infants, the respiratory symptoms can be minimal. Lethargy, irritability, and poor feeding, sometimes accompanied by apnea, may be the major manifestations. Conditions that increase the risk of severe or fatal RSV infection are cyanotic or complicated congenital heart disease (CHD); underlying pulmonary disease, especially bronchopulmonary dysplasia; prematurity; and immunodeficiency disease or immunosuppression caused by therapy. Both palivizumab (Synagis®) and RSV-IGIV (RespiGam®) have been shown to reduce hospitalization due to RSV. The American Academy of Pediatrics has published the following recommendations.

- Palivizumab or RSV-IGIV prophylaxis should be considered for infants and children younger than 2 years with chronic lung disease (CLD) who have required medical therapy for the CLD within 6 months before the anticipated RSV season. Palivizumab is preferred for most high-risk children because of its ease of administration, safety, and effectiveness.
- Infants born at 32 weeks' gestation or earlier who do not have CLD may also benefit from RSV prophylaxis.
- Palivizumab is not recommended for infants between 32 to 35 weeks' gestation, unless they have additional risk factors.

- Neither palivizumab nor RSV-IGIV is approved by the Food and Drug Administration for patients with CHD. RSV-IGIV is contraindicated in patients with cyanotic CHD. Patients who meet the above criteria regarding prematurity or CLD and who have asymptomatic, acyanotic CHD may benefit from palivizumab prophylaxis.
- Children with severe immunodeficiencies who are receiving standard IGIV may benefit from substitution of RSV-IGIV during the RSV season.
- Palivizumab or RSV-IGIV prophylaxis should be initiated before the onset of the RSV season and terminated at the end of the season. The usual time for the beginning of RSV outbreaks is between October and December, and termination is between March and May.
- Neither palivizumab nor RSV-IGIV is recommended in the hospital setting to prevent nosocomial RSV infection.
- Palivizumab does not interfere with response to vaccines; measles-mumps-rubella and varicella vaccinations should be deferred for 9 months following the last dose of RSV-IGIV.

By Michael E. Speer, MD

Home Nutrition

The available evidence on the dietary requirements of healthy preterm infants after hospital discharge is limited and controversial. Infants with CLD present a greater nutritional challenge because their growth is often negatively affected by medications, fluid restriction, and increased baseline energy requirements. Recent studies have suggested that infants with CLD may have enhanced linear growth, increased lean body mass, and improved bone density when fed an enriched formula. Such a formula has higher concentrations of protein, calcium, phosphorus, and zinc than a standard newborn formula. There are some commercially available enriched transition formulas that may benefit an infant with CLD, particularly one who may need fluid restriction. Further research is needed to determine standards for growth of all preterm infants, healthy and medically fragile, after hospital discharge.

Home nutrition is an extension of the plan begun in the hospital. When discharging infants on special diets, effective education of the parents about the reasons for dietary restriction is the best method of ensuring compliance. The clinician should schedule frequent weight checks to demonstrate continued growth and to reassure parents. The availability of special formulas in the community should be assessed. Invariably, supplies run out unexpectedly, and substitution may be required. If the child is on a formula that may not be readily available on short notice, the clinician should suggest alternatives. Vitamins and fluoride should be ordered if area water is inadequately supplemented. The clinician should order iron for anemic infants.

By Odell Wilson, MD

Suggested Readings

Discharge Criteria

Hospital discharge of the high-risk neonate. American Academy of Pediatrics, Committee on Fetus and Newborn. *Pediatrics* 1998;102:411-417.

Special Considerations

American Academy of Pediatrics Committee on Injury and Poison Prevention and Committee on Fetus and Newborn: Safe transportation of premature infants. *Pediatrics* 1991;87:120-122.

Parkins KJ, Poets CF, O'Brien LM, et al: Effect of exposure to 15% oxygen on breathing patterns and oxygen saturation in infants: interventional study. *BMJ* 1998;316:887-891.

Raddish M, Merritt TA: Early discharge of premature infants: a critical analysis. *Clin Perinatol* 1998;25:499-520.

Home Apnea, Car Seats, and RSV

Safe transportation of premature and low birth weight infants. American Academy of Pediatrics Committee on Injury and Poison Prevention and Committee on Fetus and Newborn. *Pediatrics* 1996;97:758-760.

Hospital discharge of the high-risk neonate—proposed guidelines. American Academy of Pediatrics. Committee on Fetus and Newborn. *Pediatrics* 1998;102:411-417.

Prevention of respiratory syncytial virus infections: indications for the use of palivizumab and update on the use of RSV-IGIV. American Academy of Pediatrics Committee on Infectious Diseases and Committee on Fetus and Newborn. *Pediatrics* 1998;102:1211-1216.

Changing concepts of sudden infant death syndrome: implications for infant sleeping environment and sleep position. American Academy of Pediatrics. Task Force on Infant Sleep Position and Sudden Infant Death Syndrome. *Pediatrics* 2000;105:650-656.

Daniels H, Naulaers G, Deroost F, et al: Polysomnography and home documented monitoring of cardiorespiratory pattern. *Arch Dis Child* 1999;81:434-436.

Hoffman HJ, Hillman LS: Epidemiology of the sudden infant death syndrome: maternal, neonatal, and postneonatal risk factors. *Clin Perinatol* 1992;19:717-737.

National Institutes of Health Consensus Development Conference on Infantile Apnea and Home Monitoring, Sept 29 to Oct 1, 1986. *Pediatrics* 1987;79:292-299.

Home Nutrition

Brunton JA, Saigal S, Atkinson SA: Growth and body composition in infants with bronchopulmonary dysplasia up to 3 months corrected age: a randomized trial of high-energy nutrient-enriched formula fed after hospital discharge. *J Pediatr* 1998;133:340-345.

Index

A

abdominal mass   60
abrasions   241
achondrogenesis   196, 210
achondroplasia   196
acidosis   24, 26, 111, 120, 122, 207, 303, 322
acini   4
acrocyanosis   57, 82
adenosine triphosphate (ATP)   26
adenovirus   142
agenesis   67
air block   141, 152, 153, 199, 273
air bronchograms   64, 65
air embolization   162
air leak   103, 104, 141, 155, 281, 282, 284
air trapping   136, 138, 154
airway obstruction   13, 16, 61, 186-188, 221
airway patency   230, 232, 236
airway pressure   16, 18, 74, 75
airway resistance   11-14, 17
alae nasae   58

alanine transaminase (ALT)   307
albumin   177, 307, 310, 320, 321
albuterol   172, 173
alcohol   54
alkaline phosphatase   177, 307, 321
alkalosis   24, 120, 121, 129
aluminum hydroxide   323
alveolar capillary dysplasia   116, 122, 141
alveolar ducts   2, 19
alveolar edema   136, 138
alveolar flooding   96, 126-128
alveolar gas   23, 31, 35, 38, 39
alveolar overdistention   43
alveolar oxygen tension   22, 40, 265, 272
alveolar pressure (Palv)   10, 14, 15, 68, 70, 75-77
alveolar rupture   141, 273
alveolar ventilation   9, 19-21, 38
alveolar volume   20
alveoli   3, 4, 14, 15, 19, 20, 31, 33-35, 37, 39, 40, 43, 44, 152, 188, 198

amino acids 28, 45, 303, 306, 308, 319

Aminosyn-PF® 303

amniocentesis 49

amnion nodosum 199

amniotic fluid 49, 55, 241

amniotic fluid aspiration 115

amyotonia congenita 197, 211

anemia 58, 239, 320

anencephaly 197

anesthesia bag 252

angiography 194

angiosarcoma 222

antacids 323

antibiotics 54, 118, 138, 140, 144, 207

aorta 41

aortography 192

Apgar score 55, 206

apnea 18, 60, 70, 106, 140, 143, 163, 165, 180, 217, 219, 230-236, 238, 239, 246, 247, 252, 258, 263-265, 276, 278, 280, 333-337

Arnold-Chiari malformation 218, 219

arterial blood gas 85

arterial oxygen content 26, 248, 251

arterial oxygen tension 82, 83, 86, 243, 248, 265, 271, 272

arteriography 198

arterioles 4, 198

arteriovenous fistulas 194

ascites 196

asphyxia 84, 109, 115-117, 124, 127, 128, 130, 140, 244

asphyxiating thoracic dystrophy (Jeune's syndrome) 210

aspiration 124, 130, 139, 216

aspiration pneumonia 111

aspirin 116

asthma 108, 164, 171, 172

atelectasis 34, 59, 67, 92-94, 96, 120, 136, 156, 162, 180, 187, 190, 198, 223, 279, 282, 285

atmospheric pressure (Patm) 10, 14-16

atresia 214, 215

atresia of urethra 196

atrial septal defect 193

atropine 245

auscultation 56, 61, 84

B

bacterial pneumonia 98, 111, 112, 115, 138, 143, 257

bacterial sepsis 112, 115

bag-and-mask ventilation 206, 242, 247, 252, 253

barium swallow 226

barotrauma 106, 164, 206, 279, 280, 290

Beckwith-Wiedemann syndrome 215, 217

beclomethasone 173

belly dancer's sign 209

beractant (Survanta®) 102

betamethasone 101

bethanechol 323

bicarbonate 28

bilirubin 307, 310, 320, 325

blood urea nitrogen (BUN) 177, 307, 310, 320, 321

Bohr effect 29

bradycardia 154, 236, 247, 263, 333, 334, 336

brainstem dysgenesis 219

breast hypoplasia 211

breath sounds 84, 154

British Perinatal Mortality Study 144

bronchi 2, 3, 64, 67, 225

bronchiolar metaplasia 166

bronchioles 2, 3, 19, 198

bronchogenic cysts 3, 67, 188, 190, 193

bronchography 64, 198

bronchomalacia 168, 220

bronchopleural fistula 160

bronchopulmonary dysplasia (BPD) 17, 61, 67, 100, 124, 126, 128, 129, 141, 162, 163, 165, 166,

bronchopulmonary dysplasia (BPD) *(continued)* 168, 170-172, 174, 176, 178, 180, 181, 186, 248, 278, 284, 302, 319, 322, 336, 337

bronchoscopy 188, 198, 225, 227

bronchospasm 169, 173

bronchostenosis 220

bubbly lungs 67

C

caffeine 163, 236, 238, 239

calcium 45, 48, 177, 245, 303, 304, 307, 310, 313, 318, 321

calfactant (Infasurf®) 102

camptomelic dwarfism 197

camptomelic syndrome 215

Candida 142

capillaries 4, 5

capillary blood sampling 251

capillary leak 125

capillary refilling time (CRT) 60, 61

car seats 334, 336, 337

carbohydrate 321

cardiac arrest 330

cardiac catheterization 86

cardiac output 26, 30

cardiomegaly   127

cardiomyopathy   124

cardiovascular failure   288

casein   311, 316, 319

catheter   42, 68, 72, 73, 191, 224, 307

central respiratory drive 230, 236, 238

cerebral infarction   122, 291

cerebrocostomandibular syndrome   215

cesarean (C-section)   55, 91, 108

CHARGE association   214, 222

chemical pneumonitis   136

chemoreceptor function 231

chest compressions   243, 244

chest radiograph   186, 191, 192, 194, 195, 198, 199, 223, 225, 227

chest wall   10, 11, 14, 15, 17, 58, 69, 155

chest wall compliance   9

chest wall restriction   58

chlamydia   164

Chlamydia trachomatis 142, 144

chlorothiazide   171

choanal atresia   214-217, 220

choking   218, 223

cholestasis   320, 325

cholesterol   44, 45, 311

chondrodystrophia fetalis calcificans   197

chondrodystrophy   210

chondromas   221

chondrosarcoma   222

chorioamnionitis   56, 101, 143

chromium   309

chronic pulmonary disease 166

chronic pulmonary insufficiency of prematurity (CPIP)   162

chylothorax   41, 59, 67, 131, 132, 134, 135, 243

cigarettes   54

circulatory insufficiency 244, 250

circulatory transition   243

cleft palate   216, 217

clots   291

cold stress   57

colfosceril (Exosurf®)   102

compliance   17-19, 68, 69, 71-73, 75, 102, 262, 270, 272, 278

computed tomography (CT)   64, 187, 190, 215, 219, 225

congenital absence of pericardium   193

congenital cystic adenomatoid malformation (CCAM)   3

congenital diaphragmatic hernia (CDH) 3, 4, 6, 50, 57, 60, 67, 121, 198, 203-209, 242, 287

congenital diseases 186

congenital heart defects 225

congenital heart disease (CHD) 38, 66, 83, 84, 187, 193, 214, 222, 337, 338

congenital lobar emphysema (CLE) 67, 187, 206

congenital pneumonia 56, 143

congenital pulmonary lymphangiectasia 194

congenital tracheal stenosis 225

congestive heart failure 131

continuous positive airway pressure (CPAP) 95, 104-106, 129, 140, 153, 167, 180, 187, 209, 221, 225, 232, 234, 257, 258, 264-266, 278

contrast radiography 223

control of breathing 232, 233, 236, 239

copper 309

cor pulmonale 126, 167, 169, 171, 177, 179, 216

corn oil 318

corticosteroids 54, 55, 91, 99-101, 107, 140, 169, 173, 174, 207, 217

coughing 191, 223

creatinine 310

crepitant mass 154

cricoid ring 219

croup 13

crying 215, 218

Curosurf® 102, 103, 260, 261

cyanosis 57, 82, 83, 97, 111, 117, 127, 130, 137, 180, 187, 194, 198, 215, 216, 218, 224, 236, 247, 248, 262

cyanotic congenital heart disease 84, 86

cyst 188, 197, 219

cysteine 308

cystic adenomatoid malformation (CAM) 67, 190, 191, 206

cystic fibrosis 223

cystic hygroma 128, 134

cystic kidneys 196

cystic lung diseases 41, 58, 59

cystic malformations 186

cystic periventricular leukomalacia 282

cysts 186, 187, 191, 221

cytomegalovirus 142, 164

D

dead space ventilation 21
dead space volume 9, 19
dentition 256
dexamethasone 101, 174-176
dextrose 318
diabetes 48, 54, 55, 91, 108
diaphragm 4, 14, 59, 60, 234, 238
diaphragmatic agenesis 197
diaphragmatic hernia 57, 59, 112, 116, 128, 152, 186, 191, 193, 197, 243, 253, 259, 289
diaphragmatic paralysis 206
diffusion block 29
digitalis 129
dipalmitoyl phosphatidyl-choline (DPPC) 44, 46-48
2,3-diphosphoglycerate (2,3-DPG) 24
diphtheria 220
discharge criteria 333
discharge planning 167, 319, 333
distending pressure 10, 11, 69, 72
distention 216, 224
diuresis 96, 97, 174
diuretics 112, 129

do-not-resuscitate (DNR) 330
docosahexaenoic acid (DHA) 311, 312
dopamine 105, 119, 207
doxapram 231, 238
driving pressure [P(t)] 15
drug abuse 55
ductus arteriosus 34
dwarfism 196
dynamic lung compliance 75, 76
dysphagia 224
dyspnea 191
dystrophy 197

E

E coli 142, 143
echocardiogram 86
echocardiography 177, 194
ectopia cordis 210
edema 97, 155, 164, 233
electrocardiogram 194
electrolytes 303
Ellis-van Creveld syndrome (chondroectodermal dysplasia) 196, 210
emphysema 3, 4, 41, 59, 153-155, 180, 187-189, 191, 220
encephalopathy 218, 219
end exhalation 78
end expiration 16, 72, 73

end inspiration 16, 21, 72, 73

endotracheal tube (ETT) 68, 70, 80, 242, 252-254, 256, 257, 261-263, 279, 280

EnfaCare™ 314, 317, 319, 322

Enfamil® 314, 316, 319

enriched formula 170

enteral dietary supplements 318

enteral formula 315

enteral nutrition 307, 321, 333

enteric cysts 190

Enterobacter 142

enterovirus 142

epiglottis 218

epinephrine 245

equation of motion 15, 73

erythroblastosis 130

erythromycin 144

esophageal atresia 64, 65, 222-224

esophageal cysts 193

esophageal diverticulum 193

esophageal duplication 193

esophageal reflux 65

esophagoscopy 223

esophagus 65, 68, 222, 224, 226, 227

ethical considerations 328

eventration of the diaphragm 206

exanthems 58

Exosurf® 102, 103, 260-263

expiratory time 9, 16

extracorporeal membrane oxygenation (ECMO) 46, 107, 118, 120-122, 133, 140, 141, 208, 209, 285-291, 306

extralobar pulmonary sequestration 191

F

face mask 68, 70, 80

failure to thrive 216, 218

famotidine 323

fat 321

fatty acids 311, 316

feeding intolerance 322

feeding tubes
  nasogastric 308
  orogastric 308, 310
  transpyloric 308, 310

fentanyl 119, 207

Fer-In-Sol® 319

fetal alcohol syndrome 215

fetal depression 55, 56

fetal ductal closure 116

fetal hydantoin syndrome 215

fetal hydrops 197

fetal pulmonary arteries 5

fetal trimethadione
  syndrome 215
fever 56, 143, 191
fibroblast growth factor
  (FGF) 3
fibromas 221
fibrosarcoma 222
fibrosis 164, 166, 167,
  174, 180
fibrous webs 221
F_{IO_2} 22, 29, 30, 33-36
fistulas 132, 223
foramen ovale 34, 82
forced expiratory flow 68,
  79, 80
fortified human milk 170,
  314, 319, 322
fractures 303
frequency dependence of
  lung compliance 75, 76
functional residual capacity
  (FRC) 8, 9, 11, 17, 20, 42,
  71, 75, 77-80, 154, 168,
  207, 231, 234, 270, 282
funnel chest 193
furosemide 129, 171

G

gamma glutaryl transferase
  (GGT) 307
gas exchange 249, 279
gas flow 13
gas gradients
  a-AD_{CO_2} 39
  a-AD_{N_2} 39, 40
  A-aD_{O_2} 39

gas pressures 34
gas trapping 3, 16, 43,
  110, 137, 141, 279, 286
gastroesophageal reflux
  (GER) 208, 324
gastrointestinal intolerance
  238
gastrostomy 217, 218, 224
gavage feedings 216
genital mycoplasma 142
gentle ventilation 120, 176
glossoptosis 216
glossoptosis-apnea
  syndrome 217
glucose 245, 303, 306,
  308, 310, 318
glycerol 46
glycogen storage disease
  211
goiter 220
Goldenhar's syndrome 222
Golgi apparatus 48
grainy lungs 66
group B streptococci
  (GBS) 56, 142
grunting 61, 84

H

H_2 antagonists 324
H_2 blockers 323
Haemophilus influenzae
  142
Haldane effect 29
hamartomas 193
hearing impairment 122

heart 40, 65

helium dilution 77, 78

hemangioma 194, 217, 220, 221

hematocrit 84

hemoglobin 24, 25, 27, 28, 30, 82, 83, 320

hemorrhage 55, 291

hemorrhagic edema 67

heparin 289, 308

Hering-Breuer deflation reflex 70, 80, 239

herniation 64

herpes simplex 142

high-frequency jet ventilation (HFJV) 161, 264, 281-284

high-frequency oscillatory ventilation (HFOV) 106, 120, 161, 176, 206, 264, 282-286

high-frequency ventilation 264

hyaline membrane disease (HMD) 5, 41, 48-50, 55-59, 61, 66, 67, 90-99, 102-107, 111, 112, 119, 124, 128, 137, 143, 152, 153, 158, 165, 166, 256, 259, 260, 265, 278, 284

hydrocephalus 193, 219

hydrochloride 303

hydrochlorothiazide 171

hydrops fetalis 55, 131, 132

hydrothorax 67

hygroma 220

hypercapnia 180

hypercarbia 111, 131, 137, 176, 218, 231, 256, 263

hyperinflation 111, 166

hyperoxemia 237, 251

hyperoxia 37, 118, 122, 263

hyperperistalsis 135

hypertension 54, 91, 174, 175, 238, 256, 263

hyperventilation 21, 22, 118, 119, 121, 280

hyperviscosity 119

hypocarbia 176, 263

hypoglycemia 84, 97, 105, 112, 115

hypokalemia 129

hypoparathyroidism 220

hypopharynx 232

hypophosphatasia 196, 210

hypoplasia 59, 188, 198, 225

hypoplastic left heart syndrome 194

hypoplastic lungs 66, 152, 225

hypoplastic mandible 220

hypotension 55, 105, 121, 154, 207, 263

hypothermia 112, 115, 130

hypothyroidism 217

hypoventilation 22, 29, 83-85

hypovolemia 105, 244

hypoxemia 29, 32, 33, 37-39, 57, 82, 83, 85, 86, 94, 95, 97, 106, 111, 117, 119, 131, 137, 154, 207, 236, 271

hypoxia 22, 43, 110, 112, 115, 120, 135, 137, 141, 216, 231, 247, 256, 265

I

imperforate anus 222

incubator 236

indomethacin 116, 131

indwelling catheters 250

inertance 14, 15

Infasurf® 103, 260, 261

inferior vena cava (IVC) 41

influenza virus 142

informed consent 330

inhaled nitric oxide (iNO) 118, 121, 208, 286, 287

inspiration 14

inspiratory time 9

intermittent mandatory ventilation (IMV) 95, 105, 129, 266, 279

intermittent positive pressure ventilation (IPPV) 167, 174, 264, 266

interstitial edema 93, 126, 136

intracerebral hemorrhage 288

intracranial bleeding 130, 291

intracranial hemorrhage 104, 124, 278

intrapartum amnioinfusion 139

intrauterine growth retardation 55

intraventricular hemorrhage (IVH) 100, 101, 107, 130, 162, 244, 246, 256, 281, 282, 286

intubation 139, 154, 217, 219, 232, 242, 253, 254, 256, 266, 278

ipratropium bromide 172

ischemia 118

J

jaundice 307

K

K pneumoniae 143

Klebsiella 142

L

lactic acid 26

lactic acidemia 246

lactic acidosis 161

lactoferrin 311

lactose 317

laminar gas flow 12

Laplace equation 43, 44

Laplace's law 91

laryngeal edema 220

laryngeal infection 220
laryngeal papilloma 221
laryngeal tumors 220, 221
laryngeal web 219, 220, 222
laryngitis 220
laryngomalacia 218, 220
laryngoscopy 218, 219, 225
laryngospasm 220
laryngotracheoesophageal cleft 220, 224
larynx 218, 225, 233
laser ablation 221
lecithin 49
lecithin/sphingomyelin ratio (L/S) 48, 49, 55
left superior vena cava syndrome 215
left ventricular hypertrophy 194
left-to-right shunt 95, 124, 128, 130, 192
lethargy 143
lingual thyroid 220
linoleic acids 306
lipids 47, 303
lipoprotein 45
Listeria monocytogenes 142
liver function tests 307
lobectomy 188, 194
lumbar puncture 105
lung 10, 11, 15, 20, 21, 23, 29, 34, 40, 42-44, 47, 49, 65, 69, 70, 74, 75, 195

lung biopsy 195
lung bud 3, 191
lung compliance 9, 10, 11, 59, 74, 93, 127, 130, 137
lung cyst 206
lung elasticity 10, 11, 77
lung hypoplasia 4, 124, 144
lung parenchyma 192
lung transplantation 46
lung volume 8, 11, 16, 19, 231, 233
lymphangioma 221
lymphopenia 134
lysozyme 311

M

M tuberculosis 142
macroglossia 216, 217, 220
magnesium 307
magnetic resonance imaging (MRI) 64, 190, 215, 227
malabsorption 325
maladaptation 113, 114
maldevelopment 113, 115
mandibular hypoplasia 216
maternal aspirin therapy 57
maternal history 54
mechanical ventilation 41, 43, 68, 103, 153, 159, 164, 167, 187, 221, 261, 262, 270-272, 275, 276, 278, 281, 284, 287, 307, 335

meconium 115, 241

meconium aspiration 56, 66, 67, 116, 136-138, 144, 242, 257, 259, 290

meconium aspiration pneumonia 58, 115

meconium aspiration syndrome (MAS) 50, 57, 58, 135, 137-141, 282, 285, 289

meconium staining 58, 83, 84, 112

meconium staining of the amniotic fluid (MSAF) 135-137, 139

megacolon 193

meningitis 143

metabolic acidosis 158, 245

metabolic alkalosis 171

metered dose inhaler (MDI) 172, 173

methemoglobinemia 83-85, 288

methicillin-resistant *S aureus* 144

metoclopramide 323

microatelectasis 152

micrognathia 216, 220

minute ventilation 9, 19, 30, 154

mitochondria 26

mixed arterial CO_2 tension 36

Möbius' syndrome 218

morphine 119, 207, 262

mouth, disorders of 214

mucous plugging 169

mumps virus 142

murmur 84, 194

muscle weakness 211

muscular dystrophy 211

myasthenia gravis 197, 211

myotonic dystrophy 198, 215

N

naloxone 245

nasal cavity 214

nasal continuous positive airway pressure (N-CPAP) 163, 176, 180, 238, 258, 264, 279

nasal flaring 58, 62, 127, 137

nasogastric tubes 232

nasopharynx 214

neck mass 220

necrotizing enterocolitis (NEC) 307, 315, 325

necrotizing tracheobronchitis 278

neonatal intensive care unit (NICU) 328

NeoSure® 314, 317, 319, 322

neurenteric cysts 190, 193

neurofibromas 221

neurofibrosarcoma 222

neurogenic bladder 196
neutral fat 44, 45
niacin 304, 309
nitrates 83, 84
nitric oxide 208
nitrogen washout 77, 79, 95, 159
nitroprusside 121
Noonan's syndrome 194
nose, disorders of 214
nosocomial pneumonia 107
nutrition 56, 339
nutritional support 224, 245, 302

O

O_2 consumption 32
O_2 content 25, 26, 31, 33, 36, 38
O_2 delivery 25-27, 32
O_2 saturation 23, 31, 36
O_2 tension 23, 26, 31, 32, 36, 37
oligohydramnios 57, 139, 196, 198, 199
orogastric tubes 217
osteogenesis imperfecta 196, 210
overdistention 96, 126, 154, 190, 206, 262, 265, 266, 272, 273, 275, 282
overinflation 187, 227
oxidant injury 164
oxygen 246-249, 251, 252, 262, 290

oxygen desaturation 263
oxygen monitoring 82, 237, 248
oxygen toxicity 124
oxygenation 6, 23
oxyhemoglobin dissociation curve 23-25, 31

P

palatal abnormalities 214
palatal grooving 256
palivizumab (Synagis®) 176, 337, 338
pallor 57, 97, 263
palmitic acid (hexadecanol) 46, 102
palpation 56, 60
palsy 218
pancuronium bromide 119, 207
pantothenic acid 309
paralysis of the diaphragm 209
parenchymal disease 5, 59, 67
parenchymal lung disease 29, 83, 86, 90, 119-121, 249, 265, 266, 271, 272
parental bonding 248
parenteral nutrition 303
patent ductus arteriosus (PDA) 99, 100, 107, 128, 130, 131, 164, 187, 219

peak inspiratory pressure (PIP) 160, 206, 262, 267-270, 272-275, 277, 278, 286

pectus excavatum 210

pendelluft 76, 284

penicillin 144

pericardial drain 161

perihilar markings 65

perinatal depression 57

periodic breathing 59, 84, 235

peripheral edema 96

persistent pulmonary hypertension (PPHN) 58, 66, 83-86, 112-118, 120-122, 128, 137, 141, 199, 204, 206-208, 286, 289

pharynx, disorders of 214

phosphate 46

phosphatidylcholine 44, 45, 49

phosphatidylglycerol (PG) 44, 45, 49

phosphocholine 46

phospholipids 44, 45, 47

phosphorus 177, 303, 304, 307, 313, 318, 321

phrenic nerve injury 209

physical examination 54, 84, 154

Pierre Robin sequence 215-217, 220

placenta 25

plethysmography 77-79

pleural effusions 41, 131, 134, 195, 206

pleural fissures 64

pleural fistula 160, 162

pleural peritoneal shunts 135

pleural pressure (Ppl) 10, 14, 15, 40, 41, 43, 58-60, 68, 69, 72, 73, 153

pleurocentesis 134

pneumatoceles 67, 186, 187

pneumomediastinum 137, 152-157, 160

pneumonia 50, 57, 58, 61, 66, 67, 84, 105, 112, 124, 125, 128, 141, 142, 144, 186, 192, 195, 218, 223, 285, 289, 337

pneumonitis 223

pneumopericardium 157, 161, 162

pneumoperitoneum 153

pneumotachometer 70

pneumothoraces 187

pneumothorax 41, 59, 62, 63, 137, 152, 153, 155-157, 160, 161, 191, 206, 243, 259, 263, 275

Poland's syndrome 211

poliomyelitis 211

polycose 318

polycythemia 57, 58, 84, 112, 115

polydactyly 193

polydactyly syndrome 196

polyhydramnios 57, 190, 191, 204, 222

poractant alfa (Curosurf®) 102

positive end-expiratory pressure (PEEP) 119, 129, 131, 140, 161, 165, 206, 262, 264, 267, 268, 272, 274, 275, 277

positive pressure respiratory support 252

positive pressure ventilation 4, 16, 19, 60, 224, 242, 253, 274

positive pressure ventilatory support 263, 264

Potter's syndrome 116, 196, 199

prealbumin 177

pregnancy 54

prenatal counseling 330

pressure-volume curve 10, 68, 69

preterm labor 56

prokinetic agents 324

prolonged labor 56

prophylactic surfactant therapy 103, 104

prostaglandin synthesis inhibitors 118

protein 44, 45, 306, 318, 321

prune belly syndrome 196

pseudocyst 63

pseudohyperlucent hemithorax 65

pseudohyperlucent lung 64

Pseudomonas 142

pulmonary agenesis 195

pulmonary airleak 104

pulmonary arteriovenous fistula 194

pulmonary edema 66, 67, 86, 93, 96, 99, 109, 111, 112, 124, 127-130, 144, 166, 169, 170, 195, 244, 288

pulmonary function tests 19, 68

pulmonary hemorrhage 130, 131, 144

pulmonary hypertension 4-6, 56, 57, 113, 116, 120, 171, 177, 179, 180, 206, 208, 289, 290

pulmonary hypoplasia 4, 57, 58, 61, 116, 128, 196, 198, 204, 208, 211

pulmonary interstitial emphysema (PIE) 67, 152, 153, 155, 157, 158, 160-162, 195, 263, 281, 282, 284

pulmonary lymphangiectasia 66, 99, 111, 126, 128

pulmonary parenchyma 186

pulmonary sequestration 1, 192, 193

pulmonary vascular resistance (PVR) 42, 113, 114, 116, 118, 121, 122, 130, 137, 140, 166-169, 171, 206, 247 pulse oximetry (Spo$_2$) 82, 177

pyridoxine (B$_6$) 309

R

radiograph 63, 64, 66, 155-157, 159, 186, 218

radiography 219

radiohumeral synostosis syndrome 215

rales 61, 84

ranitidine 323

rapid eye movement (REM) 162, 163

REM sleep 231-234, 237

renal agenesis 57, 191, 198, 200

renal anomalies 152

rescue surfactant therapy 103

residual volume (RV) 11

resistance 16, 18, 68, 71-73, 102

RespiGam® 337

respiratory acidosis 158

respiratory distress ix, 54, 58, 61, 84, 154, 186, 187, 190, 192, 195, 198, 215, 224-226, 302

respiratory distress syndrome (RDS) 50, 90, 100, 101, 103, 176, 207, 260, 285, 289

respiratory distress syndrome type II 108

respiratory drive 231

respiratory failure 46, 252, 284, 288

respiratory pump 230, 232, 233

respiratory rate 9, 19

respiratory syncytial virus (RSV) 142, 176, 334, 337, 338

respiratory time constant 16, 17, 70, 71

respiratory transition 241

resting lung volume 17

reticulocyte count 320

reticulonodular lungs 67

retinal vascularization 248

retinopathy of prematurity (ROP) 179, 249

retractions 180

Rh isoimmunization 48

rhabdomyomas 221

rhonchi 61

rib-gap syndrome 210

riboflavin (B$_2$) 309

rickets 303, 322

right ventricular hypertrophy 180

right-to-left shunt 29, 34, 36-40, 82, 83, 85, 94, 95, 99, 102, 105, 114, 117, 119, 137

RSV-IGIV 337, 338

rubella 142

S

S epidermidis 142, 144

safflower oil 306

salmeterol 172

sclerosing agents 135

secretory IgA 311

self-inflating bag 252, 253

sepsis 84, 124, 125, 128, 130, 144, 207, 244, 289, 291, 310, 324

septal defect 187

sexually transmitted diseases (STDs) 54

shock 57

Silverman score 55, 62

Similac® 314, 316

sirenomelia 191

skeletal deformities 199

sodium 313

sodium bicarbonate 121, 245

soy oil 306

SP-A 45, 47

SP-B 45, 46

SP-C 45, 46

SP-D 45, 47

sphingomyelin 49

spinal cord injury 211

spinal cord tumor 211

spironolactone 171

spleen 60

spondyloepiphyseal dysplasia 197

spondyloepiphyseal dysplasia congenita 215

spondylothoracic dysplasia 210

squamous cell carcinoma 222

Staphylococcus aureus 142

static compliance 76

stenosis 58, 194, 214, 217, 220, 233

stethoscope 62

Stickler syndrome 215

stillbirth 190

stridor 61, 186, 218-221, 224-226

subglottic stenosis 219, 256

subvalvular aortic stenosis 193

sucking mechanism 325

suctioning 257, 259, 262

sulfhemoglobinemia 83, 85

superior vena cava syndrome (SCV) 41, 126, 131, 132

suprasternal fossa 64

surfactant ix, 44, 45, 47-50, 90, 93, 96, 97, 100-104, 121, 127, 130, 136, 140, 165, 175, 199, 246, 256, 259, 261-263, 303

surfactant deficiency 49

surfactant proteins 45

Survanta® 102, 103, 260, 261, 263

swallowing difficulties 219

swallowing dysfunction 226

Synagis® 176

synchronized intermittent mandatory ventilation (SIMV) 264, 279

syphilis 220

systolic blood pressure 42

T

tachycardia 154, 238

tachypnea 59, 84, 92, 97, 106, 117, 127, 180

tamponade 161

telangiectasis 194

teratoma 193, 217, 220

tetanus 220

tetralogy of Fallot 187

thanatophoric dwarfism 196, 210

theophylline 236, 238, 239

thiamin (B$_1$) 304, 309

thiazide 129

thoracentesis 134

thoracic dystrophy 196, 198

thoracic volume 14

thromboxane 115

thymus 155, 156

thyroglossal cysts 220

thyroid hormone 49

thyroid-releasing hormone 102

tidal volume 9, 19, 20, 29, 39, 165, 232, 234, 238

tissue hypoxia 246

tocolytics 54, 101

tongue 216, 217

total expiratory resistance 9

total inspiratory resistance 9

total lung capacity (TLC) 11

total parenteral nutrition (TPN) 133, 303, 306, 310, 314, 320, 325

total pressure gradient 13

total resistance 14

toxemia 55

Toxoplasma gondii 142

trachea 2, 49, 64, 66, 222, 225, 226, 233

tracheal agenesis 1, 224

tracheal buckling 64

tracheal cyst 220

tracheal deviation 195

tracheal stenosis 1, 13, 220, 256

tracheal suctioning 242, 253, 256

tracheobronchomalacia 166, 225

tracheoesophageal fistula (TEF) 1, 56, 57, 60, 65, 193, 214, 220, 222-225 tracheomalacia 220

tracheoplasty 225

tracheostomy 217, 219, 221, 225

transcutaneous oxygen monitors 250

transcutaneous oxygen tension (TcPo$_2$) 177

transient tachypnea 56, 58

transient tachypnea of the newborn (TTN) 59, 66, 67, 98, 108, 110-112, 137, 138, 144, 153, 256

transillumination 62, 155

transposition of the great arteries 193

transpulmonary pressure 72, 73

Treacher Collins syndrome 214

tricuspid atresia 193

tricuspid regurgitation 177

triglycerides 306, 310

trisomy 11q 215

trisomy 13 222

trisomy 18 222

trisomy 21 217, 220, 222

Trophamine® 303

truncus arteriosus 193

tubular myelin 45, 48

tumors 193, 197, 217

turbulent gas flow 12, 13

U

ultrasound 54, 186, 190, 199

umbilical artery catheter 245

umbilical venous catheter 244, 245

unilateral lung overdistention 256

Ureaplasma 164

Ureaplasma urealyticum 142, 144

urethral valves 196

urine glucose 310

ursodiol 323

V

VACTERL 222

vancomycin 144

vascular rings 225, 226

vasoconstriction 6, 58, 95, 102, 105, 113, 119, 208, 263

vasodilators 250

ventilation-perfusion mismatch 5, 29, 31-34, 36, 37, 43, 83, 85, 110

ventricular septal defect 193

vertebral anomalies 193

viral pneumonitis 66

viscous tissue resistance 11, 13

vitamin A 176, 304, 309

vitamin B$_{12}$ 304, 309

vitamin C 309
vitamin D 304, 309
vitamin E 304, 309
vitamin K 304, 309
vitamins 54, 303
vocal cord dysfunction
  233
vocal cord paralysis 218,
  220
volume replacement 244
volutrauma 164, 290
vomiting 216, 323

W

webbed neck 134
Werdnig-Hoffman disease
  197

wheezing 61, 186, 225,
  227
whey 311, 316, 318
Wilson-Mikity syndrome
  67, 180
withdrawing life support
  331

X

x-ray 62, 63
xanthines 165, 233, 234,
  237
xeroradiography 219
xiphoid retraction 62

Z

zinc 309

NOTES

NOTES

NOTES

NOTES